BEDSIDE APPROACH TO COMMON SYMPTOMATOLOGY IN CHILDHOOD

PREMLATA PAREKH

MD, DCH, MAMS, FIAP, FNNF

Former Professor & Head
Department of Pediatrics, M.G.M. Medical College and M. Y. Hospital,
Indore, Madhya Pradesh.

FIRST EDITION

www.nationalbookdepot.com

CBS Publishers & Distributors Pvt Ltd.

First Edition : 2018

ISBN : 978-93-80206-91-2

Disclaimer

This book has been published in good faith. The author has tried her best in providing information available with her. Although, all efforts have been made by the author to ensure optimum accuracy of the material included in the book, yet it is quite possible some errors might have been left uncorrected. The publisher, the printer and the author will not be held responsible for any inadvertent errors, omissions or inaccuracies.

Published by

Vaidehi Shah-Sanghavi for

THE NATIONAL BOOK DEPOT

Opp. Wadia Children's Hospital, Parel, Mumbai - 400 012.

Tel : 2416 5274 / 2413 1362 / 2413 2411 | Fax : 2413 0877

E-mail : nationalbook55@gmail.com

Website : nationalbookdepot.com

and

Satish Kumar Jain for

CBS Publishers & Distributors Pvt Ltd

4819/XI Prahlad Street, 24 Ansari Road, Daryaganj, New Delhi - 110 002, India.

Ph : 23289259, 23266861, 23266867 | Fax : 011-23243014

Website: www.cbspd.com | e-mail: delhi@cbspd.com; cbspubs@airtelmail.in.

Corporate Office: 204 FIE, Industrial Area, Patparganj, Delhi - 110 092.

Ph: 4934 4934 | Fax: 4934 4935 | e-mail: publishing@cbspd.com; publicity@cbspd.com

Printed by : Neel Graphics

PREFACE

The medical profession today is facing many problems; the biggest malady being churning out medical graduates with poor clinical skills. Most of the medical students graduating today are unable to take proper medical history, cannot perform appropriate physical examination, cannot advise pertinent investigations, cannot critically analyze the information they gather and hence cannot create a sound management plan for the ailing patient. Such graduates are termed as "hyposkilliacs". The main reason for the situation is the falling standards of bedside teaching. Also the current day medical students are neglecting the clinical postings due to the pressure of the forthcoming entrance examinations for admission to postgraduate courses. They take recourse to skipping bedside clinics in favor of acquiring theoretical knowledge that ultimately enables them an admission to a course of choice. The newer advanced diagnostic techniques that enable short cuts to instant diagnosis are also gradually replacing the art and science of clinical medicine.

Medical Educationists everywhere are sincerely concerned about the situation and are pleading for the revival of the clinical craft to generate competent physicians. Teaching clinical skills should be a continuous lifelong learning process from the medical school through training and into practice. Modern technology is to complement and not to replace bedside teaching and the patient should always remain the best teacher for the physician. Textbooks provide exhaustive information which is system based whereas in clinical practice, the parents bring their sick children with symptoms or obvious signs. In order to facilitate the process of bedside diagnosis, a 'symptom-complex approach' is beneficial and the same has been chosen in this book. The suggested approach is more direct, rationale and time saving. The book would be useful for Medical students, Pediatric Residents and Family Physicians who cater to a large number of sick children. It is presented in simple symptom/sign based format. Important points in history taking, clinical examination and investigations required to arrive at a logical conclusion towards a clinical diagnosis have been described in a methodical way. An attempt has been made consistently to adopt a learner friendly style throughout the book. The author hopes the book will benefit the clinician in his/her day-to-day clinical practice.

Premlata Parekh

DEDICATED TO

Professor K. K. Kaul

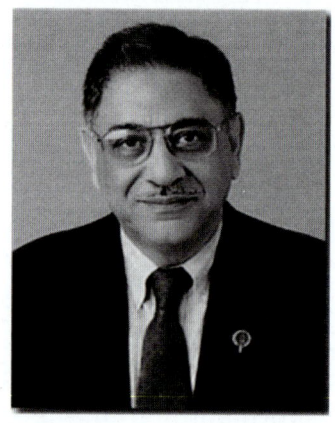

*An Excellent Clinician, a Teacher par Excellence
And above all a Great Human Being*

ACKNOWLEDGEMENTS

I am grateful to my erstwhile colleagues Prof. Jyotsana Shrivastava, Dr. Preeti Malpani, Dr. Nirbhay Mehta and Dr. Sudeep Verma for their efforts, useful suggestions and inputs for the book.

I am greatly indebted to my husband Prof. B. R. Parekh for his constant support, guidance and encouragement and also for providing a number of clinical photographs. Thanks to my daughters Deepika and Preeti for their love and inspiration.

My thanks are due to my grandson Aryan who has helped me with the compilation of photographs in this book.

I sincerely appreciate the secretarial assistance of Mr. Kiran Rao for preparation of the manuscript. His dedication, competence and skills are noteworthy.

My special thanks are due to Mr. Raju Shah & Vaidehi Shah-Sanghavi of The National Book Depot and Mr. Viren Shah, for their enthusiasm and commitment to bring out this book.

Premlata Parekh

NO SHORT CUTS

"There are no short cuts on physical diagnosis.

It is learnt by all the five senses alert.

Eyes, ears, nose and palpating

fingers are the Gems of physician and intact

brain is the necklace"

- Hippocrates

CONTENTS

Chapter

1

SHORT STATURE

INTRODUCTION

Short stature is one of the common pediatric problems encountered by practicing pediatricians. Short stature is not a diagnosis by itself, but a presenting symptom of a variety of systemic, genetic and hormonal disorders. It can sometimes be the only symptom of systemic or endocrine disease. Normal variation accounts for majority of cases. Pathological causes are numerous but rare and constitute 20% of the cases presenting with short stature and require comprehensive evaluation. Approximately 3% children in any population will be short, amongst which half will be physiological (familial or constitutional) and half will be pathological. A systematic approach is the key to reduce the need for a whole battery of tests, which are often expensive and unnecessary.

DEFINITION

A child is considered short if:
- The child's height is below the third percentile or two standard deviations below the mean height for that age on a growth chart for the specific population.
- If the growth velocity is consistently below 25th percentile over 6 to 12 months of observation (i.e. growth velocity less than 5 cm/year) from the age of 3 years to onset of puberty.
- If there is significant discrepancy between midparental target centile and the child's percentile.

It should be remembered that 80 percent of children with height less than 3 standard deviation (SD) below mean have pathologic short stature, whereas 80 percent of the children with height less than 2 standard deviation (SD) usually have normal variant of short stature. The latter may be categorized as familial short stature (FSS) or constitutional growth delay (CGD).

AETIOLOGY

Normal growth requires adequate nutrition along with various hormonal stimuli. The important hormones are: growth hormone (GH), insulin-like growth factor (IGF)1, thyroid hormones, sex steroids and other growth factors. Short stature could be due to constitutive intrinsic growth defect or because of any of the extrinsic factors which are required for normal growth.

Table: Causes of short stature

1. **Physiological or normal short stature:**
   a. Familial
   b. Constitutional delay of growth and puberty.

2. **Pathological short stature:**
   a. Chronic malnutrition.
   b. Systemic disease:
      - Chronic anemia: Sickle cell, thalassemia
      - Chronic renal failure
      - Chronic asthma

- Congenital heart disease
- Chronic severe infection (tuberculosis)
- Malabsorption
- Chronic liver disease
- Renal tubular acidosis.

c. Endocrine disorders:
- Hypothyroidism
- Growth hormone deficiency
- Cushing syndrome
- Pseudohypoparathyroidism.

d. Intrauterine growth retardation.

e. Skeletal dysplasias and rickets.

f. Chromosomal abnormalities and genetic syndromes:
- Turner syndrome
- Noonan syndrome
- Russel Silver syndrome
- Down's syndrome
- Seckel syndrome

g. Inborn errors of metabolism:
- Mucopolysaccharidosis
- Glycogen storage disease
- Galactosemia

The proportion of etiologies for short stature in Indian referral centers is FSS (20%), systemic disease syndromes (10-20%) and skeletal dysplasias (10-19%). Turner syndrome (7-10%), growth hormone deficiency (15%), hypothyroidism (5-10%) and constitutional delay of growth and puberty is 10% to 15%.

CLINICAL EVALUATION

A. History

While recording a detail history points given in the box must be specifically asked.

Points in history

- Family history of short stature
- Birth history
- Dietary history
- Developmental history
- Symptoms of illness
- Psychosomatic illness
- Receiving any drugs

Family history:

Enquire about the height of parents, siblings and cousins. Is there any history of short stature amongst family members? Short stature amongst other family members would point towards familial short stature. Such a child is short for the general population, but is normal for family pedigree. Puberty is achieved at normal age. In constitutional growth delay there is a history of short stature with delayed maturation in other family members. Although the final adult height and sexual development are normal.

Since majority (80%) of the cases of short stature are normal variants the following are distinguishing features between familial short stature and constitutional delay.

Table: Comparison between familial short stature and constitutional delay

	Features	Familial short stature	Constitutional delay
1.	Sex	Both equally affected	More common in boys
2.	Length at birth	Normal	Normal (starts falling <5th percentile in 1st three years of life)
3.	Family history	Short stature	Delayed puberty
4.	Parents stature	Short (one or both)	Average
5.	Height velocity	Normal	Normal
6.	Puberty	Normal	Delayed
7.	Bone age (BA) and chronological age (CA)	BA = CA > Height age	CA > BA = Height age
8.	Final height	Short but normal for target height	Normal

Birth history:

Enquire about the birth weight, length and gestation of the child. Low birth weight would suggest an intrauterine growth retardation.

Arrest of foetal growth in early embryonic life causes reduction in total number of cells, leading to diminished growth potential in postnatal life. Although majority of small-for-gestational age (SGA) infants show catch-up-growth, about 20% may follow a life-long pattern of short stature. In comparison, appropriate-for-gestational-age premature infants usually catch-up to the normal range of height and weight by 1-2 years of age. Bone age, age of onset of puberty and yearly growth rate are normal in SGA patients, and the parents are characteristically thin.

Perinatal complications such as hypoglycemia or micropenis, are suggestive of growth hormone (GH) deficiency.

Dietary history:

History of nutritional intake must be recorded. Inadequate intake, especially during infancy and early childhood can lead to stunting. Enquire about failure of lactation in the mother. It is an important cause of growth failure in infancy.

Psychosocial deprivation:

Enquire whether the child has any emotional problem as emotional deprivation can lead to growth failure. Commonly seen in abandoned children and those subjected to child abuse, or emotional trauma due to death of a parent.

Developmental history:

Enquiry must be made regarding the milestones of development. Global developmental delay is seen in hypothyroidism and in various genetic and chromosomal aberrations.It may also be delayed in severe case of psychosocial deprivation.

Medication history:

Chronic corticosteroid treatment may lead to iatrogenic short stature. A diabetic child on insulin therapy and the children receiving drugs for attention deficit hyperactivity disorders can also remain short.

Symptoms of illness:

The most common post-natal cause of short stature in our country is protein energy malnutrition followed by chronic systemic illnesses viz. anaemia, heart diseases, chronic renal diseases, malabsorption. One must enquire about these illnesses.

History of recurrent fever, anorexia and failure to thrive would suggest a chronic infection such as tuberculosis and urinary tract infection, usually due to anomalies of urinary tract.

If there is a history of recurrent or chronic diarrhea, large bulky foul smelling stools the possibility of malabsorption should be kept in mind. Recurrent or chronic cough, respiratory distress or cyanosis would suggest asthma, tuberculosis or congenital heart disease. If there is a history of polyuria, polydypsia one must consider diabetes insipidus, diabetes mellitus or renal tubular acidosis. Headache, vomiting and diplopia points towards craniopharyngioma.History of recent weight gain, acne, mood swings, headache and obesity consider Cushing syndrome, while seizures would indicate glycogen storage disorder.

Table: **Clues to aetiology of short stature from history**

History	Aetiology
H/O delayed puberty in parents	Constitutional delay of growth
Low birth weight	SGA
Neonatal hypoglycemia, jaundice, micropenis	GH deficiency
Poor dietary intake	Undernutrition
Headache, vomiting, visual problem	Pituitary, hypothalamic SOL
Lethargy, constipation, weight gain	Hypothyroidism
Polyuria	CRF, RTA
Social history	Psychosocial dwarfism
Diarrhea, greasy stools	Malabsorption

CRF – Chronic renal failure, RTA – Renal tubular acidosis

B. Physical Examination

A detailed history and physical examination are the cornerstones for the aetiological diagnosis of short stature. Fatigue, cold intolerance, dry skin, hair loss, constipation, lethargy and weight gain suggest hypothyroidism. The key issues which help in deciding the cause are enumerated in the box:

Physical findings to be looked for

- Is the child really short?
- Assess the height velocity
- Determine the midparental height
- Check body proportions
- Measure head circumference and weight
- Size of anterior fontanelle
- Dysmorphism
- Look for pallor/cyanosis
- Hypertension

- Goiter, coarse skin
- Central obesity, striae
- Clubbing
- Skeletal deformities
- Genitalia
- Record the blood pressure
- Assess pubertal status

Is the child really short?

It is essential at the outset to determine whether the child is short. This is done by accurately measuring the height of the child on a Stadiometer. The height is then plotted on a centile chart. If the child's height is below the third percentile or 2 SD below the mean height for that age he should be considered to have a short stature. In children below 2 years of age supine length with an infantometer is recorded. Height is then recorded on appropriate growth charts and expressed as centile or D score.

The reference values used for height and weight are the WHO published growth charts in 2006, upto the age of five years. They are used as single uniform global standard. For children between 5 to 18 years. Revised IAP growth charts for height and weight are used (2015).

Longitudinal growth assessment is essential in child care. Short stature can be promptly recognized only with accurate measurements of growth and critical analysis of growth data.

Assess the height velocity:

Enquire from the parents whether they have a record of serial height measurements of the child. One time measurement of height is not enough. Height velocity is the most important aspect of assessment of short stature. Height velocity is the rate of increase in height over a period of time, expressed as cm/year.

Retardation of growth velocity is the hallmark of postnatal pathological short stature. Serial height measurements at 3 to 6 monthly intervals should be done to know the growth velocity. Between the ages of 5 years until onset of puberty, average growth velocity is 5 cm/year.

Determine the midparental height (MPH):

Short stature optimally defined relative to the genetic endowment of the individual, is recognized by comparing an individual child's height with that of a large population of a similar genetic background and more particularly, using the mid-parental target height.

After having confirmed that the child is short the next step is to determine the midparental height (MPH). This is done to estimate child's probable inherited growth potential.

The height of father and mother are recorded in centimeters and the following formula is applied to calculate the MPH:

$$\text{MPH range for boys (in cms)} = \frac{[\text{Mother's height (cms)} + \text{Father's height (cms)}] + 13}{2}$$

$$\text{MPH range for girls (in cms)} = \frac{[\text{Mother's height (cms)} + \text{Father's height (cms)}] + 13}{2}$$

The MPH calculated is then plotted as adult height at 18 years and the spread is 8 cm on either side of MPH. This then becomes the midparental range. If the child's height is within these percentiles, it is taken as normal for that child.

Sample calculations:

Midparental height calculations for a son and a daughter of parent with the following heights = Father is 172.72 cms, mother is 157.48 cms.

Son: [172.72 cms (157.48 cms + 13 cms)] / 2 = 171.6 cms.

Daughter : [172.72 cms (157.48 cms - 13 cms)] / 2 = 158.6 cms.

A rough estimate of the child's projected height, can be determined by extrapolating the child's growth along his or her own height percentile to the corresponding 18 year point. If the estimated final height is within 8 cms of the mid parental height, the child's current height is appropriate for the family. However, if the projected height differ from the mid parental height by more than 8 cms a variant growth pattern or a pathologic cause should be considered.

A short child who is growing close to his/her target height centile is likely to have familial short stature. Growth deceleration during the first 2 years followed by a normal growth velocity, with acceleration late in adolescence, leading to a final height that is close to the target height suggests constitutional delay in growth and development.

Check the body proportion:

Determine the crown to rump (CR): Rump to heel (RH) ratio, i.e.

The proportion between the upper and lower segments of the body. Normally the ratio is 1.7 : 1 at birth; 1.3 : 1 at 3 years and 1.0 : 1 at 7 years.

Infantile upper segment to lower segment ratio is seen in cretinism, achondroplasia and short limb dwarfism.

Upper segment lower segment ratio is increased in – Rickets, achondroplasia, untreated hypothyroidism. A decreased ratio is seen inspondyloepiphyseal dysplasia, vertebral anomalies.

Arm span:

The relation between arm span, i.e. (arm length from middle finger tip to opposite finger tip in fully outstretched arms) and standing height is determined.
In toddlers arm span is 1 to 2 cm smaller than body length, by 10 years of age arm span is equal to height. After the age of 14 years span is more than height by 2 cm. Arm span is short as compared to height in patients with short limb dwarfism, cretinism and achondroplasia.

Circumference of skull:

Macrocephaly would suggest mucopolysaccharidosis. Microcephaly would be seen in various chromosomal, genetic disorders and also in cases of IUGR due to intrauterine infections.

Weight:

In case of malnutrition weight for height would be decreased.

Weight gain with central obesity would suggest Cushing syndrome.

Anterior fontanelle:

The anterior fontanelle should be felt to assess, whether it is open or closed and its size. Wide fontanelle with delayed closure is a feature of hypothyroidism, rickets and Russell-Silver syndrome.

Facies:

A lot of information can be obtained from the facial appearance. One should also look for facial dysmorphism.

Coarse facies in a child with short stature would be seen in hypothyroidism and mucopolysaccharidosis. Triangular face is seen in Noonan and Russell-Silver syndrome. Moon face is a feature of Cushing syndrome.

Doll-like face is seen in glycogen storage disorder, while a child with growth hormone deficiency has an immature facies. Mongoloid facies with brachycephaly is seen in Down syndrome.

Pallor/cyanosis:

Pallor in a child with short stature would indicate chronic renal failure, chronic anemia, hypothyroidism and malabsorption. Presence of central cyanosis with clubbing is seen in congenital cyanotic heart disease. Clubbing can also be present in cases with malabsorption.

Vital signs:

Vital signs should be recorded.
In the presence of tachypnea/dyspnea, one must consider congenital heart disease and in born errors of metabolism. If the child has hypertension look for chronic renal disease, Cushing syndrome or central nervous system (CNS) tumors.

Skeletal deformities:

It is important to examine the skeletal system. In case of rickets, both nutritional and resistant look for frontal bossing, widening of wrists, rachitic rosary and bowing of legs. Webbed neck seen in Turner and Noonan syndrome. cubitus valgus in Turner syndrome.

Examination of the eyes:

In the presence of papilledema and visual field defects one must suspect an intracranial tumour especially craniopharyngioma.

Pubertal examination:

Pubertal status needs to be carefully assessed because it indicates skeletal maturation and growth potential. Pubertal delay points to a possibility of constitutional delay of growth and development or hypogonado-trophinhypogonadism due to hypopituitarism.

Table: Tanner staging of sexual maturity rating

GIRLS Stage	Breast	Pubic hair
1	No breast tissue	Same as abdominal hair
2	Breast bud, enlargement of areola	Minimally pigmented, mainly labia
3	Further enlargement of breast and areola	Darker and coarser hair in mons pubis
4	Secondary mound formed by papilla and areola	Adult type, less distribution
5	Adult contour with projection of papilla alone	Adult feminine distribution

BOYS Stage	Genital	Testicular volume	Pubic hair
1	Prepubertal	< 4 mL	Same as abdominal hair
2	Early penile growth scrotum-thinning, redness	4-10 mL	Fine pubic hair at base of penis
3	Increase in penile length, scrotal growth	10-15 mL	Increase in number, darkening
4	Increase in penile length and width, pigmented scrotum	15-20 mL	Spread around thighs, less than adult distribution
5	Adult size	>20 mL	Adult male distribution

Table: Clues to aetiology of short stature

Clue	Etiology
Disproportion	Skeletal dysplasia, rickets, hypothyroidism
Dysmorphism	Congenital syndrome
Rickets	Renal failure, malabsorption, renal tubular acidosis
Hypertension	Chronic renal failure, cushing syndrome, CNS tumor
Anaemia	Malabsorption, renal failure
Goiter coarse skin	Hypothyroidism
Central obesity striae	Cushing's syndrome
Midline defect	Hypopituitarism
Cataract	Intrauterine infection
Developmental delay	Genetic syndrome with hypothyroidism

C. Investigations

List of investigations

- Complete hemogram
- Bone age
- Urine examination
- Stool examination
- Blood chemistry
- Serum thyroxine and thyroid stimulating hormone
- Skeletal survey
- Karyotype
- Antigliadin antibodies
- Growth hormones stimulation tests and serum insulin-like growth factor-1
- MRI brain

All the investigations enumerated in the box are not indicated in all cases of short stature. After a careful history and physical examination choice of tests are based on potential aetiology. The tests have been divided into three groups:

Level 1 investigations also termed as essential investigations need to be done in nearly all cases of short stature. Level 2 and 3 are indicated only in selected cases depending upon the clinical cause.

Level 1 (Essential investigations):
- Complete blood count
- ESR – to rule out underlying undiagnosed chronic inflammatory illness

- Urine examination for pH, microscopy, osmolality. This would help to rule out urinary infection. If the proteinuria is present it would indicate chronic renal disease and pH would point towards normal tubular acidosis.

Assessment of bone age:

It must be done in all children with short stature. Appearance of various epiphyseal centres and fusion of epiphysis with metaphysis tells about skeletal maturity of the child. Conventionally bone age is assessed from X-ray of hand and wrist using Grulich-Pyle atlas or by Tanner Whitehouse method. Bone age gives an idea as to what proportion of adult height has been achieved by the child and what is the remaining potential for height gain. Bone age is delayed compared to chronological age in almost all causes of pathological short stature. When bone age is retarded by 2 years or more it is abnormal and usually suggests an endocrine disease such as hypothyroidism, growth hormone deficiency or Cushing disease. In children who have chronic systemic disease, malnutrition or delayed puberty bone age is delayed but not as much as in endocrine deficiency. In familial short stature bone age equal chronological age. In constitutional delay, bone age is less than chronological age and equals height age.

Blood biochemistry:

Biochemical tests are done based on the probable cause of short stature, renal and liver function tests are done. Following are some of the tests indicated in systemic illnesses – blood urea, serum creatinine, serum calcium, phosphorus, alkaline phosphatase, venous blood gas analysis, fasting blood sugar, albumin, transaminases.

Level 2 investigations:

- Serum thyroxine, thyroid stimulating hormone (TSH) in a case of hypothyroidism.
- Karyotyping to rule out Turner's syndrome in girls with short stature especially if there are any pointers to suggest Turner's syndrome.
- Radiological investigations:
  - Skeletal survey: X-ray chest is done as routine, but X-ray of pelvis, upper and lower limbs are indicated in children with disproportionate short stature to rule out skeletal dysplasias and rickets.
  - MRI brain: Indicated where cause of short stature could be due to pathology in the pituitary or hypothalamus.
  - X-ray skull: Helpful in cases with suprasellar calcification.

If all of the above investigations are normal and height of the child is between -2 to -3SD then observe height velocity for 6-12 months. If height is <3 SD, proceed to level 3 investigations.

Level 3 investigations:

- Celiac serology (anti-endomyrial or anti-tissue transglutaminase antibodies)
- Duodenal biopsy
- Evaluation for growth hormone deficiency should be done only after common causes of growth retardation have been excluded. IGF-1 and its binding protein 3 are screening tests for GH deficiency. Low levels should be followed by a GN stimulation test.

The algorithm describes how to approach a child with short stature. If the child's height is >2SD, he is normal and just needs to be followed up for growth velocity. If the child's height is below the 3rd centile, it is pathological then see whether he has dysmorphicfeatures, which are suggestive of genetic syndromes. Again they can be with proportionate or disproportionate based on upper to lower segment ratio.

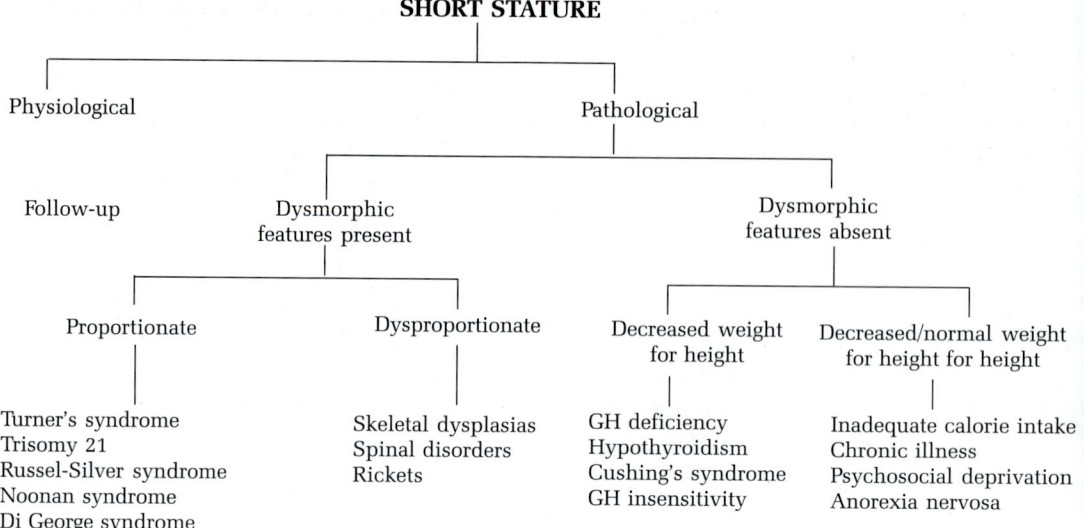

SHORT STATURE

- Physiological
  - Follow-up
- Pathological
  - Dysmorphic features present
    - Proportionate
      - Turner's syndrome
      - Trisomy 21
      - Russel-Silver syndrome
      - Noonan syndrome
      - Di George syndrome
      - Fetal alcohol syndrome
    - Dysproportionate
      - Skeletal dysplasias
      - Spinal disorders
      - Rickets
  - Dysmorphic features absent
    - Decreased weight for height
      - GH deficiency
      - Hypothyroidism
      - Cushing's syndrome
      - GH insensitivity
    - Decreased/normal weight for height for height
      - Inadequate calorie intake
      - Chronic illness
      - Psychosocial deprivation
      - Anorexia nervosa

SUMMARY

Short stature is a common problem for which a child is brought to a pediatrician. A thorough history followed by a complete review of systems needs to be undertaken in order to help exclude an undiagnosed syndrome or chronic medical condition responsible for the short stature. Investigations will depend upon the clinical diagnosis. The first step is to confirm whether the child is really short by plotting his height on a centile chart, assessing his growth velocity and comparing his present centile with mid-parental target centile.

SUGGESTED READING

1. Gardener DJ, Shoback D. Greenspan's Basic and Clinical Endocrinology, 8th Ed. Columbus OH: McGraw-Hill Professional, 2007.

2. PreetamNath, Jitendra Kumar, SK HammardeusRahman, M. Rai. Short Stature: Evaluation and Management apindia.org.

3. Revised IAP Growth charts for Height, Weight and Body Mass Index for 5-18 years old. Indian Children. http://www.indianpediatrics.net.

4. Short stature: Background, pathophysiology. http://www.Epidemiology. emedicine. mediscape.com.

5. Short stature (Assessment) Step-by-Step Diagnostic approach. http://www. bestpractice. bmj.com.

6. Dubey AP, PandhkarNagroy: Approach to a child with short stature 164-169. Pediatrics for Practitioners. Jaypee Brothers Medical Publishers Pvt. Ltd., 2014.

0 to 5 years: WHO Girls Length / Height, Weight and Head Circumference Charts

Name: ──────────────

DOB : ──────────────

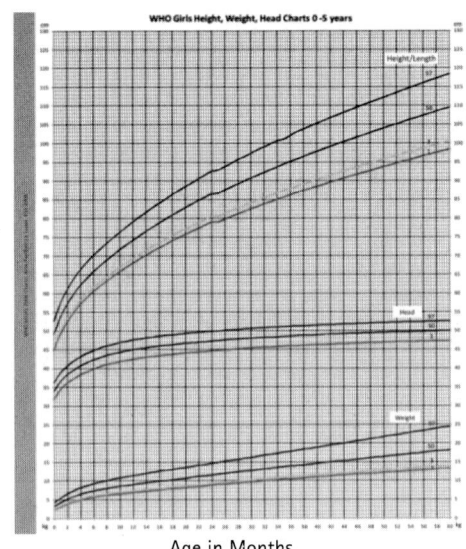

Age in Months

Graph 1 : Showing 0-5 years : WHO girls length / height, weight and head circumference chart

5 to 18 years: IAP Girls Height and Weight Charts

Father's Height:_____ Mother's Height::_____ Target Height:_____

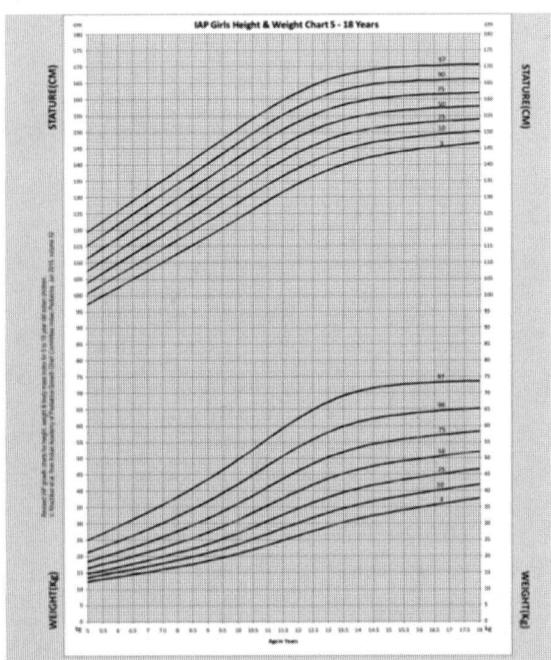

Graph 2 : Showing 5 to 18 years : IAP Girls Height and Weight Charts

0 to 5 years: WHO Boys Length / Height, Weight and Head Circumference Charts

Name: _____

DOB : _____

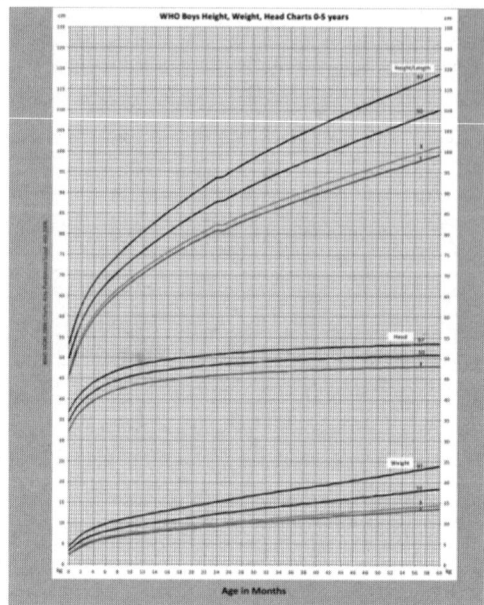

Graph 3 : Showing 0-5 years : WHO boys length / height, weight and head circumference chart

5 to 18 years: IAP Boyls Height and Weight Charts

Father's Height:_____ Mother's Height::_____ Target Height:_____

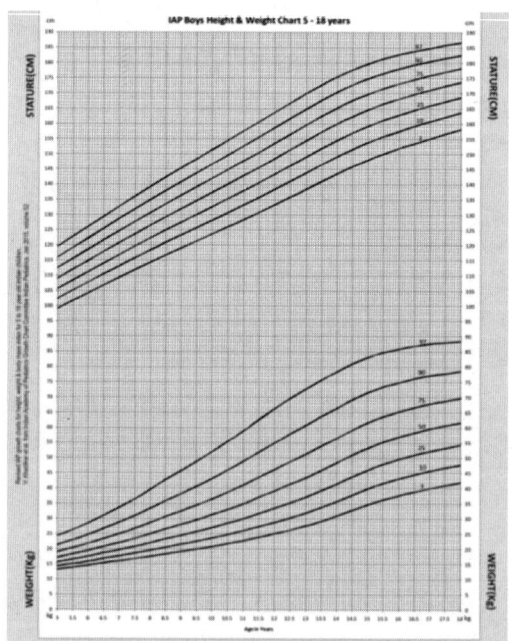

Graph 4 : Showing 5 to 18 years : IAP Boys Height and Weight Charts

Chapter

2

FAILURE TO THRIVE

INTRODUCTION

Failure to thrive or growth failure is a descriptive term and not a specific diagnosis. It is a result of inadequate usable calorie necessary for a child's metabolic and growth demands and it manifests as physical growth that is significantly less than that of peers.

This term is widely used to describe inadequate growth in early childhood. However, no consensus has been reached concerning the specific anthropometric criteria to define this description. Although definitions vary, most authors use the term only when growth has been noted to be below 3rd percentile for age or if growth has decreased over time (measurements falling two major percentiles) using the standard growth charts. However, all authorities agree that only by comparing height and weight on a growth chart over time, can failure to thrive be accurately assessed.

Markowitz emphasized that FTT is "failure to reach one's growth potential". This allows that small for gestational age (SFD) infants, very small premature babies, children of short parents or very thin parents, as well as those with congenital syndromes characterized by short stature are not necessarily failing to thrive. These children may appear to have growth failure based on anthropometric screening measurements (e.g. growing below the third percentile) but as Markowitz notes, one should not confuse "screens for FTT" with failing growth potential.

ETIOLOGY

Causes of failure to thrive can be organic, inorganic or a combination of the two.

Table: Causes of failure to thrive

1. *Organic causes*

   - Prenatal: Intrauterine growth retardation, intrauterine infections.
   - Gastrointestinal: Persistent or recurrent vomiting as in gastroesophageal reflux disease, pyloric stenosis.
   - Defects in absorption: Celiac disease, cystic fibrosis, lactose intolerance.
   - Cardiovascular: Congenital heart disease, cardiomyopathy, congestive cardiac failure.
   - Renal: Chronic renal failure, renal tubular acidosis, chronic pyelonephritis.
   - Metabolic disease: Diabetes, in-born errors of metabolism, adrenal hyperplasia.
   - Occult infection: Tuberculosis, urinary tract infection, human immunodeficiency virus infection.
   - Central nervous system: Mental retardation, cerebral palsy.

2. *Inorganic causes*

   - Poor nutritional intake: poverty, maternal ignorance, failure of lactation, prematurity, cleft lip and palate.
   - Emotional deprivation syndrome: abandoned child, single parent, parenteral rejection, child abuse.

Causes of failure to thrive based on pathophysiology:

1. Inadequate calorie intake

2. Inadequate absorption of nutrients

3. Increased caloric requirement

4. Defective utilization of calories (defect in assimilation)

EVALUATION

A. History

The most important part of evaluation of a child with failure to thrive is to obtain a careful detail history and to determine whether the cause is organic, inorganic or mixed.

Points to be enquired in history

- Age at onset

- Antenatal history

- What was the birth weight and length?

- Feeding history in detail

- History of vomiting

- History of recurrent diarrhea

- History of recurrent respiratory infections

- History of breathlessness, palpitation, easy fatigability

- Record of previous weight and height

- Family history

Age at onset:

Causes of failure to thrive vary with age. In early infancy the commonest cause is failure of lactation, especially if it occurs in women who are illiterate and belonging to the underpriviledged society as they tend to use overdiluted top milk. Other causes are intrauterine growth retardation (IUGR), intrauterine infections, renal tubular acidosis and inborn errors of metabolism. Beyond infancy the cause could be poor nutritional intake, occult infections such as urinary tract infection (UTI), tuberculosis, persistent diarrhea, chronic systemic disease such as congenital heart disease with congestive cardiac failure, chronic renal failure.

Antenatal history:

A detail antenatal history must be recorded. Did the mother suffer any illnesses or infections during pregnancy such as hypertension, oligohydramnios? Did she have fever and exanthems? Any history of drug ingestion. How was the weight gain during pregnancy?

Birth history:

What was the weight and length of the baby at birth? This would help in determining whether there was IUGR. IUGR babies are slow growers. History of any illness in the neonatal period should also be enquired.

Feeding history:

Failure to thrive in infancy is commonly due to faulty feeding. Therefore, feeding history is extremely important. A detail lactation history should be enquired. Is there lactation failure? If the baby is receiving top milk, which milk is he receiving? Whether it is diluted with water? Are there any taboos regarding feeding? Any obvious feeding difficulty such as cleft lip or palate. In certain metabolic disorders, growth is poor inspite of good appetite, e.g. diabetes and thyrotoxicosis.

History of recurrent or chronic illnesses:

Persistent or recurrent vomiting in infancy with failure to thrive is suggestive of gastroesophageal reflux disease, pyloric stenosis or metabolic disease.

Babies with chronic diarrhea may fail to grow properly. Frequency and nature of stool should be enquired. Bulky, foul smelling sticky stools are seen in cystic fibrosis and celiac disease. Large watery stools may suggest lactose intolerance.

In cases of mucoviscidosis a history of recurrent respiratoryinfection is present.

Presence of breathlessness, palpitation, excessive sweating, feeding difficulty with failure to thrive points towards cardiac failure.

Does the child get recurrent fever? Such a history points towards a chronic infective process such as UTI, tuberculosis, HIV, etc.

Record of previous weight and height:

Record of previous weight and height should be seen. It helps to assess whether the child was born normal or whether it was an IUGR baby. Babies with IUGR grow slowly. If the baby was normal at birth and subsequently growth decelerated, one has to look out for a cause.

Family history:

If the parents are thin then the cause could be genetic. If the cause appears to be inorganic, one must enquire whether the child has been abandoned by his parents? Is the infant mother bonding poor? Is it an unwanted child? Infants staying in orphanages, if not given adequate love and affection fail to thrive.

B. Examination

Specific signs to be looked for
● Assessment of growth
● Does the child look ill or well?
● Dysmorphic features
● Dyspnea/tachypnea
● Blood pressure
● Pallor
● Signs of vitamin deficiencies
● Presence of edema
● Skin changes
● Systemic examination

First thing to assess in a child with failure to thrive is growth.

Screens used to detect possible FTT:

1. Weight for age below the third centile.
2. Height for age below the third centile.
3. Weight < 80% of ideal weight for height (BMI after 3 years).
4. Weight below 5th centile more than once.
5. Weight crosses down 2 percentiles.
6. Failing to gain grams per day at expected rate.

The above shows a variety of screens that have been used to assess for FTT. Most commonly used is growth occurring below the 3rd centile on height/weight falling through 2 percentiles lines. None of the screens are perfect.

This is done to make sure that the child definitely has failure to thrive. The first thing that should be done is to plot the head circumference, height and weight on a growth chart. Effort should be made to obtain as many previous growth parameters as possible to detect trends in growth rather than to rely on measurements of one particular visit.

If all the three anthropometric measurements, i.e. weight, height and head circumference are less than expected for age this indicates organic etiology that occurred in utero viz. chromosomal, genetic or intrauterine infection.

If weight and height are affected with normal head circumference one must suspect endocrinopathies such as growth hormone deficiency, acquired hypothyroidism or constitutional delay. When only weight gain is affected it indicates recent caloric deprivation or acute illness.

Normal growth in infants

Average birth weight – 3.3 kg
Weight drops as much as 10% in first few days of life.
Birth weight regained by D10–D15 of life.
Birth weight doubles by 4 months of age.Birth weight triples by 1 year of age.

Appearance of child

It is important to assess from general appearance whether the child looks ill or well. If the child looks sick one must think of a chronic infection, in-born error of metabolism, chronic renal failure, renal tubular acidosis, cardiac disease or an intrauterine infection.

If the child appears well one must consider constitutional/ genetic cause, IUGR, pituitary deficiency or feeding problem.

Dysmorphicfeatures:

Presence of dysmorphology would suggest certain syndromes or chromosomal aberrations such as in Turner's syndrome, there could be a low hair line, webbing of neck, wide carrying angle. Micropenis would be a feature of hypopituitarism.Other features such as hypo-hypertelorism, cataracts, high arched palate, clinodactyl, abnormal dermatoglyphics, may point to specific syndrome.Presence of cleft lip and palate may give rise to feeding difficulty and thereby failure to thrive.

Vital signs:

Assessment of vital signs would be informative. Dyspnea would point towards long standing congestive cardiac failure due to heart disease or interstitial lung disease.Persistent tachypneaindicates an in-born error of metabolism or renal tubular acidosis. Blood pressure should be recorded. Hypertension is an important feature of chronic renal failure, while hypotension is seen in Addison's disease.

General examination:

Pallor would be seen in chronic renal failure. Addison's disease, chronic infective processes, malabsorption and caloric deprivation.

Clubbing would suggest interstitial lung disease, celiac disease, cystic fibrosis, cyanotic congenital heart disease.

One must carefully look for signs of vitamin deficiencies. Presence of deficiency signs would suggest either malabsorption or poor intake.

Examination of the skin will reveal a lot of information, dry, rough skin with dermatosis is seen in protein energy malnutrition. Sparse dry hair with dyschromotrichia is also a feature of malnutrition. Increased pigmentation is a feature of Addison's disease.

If there is lymphadenopathy in a child with failure to thrive one must keep in mind tuberculosis and HIV.

Presence of pitting edema is seen in Kwashiorkor.

Systemic examination:

Examination of abdomen: A generalized distended abdomen would suggest a disorder of malabsorption such as celiac disease. In infants, hepatosplenomegaly and petechiae may suggest intrauterine infections, chronic liver disease. In older children, if there is hepatosplenomegaly with failure to thrive one must keep in mind tuberculosis and HIV.

Examination of cardiovascular system (CVS): One must look for evidence of heart disease, murmur and signs of congestive cardiac failure, which could hamper growth.

Examination of central nervous system (CNS): Cerebral palsy, mental retardation do give rise to growth failure due to feeding difficulty.

> **Red flag signs and symptoms suggesting medical emergency needing urgent attention**
> - Cardiac findings suggesting congenital heart disease or heart failure (e.g. murmur, oedema, jugular venous distension)
> - Severe infection
> - Respiratory distress, acidosis
> - Failure to gain weight despite adequate caloric intake
> - Organomegaly, lymphadenopathy
> - Recurrent severe respiratory, mucocutaneous or urinary infection
> - Recurrent vomiting, diarrhoea, dehydration
> - Patient in shock

C.   Investigations

What investigations are needed?

Poor nutrition and psychosocial factors are the most frequent causes of growth failure, therefore laboratory tests would yield very little. If history and physical findings indicate an organic cause or there are red flags signs or symptoms, then investigations are necessary.

First line of investigations are done in all cases. When first line of investigations are inconclusive then one should proceed to the second line again based on clinical findings.

First line of investigations:
- CBC
- ESR
- Urine analysis including culture
- Biochemical tests – glucose, creatinine, serum calcium, liver function tests

Second line of investigations:
- Serum amino acids
- Urine amino acids and organic acids
- Serum electrolytes
- Stool fat
- Sweat test
- HIV screening
- Anti-endomysial antibodies
- TCG
- Bone age
- Skeletal survey
- Milk scan
- Endoscopy with mucosal biopsies
- ECG, echocardiogram
- Thyroid profile

Table: Probable diagnosis based on investigations

	Investigations	Probable Diagnosis
1.	Complete blood count:Normocytic normochromic anaemia	Chronic renal failure
2.	Urine examination:	
	• Pyuria	Urinary tract infection
	• Urine culture positive	Urinary tract infection
	• Hematuria and proteinuria	Chronic renal failure due to glomerulonephritis
3.	Blood biochemistry altered:	
	• Serum creatinine	
	• Serum sodium	
	• Serum potassium	Chronic renal failure
	• Serum calcium	
	• Serum phosphorus	
	• Arterial blood gas analysis altered	Inborn errors of metabolism Renal tubular acidosis
4.	Stool examination:	
	• Fat estimation increased	Malabsorption
	• Reducing substance present	Lactose intolerance
5.	Antigliadin antibodies – present	Coeliac disease
6.	Jejunal biopsy – atrophy of villi	Coeliac disease
7.	Sweat chloride test	Cystic fibrosis
8.	X-ray chest:	
	• Cardiomegaly	Heart disease
	• Parenchymal lesion	Tuberculosis
	• Lymphadenopathy	Tuberculosis
9.	Virological assay:	
	• Detection of HIV by PCR, P24 antigen if positive	AIDS
10.	Karyotyping	Chromosomal abnormalities
11.	Thyroid profile	Thyroid disorders

ALGORITHM FOR EVALUATION OF FAILURE TO THRIVE

ARE RED FLAG SIGNS OR SYMPTOMS PRESENT?

No | Yes

No → Proceed with evaluation and management of appropriate caloric intake

Yes → Consider CBC, serum electrolytes, BUN, urine analysis and culture, ESR, thyroid function tests, LFT

If indicated by history, physical examination, or initial lab testing consider complement levels, echocardiography, HIV testing, immunoglobulin levels, MT, stool for ova, Cyst, fat content, reducing substances

SUMMARY

Failure to thrive is because of:

Too little in

Too much out

Too little utilized

Too much required

Wasting and stunting is due to metabolic, renal or cardiac cause.

Whenever a child is brought with the complaints of 'poor growth' or 'child not growing' one must first ascertain, if this is really so or is it merely parental anxiety.

Psychosocial and nutritional causes are commonly responsible but significant organic pathology requires appropriate investigations.

Initial hospital observation of about 2 weeks is often necessary to get at the cause. A calculated regular diet is given and the daily intake and weight are carefully plotted.

The following results enable a categorization:

a. If intake is adequate and weight gain is satisfactory, it may indicate improper feeding technique at home or disturbed relationship with the mother. Such children need no investigations.

b. Adequate intake, poor or no weight gain despite increased calories indicates malabsorption, which should be investigated.

c. If intake is inadequate the cause can be organic and needs investigation.

After a careful history thorough physical examination and a 2 week hospital observation relevant diagnostic tests should be carried out.

SUGGESTED READING

1. Failure to thrive: Causes, symptoms and diagnosis. www.healthline.com

2. Failure to thrive: Background, epidemiology. Medscape emedicine.medscape.com

OBESITY

INTRODUCTION

Obesity in childhood is a complex disorder and is becoming an increasing problem in developing countries like India, where both malnutrition as well as obesity occur side by side. This is because we as an emerging nation, have both poor as well as rich populations, with the middle class getting progressively prosperous.

Childhood obesity predisposes to insulin resistance and type-2 diabetes, hypertension, hyperlipidemia, liver and renal disease and reproductive dysfunction. This condition also increases the risk of adult onset obesity and cardiovascular disease.

DEFINITION

Obesity denotes overweight as a result of excessive accumulation of fat in the subcutaneous and other tissues. It is not merely excess weight.

ETIOLOGY

Many factors including genetics, environment, metabolism, lifestyle and eating habits are believed to play a role in the development of obesity. However, more than 90% of the cases are idiopathic, less than 10% are associated with hormonal or genetic causes.

Table: Causes of obesity

- Environmental factors: Excessive energy intake, sedentary life style, TV viewing, playing computer games.
- Genetic factors: Obesity in parents and other family members.
- Endocrine cause: Hypothyroidism, pseudoparathyroidism, Cushing syndrome.
- Hypothalamic dysfunction: Central nervous system injury—encephalitis, meningitis, head trauma, neurosurgery, craniopharyngioma.
- Others: Albright syndrome, polycystic ovarian disease, Prader- Willi syndrome, Laurence-Moon-Biedl syndrome.
- Drugs: Steroids, anticonvulsants—valproate, clonazepam.

CLINICAL EVALUATION

A. History

Since in majority of cases the cause of obesity is environmental or genetic, a good history and examination will help in arriving at the cause of obesity.

Points to be elicited in the history
- Family history of obesity
- Dietary intake
- Outdoor activities
- TV viewing/computer games
- History of central nervous system infection
- History of head injury, neurosurgery
- History of headache, vomiting
- Developmental history.

Family history:

Enquire whether parents and other family members are obese. Obesity tends to run in families partly because of genetic reasons and partly because of same lifestyle and food habits.

Dietary intake:

The parents must be asked about total diet recall of the child for the past 3 to 5 days. What type of food does the child take? Frequency of meals. How often does he take fast food? Child's liking for sweets and fatty food? Does he indulge in overeating? Dietary factor is the most important cause of obesity. Energy intake exceeds expenditure leading to increased body fat store. Consumption of carbohydrate and fat rich high density foods lead to obesity.

Activities of the child:

How much time does the child devote for outdoor activities? Does he regularly play outdoor games? How much time does he spend for TV viewing and playing computer games? Children are increasingly spending a lot of time viewing the television and playing computer games, resulting in sedentary life style and eating junk food, leading ultimately to obesity.

History of excessive appetite:

Has the child's appetite recently increased? Such a history would suggest a hypothalamic lesion.

History of central nervous system involvement:

Had the child suffered from encephalitis or meningitis in the past? Any history of head injury? Has the child undergone any neurosurgical procedure? Does he complain of headache, vomiting, visual disturbance? How is the school performance? Has there been a recent deterioration in scholastic performance? Infections, trauma, tumor or neurosurgery affecting the pituitary hypothalamic region can lead to obesity due to destruction of the satiety center.

History of listlessness:

Does the child complaint of tiredness, dullness, constipation, since the time he has put on weight? Such a history would suggest hypothyroidism.

History of drug intake:

Is the child receiving any drugs? Drugs such as steroids, clonazepam and sodium valproate are known to give rise to obesity.

Developmental history:

Has the development of the child been normal or delayed? Delayed development is a feature of hypothyroidism and genetic syndromes.

B. Examination

> **Points on examination**
> - Anthropometric measurements
> - Fat distribution
> - Facies
> - Congenital malformations
> - Vitals
> - Skin
> - Secondary sex characters
> - Systemic examination

Assessment of obesity:

Obesity can be assessed by the following parameters:
a. Calculation of BMI: For this the height and weight of the child is recorded and body mass index (BMI) is calculated, according to the following formula:

$$BMI = Weight\ (kg)\ /\ Height\ (m)^2$$

Normal values for BMI vary with age, sex and pubertal status. Consensus committees have recommended that children and adolescents be considered overweight or obese if BMI exceeds the 95th percentile or exceeds 30 kg/m² at any age.

Weight for height:

If weight for height is greater than 120% the child is considered to be obese.

Skin fold thickness:

Skin fold thickness is measured over the subscapular, triceps and biceps region. The readings are plotted on age specific percentile charts. Values greater than 85th percentile are abnormal.

The fat distribution is also assessed whether it is generalized or truncal. Selective accumulation of fat in the neck and trunk suggests excess cortisol. Buffalo hump is characteristic of Cushing syndrome. Children with constitutional obesity are tall for age. Reduced rate of linear growth in a child with obesity is seen in growth hormone deficiency, hypothyroidism, pseudoparathyroidism, cortisol excess and genetic syndromes such as Prader-Willi syndrome.

Secondary sex characters:

Sexual maturation should also be assessed. In case of familial and diet induced obesity growth rate is normal or excessive. These children enter puberty at appropriate age. Many of them mature more quickly than children with normal weight. Bone age is usually advanced.

Growth rate and pubertal development is delayed in conditions with hormone deficiency viz. hypothyroidism, cortisol excess and various genetic syndromes.

If growth rate and pubertal development are accelerated one should consider precocious puberty and in girls polycystic ovarian syndrome.

Facies:

Coarse facies would be a feature of hypothyroidism. Moon face is typical of Cushing syndrome. Almond-shaped eyes are seen in Prader-Willi syndrome.

Congenital malformations:

Children with obesity should be thoroughly examined for the presence of congenital anomalies viz. polydactyl, syndactyl, short extremities, metacarpal shortening and hypogonadism.

Polydactyl is seen in case of Laurence-Moon-Biedl syndrome and Alstrom syndrome. In Prader-Willi syndrome hands and feet are short. Metacarpals of the 3rd, 4th and 5th digit are short in pseudoparathyroidism. Ear lobe creases are seen in Beckwith-Weidemann syndrome. Hypogonadism is a feature of Laurence-Moon-Biedl syndrome and Prader-Willi syndrome.

Other features:

Presence of striae and hirsutism is seen in case of Cushing syndrome. Hypoplasia of dental enamel would suggestpseudohypoparathyroidism. Blood pressure should be recorded in all cases of obesity. Hypertension is present in Cushing syndrome.

Systemic examination:

Hepatosplenomegaly would suggest glycogenosis. Generalized hypotonia is a feature of Prader-Willi syndrome. Presence of mental subnormality is a feature of hypothyroidism, Prader-Willi syndrome and pseudohypoparathyroidism. The fundus should be examined for retinitis pigmentosa. It is present in cases of Laurence-Moon-Biedl syndrome and Alstrom syndrome.

C. Investigations

Relevant investigations should be done depending upon the clinical causes.

Most cases of obesity in children are due to constitutional and environmental factors for which a good history and examination is all that is required. A very small number of cases would need investigations.

Table: Investigations in obesity

Investigations	Indication
• Bone age	Advanced BA – healthy childrenDelayed BA – hypothyroidism, hypopituitarism
• Blood glucose- fasting and post meal	Diabetes
• Altered lipid profile	Dyslipidemia
• Serum calcium phosphorus, alkaline phosphatase, parathormone levels	Pseudoparathyroidism
• Thyroid hormones (FT4 &TSH)	Hypothyroidism
• Growth hormone assay	Growth hormone deficiency
• Adrenal functions, urinary cortisol, ACTH, CRH	Cushing's syndrome
• Karyotyping	Chromosomal anomalies
• MRI brain and abdomen	Hypothalamus / pituitary lesion, adrenal tumor

SUMMARY

Childhood obesity affects both developed and developing countries of all socioeconomic groups irrespective of age, sex or ethnicity.

Whenever a child is brought to a clinician for obesity the first step would be to confirm that the child is really obese. This is done by calculating the Body Mass Index (BMI). Normal values for BMI vary with age, sex and pubertal status. For a 13-year-old, a BMI greater than 25 constitutes obesity whereas in adolescents over 18, BMI greater than 30 is obesity. Most children with obesity do not have an organic cause. It is usually due to imbalance in energy intake and expenditure. Such an imbalance results due to excessive consumption of energy dense food and sedentary life style.

If an adolescent is healthy and has no delay of growth or sexual maturation an underlying endocrinologic, neurologic or genetic cause is unlikely.

SUGGESTED READING

1. Obesity in children work up: Approach considerations. emedicinemedscape.com Mar 29, 2016. Steven M. Schwarz.

2. Obesity in children & adolescents: Manju Ray & R. Krishna Kumar. Indian J Med Res 132, 2010, 598-607.

3. Obesity in children and adolescents – NCBI – National Institute of Health. www. ncbi. nim. nih. gov >NCBI>Pubmed Central by M. Ray, 2010.

Table: Body Mass Index - Boys - 0-5 Years (WHO Standard)

Year	Month	Percentiles					Z (SD) Score					
		5th	15th	50th	85th	95th	-3Z	-2Z	-1Z	. +1Z	+2Z	+3Z
0	0	11.5	12.2	13.4	14.8	15.8	10.2	11.1	12.2	14.8	16.3	18.1
	1	12.8	13.6	14.9	16.4	17.3	11.3	12.4	13.6	16.3	17.8	19.4
	2	14.1	14.9	16.3	17.8	18.8	12.5	13.7	15.0	17.8	19.4	21.1
	3	14.7	15.5	16.9	18.5	19.4	13.1	14.3	15.5	18.4	20.0	21.8
	4	15.0	15.7	17.2	18.7	19.7	13.4	14.5	15.8	18.7	20.3	22.1
	5	15.1	15.9	17.3	18.9	19.8	13.5	14.7	15.9	18.8	20.5	22.3
	6	15.2	15.9	17.3	18.9	19.9	13.6	14.7	16.0	18.8	20.5	22.3
	7	15.2	15.9	17.3	18.9	19.9	13.7	14.8	16.0	18.8	20.5	22.3
	8	15.1	15.9	17.3	18.8	19.8	13.6	14.7	15.9	18.7	20.4	22.2
	9	15.1	15.8	17.2	18.7	19.7	13.6	14.7	15.8	18.6	20.3	22.1
	10	15.0	15.7	17.0	18.6	19.5	13.5	14.6	15.7	18.5	20.1	22.0
	11	14.9	15.6	16.9	18.4	19.4	13.4	14.5	15.6	18.4	20.0	21.8
1	0	14.8	15.5	16.8	18.3	19.2	13.4	14.4	15.5	18.2	19.8	21.6
1	1	14.7	15.4	16.7	18.1	19.1	13.3	14.3	15.4	18.1	19.7	21.5
1	2	14.6	15.3	16.6	18.0	18.9	13.2	14.2	15.3	18.0	19.5	21.3
1	3	14.5	15.2	16.4	17.9	18.8	13.1	14.1	15.2	17.8	19.4	21.2
1	4	14.4	15.1	16.3	17.8	18.7	13.1	14.0	15.1	17.7	19.3	21.0
1	5	14.3	15.0	16.2	17.6	18.6	13.0	13.9	15.0	17.6	19.1	20.9
1	6	14.2	14.9	16.1	17.5	18.5	12.9	13.9	14.9	17.5	19.0	20.8
1	7	14.2	14.8	16.1	17.4	18.4	12.9	13.8	14.9	17.4	18.9	20.7
1	8	14.1	14.8	16.0	17.4	18.3	12.8	13.7	14.8	17.3	18.8	20.6
1	9	14.1	14.7	15.9	17.3	18.2	12.8	13.7	14.7	17.2	18.7	20.5
1	10	14.0	14.6	15.8	17.2	18.1	12.7	13.6	14.7	17.2	18.7	20.4
1	11	14.0	14.6	15.8	17.1	18.0	12.7	13.6	14.6	17.1	18.6	20.3
2	0	13.9	14.5	15.7	17.1	18.0	12.7	13.6	14.6	17.0	18.5	20.3
2	1	14.1	14.8	16.0	17.4	18.3	12.8	13.8	14.8	17.3	18.8	20.5
2	2	14.1	14.7	15.9	17.3	18.2	12.8	13.7	14.8	17.3	18.8	20.5
2	3	14.0	14.7	15.9	17.3	18.2	12.7	13.7	14.7	17.2	18.7	20.4
2	4	14.0	14.7	15.9	17.2	18.1	12.7	13.6	14.7	17.2	18.7	20.4
2	5	14.0	14.6	15.8	17.2	18.1	12.7	13.6	14.7	17.1	18.6	20.3
2	6	13.9	14.6	15.8	17.2	18.0	12.6	13.6	14.6	17.1	18.6	20.2
2	7	13.9	14.5	15.8	17.1	18.0	12.6	13.5	14.6	17.1	18.5	20.2
2	8	13.9	14.5	15.7	17.1	18.0	12.5	13.5	14.6	17.0	18.5	20.1
2	9	13.8	14.5	15.7	17.0	17.9	12.5	13.5	14.5	17.0	18.5	20.1

2	10	13.8	14.4	15.7	17.0	17.9	12.5	13.4	14.5	17.0	18.4	20.0
2	11	13.8	14.4	15.6	17.0	17.9	12.4	13.4	14.5	16.9	18.4	20.0
3	0	13.7	14.4	15.6	17.0	17.8	12.4	13.4	14.4	16.9	18.4	20.0
3	1	13.7	14.4	15.6	16.9	17.8	12.4	13.3	14.4	16.9	18.3	19.9
3	2	13.7	14.3	15.5	16.9	17.8	12.3	13.3	14.4	16.8	18.3	19.9
3	3	13.6	14.3	15.5	16.9	17.7	12.3	13.3	14.3	16.8	18.3	19.9
3	4	13.6	14.3	15.5	16.8	17.7	12.3	13.2	14.3	16.8	18.2	19.9
3	5	13.6	14.2	15.5	16.8	17.7	12.2	13.2	14.3	16.8	18.2	19.9
3	6	13.6	14.2	15.4	16.8	17.7	12.2	13.2	14.3	16.8	18.2	19.8
3	7	13.5	14.2	15.4	16.8	17.7	12.2	13.2	14.2	16.7	18.2	19.8
3	8	13.5	14.2	15.4	16.8	17.7	12.2	13.1	14.2	16.7	18.2	19.8
3	9	13.5	14.2	15.4	16.8	17.6	12.2	13.1	14.2	16.7	18.2	19.8
3	10	13.5	14.1	15.4	16.7	17.6	12.1	13.1	14.2	16.7	18.2	19.8
3	11	13.5	14.1	15.3	16.7	17.6	12.1	13.1	14.2	16.7	18.2	19.9
4	0	13.4	14.1	15.3	16.7	17.6	12.1	13.1	14.1	16.7	18.2	19.9
4	1	13.4	14.1	15.3	16.7	17.6	12.1	13.0	14.1	16.7	18.2	19.9
4	2	13.4	14.1	15.3	16.7	17.6	12.1	13.0	14.1	16.7	18.2	19.9
4	3	13.4	14.0	15.3	16.7	17.6	12.1	13.0	14.1	16.6	18.2	19.9
4	4	13.4	14.0	15.3	16.7	17.6	12.0	13.0	14.1	16.6	18.2	19.9
4	5	13.3	14.0	15.3	16.7	17.6	12.0	13.0	14.1	16.6	18.2	20.0
4	6	13.3	14.0	15.3	16.7	17.6	12.0	13.0	14.0	16.6	18.2	20.0
4	7	13.3	14.0	15.2	16.7	17.6	12.0	13.0	14.0	16.6	18.2	20.0
4	8	13.3	14.0	15.2	16.7	17.6	12.0	12.9	14.0	16.6	18.2	20.1
4	9	13.3	14.0	15.2	16.7	17.6	12.0	12.9	14.0	16.6	18.2	20.1
4	10	13.3	13.9	15.2	16.7	17.6	12.0	12.9	14.0	16.6	18.3	20.2
4	11	13.3	13.9	15.2	16.7	17.7	12.0	12.9	14.0	16.6	18.3	20.2
5	0	13.3	13.9	15.2	16.7	17.7	12.0	12.9	14.0	16.6	18.3	20.3

Table: Body Mass Index – Girls – 0–5 Years (WHO Standard)

Year	Month	Percentiles					Z (SD) Score					
		5th	15th	50th	85th	95th	–3Z	–2Z	–1Z	. +1Z	+2Z	+3Z
		5th	15th	50th	85th	95th	–3Z	–2Z	–1Z	. +1Z	+2Z	+3Z
	0	11.5	12.1	13.3	14.7	15.8	10.2	11.1	12.2	14.8	16.3	18.1
	1	12.4	13.2	14.6	16.1	17.3	11.3	12.4	13.6	16.3	17.8	19.4
	2	13.5	14.3	15.8	17.4	18.8	12.5	13.7	15.0	17.8	19.4	21.1
	3	14.0	14.9	16.4	18.0	19.4	13.1	14.3	15.5	18.4	20.0	21.8
	4	14.3	15.2	16.7	18.3	19.7	13.4	14.5	15.8	18.7	20.3	22.1
	5	14.5	15.3	16.8	18.5	19.8	13.5	14.7	15.9	18.8	20.5	22.3
	6	14.6	15.4	16.9	18.6	19.9	13.6	14.7	16.0	18.8	20.5	22.3
	7	14.6	15.4	16.9	18.6	19.9	13.7	14.8	16.0	18.8	20.5	22.3
	8	14.6	15.4	16.8	18.5	19.8	13.6	14.7	15.9	18.7	20.4	22.2
	9	14.5	15.3	16.7	18.4	19.7	13.6	14.7	15.8	18.6	20.3	22.1
	10	14.4	15.2	16.6	18.2	19.5	13.5	14.6	15.7	18.5	20.1	22.0
	11	14.3	15.1	16.5	18.1	19.4	13.4	14.5	15.6	18.4	20.0	21.8
1	0	14.2	15.0	16.4	17.9	19.2	13.4	14.4	15.5	18.2	19.8	21.6
1	1	14.1	14.8	16.2	17.8	19.1	13.3	14.3	15.4	18.1	19.7	21.5
1	2	14.0	14.7	16.1	17.7	18.9	13.2	14.2	15.3	18.0	19.5	21.3
1	3	13.9	14.6	16.0	17.5	18.8	13.1	14.1	15.2	17.8	19.4	21.2
1	4	13.8	14.6	15.9	17.4	18.7	13.1	14.0	15.1	17.7	19.3	21.0
1	5	13.8	14.5	15.8	17.3	18.6	13.0	13.9	15.0	17.6	19.1	20.9
1	6	13.7	14.4	15.7	17.2	18.5	12.9	13.9	14.9	17.5	19.0	20.8
1	7	13.6	14.3	15.7	17.2	18.4	12.9	13.8	14.9	17.4	18.9	20.7
1	8	13.6	14.3	15.6	17.1	18.3	12.8	13.7	14.8	17.3	18.8	20.6
1	9	13.6	14.2	15.5	17.0	–18.2	12.8	13.7	14.7	17.2	18.7	20.5
1	10	13.5	14.2	15.5	17.0	18.1	12.7	13.6	14.7	17.2	18.7	20.4
1	11	13.5	14.2	15.4	16.9	18.0	12.7	13.6	14.6	17.1	18.6	20.3
2	0	13.5	14.1	15.4	16.9	18.0	12.7	13.6	14.6	17.0	18.5	20.3
2	1	13.7	14.4	15.7	17.1	18.1	12.4	13.3	14.4	17.1	18.7	20.6
2	2	13.7	14.4	15.6	17.1	18.1	12.3	13.3	14.4	17.0	18.7	20.6
2	3	13.7	14.3	15.6	17.1	18.0	12.3	13.3	14.4	17.0	18.6	20.5
2	4	13.6	14.3	15.6	17.0	18.0	12.3	13.3	14.3	17.0	18.6	20.5
2	5	13.6	14.3	15.6	17.0	18.0	12.3	13.2	14.3	17.0	18.6	20.4
2	6	13.6	14.3	15.5	17.0	17.9	12.3	13.2	14.3	16.9	18.5	20.4
2	7	13.6	14.2	15.5	17.0	17.9	12.2	13.2	14.3	16.9	18.5	20.4
2	8	13.5	14.2	15.5	16.9	17.9	12.2	13.2	14.3	16.9	18.5	20.4

2	9	13.5	14.2	15.5	16.9	17.9	12.2	13.1	14.2	16.9	18.5	20.3
2	10	13.5	14.2	15.4	16.9	17.9	12.2	13.1	14.2	16.8	18.5	20.3
2	11	13.5	14.1	15.4	16.9	17.8	12.1	13.1	14.2	16.8	18.4	20.3
3	0	13.5	14.1	15.4	16.9	17.8	12.1	13.1	14.2	16.8	18.4	20.3
3	1	13.4	14.1	15.4	16.8	17.8	12.1	13.1	14.1	16.8	18.4	20.3
3	2	13.4	14.1	15.4	16.8	17.8	12.1	13.0	14.1	16.8	18.4	20.3
3	3	13.4	14.1	15.3	16.8	17.8	12.0	13.0	14.1	16.8	18.4	20.3
3	4	13.4	14.0	15.3	16.8	17.8	12.0	13.0	14.1	16.8	18.4	20.3
3	5	13.3	14.0	15.3	16.8	17.8	12.0	13.0	14.1	16.8	18.4	20.4
3	6	13.3	14.0	15.3	16.8	17.8	12.0	12.9	14.0	16.8	18.4	20.4
3	7	13.3	14.0	15.3	16.8	17.8	11.9	12.9	14.0	16.8	18.4	20.4
3	8	13.3	14.0	15.3	16.8	17.8	11.9	12.9	14.0	16.8	18.5	20.4
3	9	13.3	14.0	15.3	16.8	17.8	11.9	12.9	14.0	16.8	18.5	20.5
3	10	13.2	13.9	15.3	16.8	17.8	11.9	12.9	14.0	16.8	18.5	20.5
3	11	13.2	13.9	15.3	16.8	17.9	11.8	12.8	14.0	16.8	18.5	20.5
4	0	13.2	13.9	15.3	16.8	17.9	11.8	12.8	14.0	16.8	18.5	20.6
4	1	13.2	13.9	15.3	16.8	17.9	11.8	12.8	13.9	16.8	18.5	20.6
4	2	13.2	13.9	15.3	16.8	17.9	11.8	12.8	13.9	16.8	18.6	20.7
4	3	13.2	13.9	15.3	16.8	17.9	11.8	12.8	13.9	16.8	18.6	20.7
4	4	13.1	13.9	15.2	16.9	17.9	11.7	12.8	13.9	16.8	18.6	20.7
4	5	13.1	13.9	15.3	16.9	17.9	11.7	12.7	13.9	16.8	18.6	20.8
4	6	13.1	13.9	15.3	16.9	18.0	11.7	12.7	13.9	16.8	18.7	20.8
4	7	13.1	13.9	15.3	16.9	18.0	11.7	12.7	13.9	16.8	18.7	20.9
4	8	13.1	13.8	15.3	16.9	18.0	11.7	12.7	13.9	16.8	18.7	20.9
4	9	13.1	13.8	15.3	16.9	18.0	11.7	12.7	13.9	16.9	18.7	21.0
4	10	13.1	13.8	15.3	16.9	18.0	11.7	12.7	13.9	16.9	18.8	21.0
4	11	13.1	13.8	15.3	16.9	18.1	11.6	12.7	13.9	16.9	18.8	21.0
5	0	13.1	13.8	15.3	17.0	18.1	11.6	12.7	13.9	16.9	18.8	21.1

Table: Body Mass Index – Boys – 5–19 Years (WHO Standard)

Age (Year)	Percentiles					Z (SD) Score					
	5th	15th	50th	85th	95th	−3Z	−2Z	−1Z	. +1Z	+2Z	+3Z
Boys											
5.0	13.3	13.9	15.2	16.7	17.7	12.1	13.0	14.1	16.6	18.3	20.2
5.5	13.4	14.0	15.3	16.7	17.7	12.1	13.0	14.1	16.7	18.4	20.4
6.0	13.4	14.0	15.3	16.8	17.9	12.1	13.0	14.1	16.8	18.5	20.7
6.5	13.4	14.1	15.4	16.9	18.0	12.2	13.1	14.1	16.9	18.7	21.1
7.0	13.5	14.2	15.5	17.1	18.3	12.3	13.0	14.2	17.0	19.0	21.6
75.0	13.6	14.3	15.6	17.3	18.5	12.3	13.2	14.3	17.2	19.3	22.1
8.0	13.7	14.4	15.7	17.5	18.8	12.4	13.3	14.4	17.4	19.7	22.8
8.5	13.8	14.5	15.9	17.7	19.1	12.5	13.4	14.5	17.7	20.1	23.5
9.0	13.9	14.6	16.0	18.0	19.5	12.6	13.5	14.6	17.9	20.5	24.3
9.5	14.0	14.7	16.2	18.3	19.8	12.7	13.6	14.8	18.2	20.9	25.1
10.0	14.1	14.9	16.4	18.6	20.2	12.8	13.7	14.9	18.5	21.4	26.1
10.5	14.3	15.1	16.7	18.9	20.7	12.9	13.9	15.1	18.8	21.9	27.0
11.0	14.5	15.3	16.9	19.3	21.1	13.1	14.1	15.3	19.2	22.5	28.0
11.5	14.7	15.5	17.2	19.6	21.6	13.2	14.2	15.5	19.5	23.0	29.0
12.0	14.9	15.7	17.5	20.1	22.1	13.4	14.5	15.8	19.9	23.6	30.0
12.5	15.1	16.0	17.9	20.5	22.6	13.6	14.7	16.1	20.4	24.2	30.9
13.0	15.4	16.3	18.2	20.9	23.1	13.8	14.9	16.4	20.8	24.8	31.7
13.5	15.7	16.6	18.6	21.4	23.7	14.0	15.2	16.7	21.3	25.3	32.4
14.0	16.0	16.9	19.0	21.9	24.2	14.3	15.5	17.0	21.8	25.9	33.1
14.5	16.3	17.3	19.4	22.4	24.7	14.8	15.7	17.3	22.2	26.5	33.6
15.0	16.5	17.6	19.8	22.8	25.2	14.7	16.0	17.6	22.7	27.0	34.1
15.5	16.8	17.9	20.1	23.2	25.7	14.9	16.3	18.0	23.1	27.4	34.5
16.0	17.1	18.2	20.5	23.7	26.1	15.1	16.5	18.2	23.5	27.9	34.8
16.5	17.3	18.5	20.8	24.0	26.5	15.3	16.3	18.5	23.9	28.3	35.0
17.0	17.5	18.7	21.1	24.4	26.9	15.4	16.9	18.8	24.3	28.6	35.2
17.5	17.7	18.9	21.4	24.7	27.2	15.6	17.1	19.0	24.6	29.0	35.3
18.0	17.9	19.2	21.7	25.0	27.5	15.7	17.3	19.2	24.9	29.2	35.4
18.5	18.1	19.4	22.0	25.3	27.8	15.8	17.4	19.4	25.2	29.5	35.5
19.0	18.2	19.5	22.2	25.6	28.1	15.9	17.6	19.6	25.4	29.7	35.5

Obesity

Table: Body Mass Index – Girls – 5–19 Years (WHO Standard)

Age (Year)	Percentiles					Z (SD) Score					
	5th	15th	50th	85th	95th	–3Z	–2Z	–1Z	. +1Z	+2Z	+3Z
Girls											
5.0	13.1	13.8	15.3	17.0	18.1	11.8	12.7	13.9	16.9	18.9	21.3
5.5	13.1	13.8	15.3	17.0	18.2	11.7	12.7	13.9	16.9	19.0	21.7
6.0	13.1	13.8	15.3	17.1	18.4	11.7	12.7	13.9	17.0	19.2	22.1
6.5	13.1	13.8	15.3	17.2	18.6	11.7	12.7	13.9	17.1	19.5	22.7
7.0	13.1	13.9	15.4	17.4	18.8	11.8	12.7	13.9	17.3	19.8	23.3
7.5	13.2	14.0	15.5	17.6	19.1	11.8	12.8	14.0	17.5	20.1	24.0
8.0	13.3	14.1	15.7	17.8	19.4	11.9	12.9	14.1	17.7	20.6	24.8
8.5	13.4	14.2	15.9	18.1	19.8	12.0	13.0	14.3	18.0	21.0	25.6
9.0	13.6	14.4	16.1	18.4	20.2	12.1	13.1	14.4	18.3	21.5	26.5
9.5	13.7	14.6	16.3	18.8	20.7	12.2	13.3	14.6	18.7	22.0	27.5
10.0	13.9	14.8	16.6	19.1	21.1	12.4	13.5	14.8	19.0	22.6	28.4
10.5	14.1	15.0	16.9	19.5	21.6	12.5	13.7	15.1	19.4	23.1	29.3
11.0	14.4	15.3	17.2	20.0	22.2	12.7	13.9	15.3	19.9	23.7	30.2
11.5	14.6	15.6	17.6	20.4	22.7	12.9	14.1	15.6	20.3	24.3	31.1
12.0	14.9	15.9	18.0	20.9	23.3	13.2	14.4	16.0	20.8	25.0	31.9
12.5	15.2	16.2	18.4	21.4	23.9	13.4	14.7	16.3	21.3	25.6	32.7
13.0	15.5	16.5	18.8	21.9	24.4	13.6	14.9	16.6	21.8	26.2	33.4
13.5	15.8	16.9	19.2	22.4	25.0	13.8	15.2	16.9	22.3	26.8	34.1
14.0	16.0	17.2	19.6	22.9	25.5	14.0	15.4	17.2	22.7	27.3	34.7
14.5	16.3	17.4	19.9	23.3	25.9	14.2	15.7	17.5	23.1	27.8	35.1
15.0	16.5	17.7	20.2	23.7	26.3	14.4	15.9	17.8	23.5	28.2	35.5
15.5	16.7	17.9	20.5	24.0	26.7	14.5	16.0	18.0	23.8	28.6	35.8
16.0	16.8	18.1	20.7	24.2	27.0	14.6	16.2	18.2	24.1	28.9	36.1
16.5	16.9	18.2	20.9	24.5	27.2	14.7	16.3	18.3	24.3	29.1	36.2
17.0	17.0	18.3	21.0	24.7	27.4	14.7	16.4	18.4	24.5	29.3	36.3
17.5	17.1	18.4	21.2	24.8	o27.5	14.7	16.4	18.5	24.6	29.4	36.3
18.0	17.1	18.5	21.3	24.9	27.7	14.7	16.4	18.6	24.8	29.5	36.3
18.5	17.2	18.5	21.3	25.0	27.7	14.7	16.5	18.6	24.9	29.6	36.2
19.0	17.2	18.6	21.4	25.1	27.8	14.7	16.5	18.7	25.0	29.7	36.2

MACROCEPHALY

INTRODUCTION

Majority of children have head size that is appropriate for age and gender. But a few have either too small or too large head at birth or may be of post-natal acceleration. Abnormality of head circumference is determined by brain size.

Most cases of large head are picked up by the pediatrician on examination. Only a few are noticed by parents and brought to the physician for evaluation.

DEFINITION

Macrocephaly is defined as a large head greater than 2 standard deviation above the mean for age, height and sex or above 99.6th centile for age. Normally, occipitofrontal circumference is greater than 1 to 2 cm in males, it ranges ± 2.5 cm around mean and increases linearly with height. The normal growth velocity of head circumference is shown in Table.

Table: Normal growth velocity of head circumference

Duration	Normal growth velocity
< 3 month	2 cm/month
3 to 6 month	1 cm/month
6 month to 1 year	0.5 cm/month
1 year to 3 year	1 cm/6 month
3 year to 5 year	1 cm/year
5 year to 6 year	Adult head size is achieved

In premature infants, catch up growth in head circumference can exceed predicted growth rates and catches up at 18 months postnatal age with a term infant.

ETIOLOGY

Usually it is due to benign isolated macrocephaly or familial macrocephaly where some close family members are similarly affected; neither condition requires any further intervention. However, there are a few important underlying causes which need to be actively considered and investigated when indicated before reassuring parents. These considerations include whether there is any associated developmental disorder or suggestion of a syndromic association or evidence of raised intracranial tension.

Table: Causes of macrocephaly

1. **Excessive volume of cerebrospinal fluid (Hydrocephalus)**
   a. Communicating-meningitis, posthemorrhagic, achondroplasia
   b. Non-communicating-aqueductal stenosis, Arnold-Chiari malformation, Dandy-Walker malformation, Klippel-Feil syndrome, mass lesions-tumors
   c. Hydrancephaly-Holoprosencephaly, porencephaly.

2. **Megalencephaly**
   a. Anatomical-Benign familial macrocephaly, achondroplasia, Soto syndrome, Fragile X syndrome, neurocutaneous disorders, tuberous sclerosis, neurofibromatosis, incontinentiapigmenti, hypomelanosis of Ito.
   b. Metabolic megalencephaly-Alexander disease, Canavan disease, gangliosidosis,mucopolysaccharidosis, metachromaticleukodystrophy, Maple syrup urine disease.

3. **Subdural space occupation**
   Subdural effusion, subdural empyema, hematoma.

4. **Conditions associated** with thickened skull-rickets, cleidocranialdysostosis, osteopetrosis, osteogenesisimperfecta, pyknodysostosis, hyperphosphatemia, thalassemia, Russel-Silver dwarf.

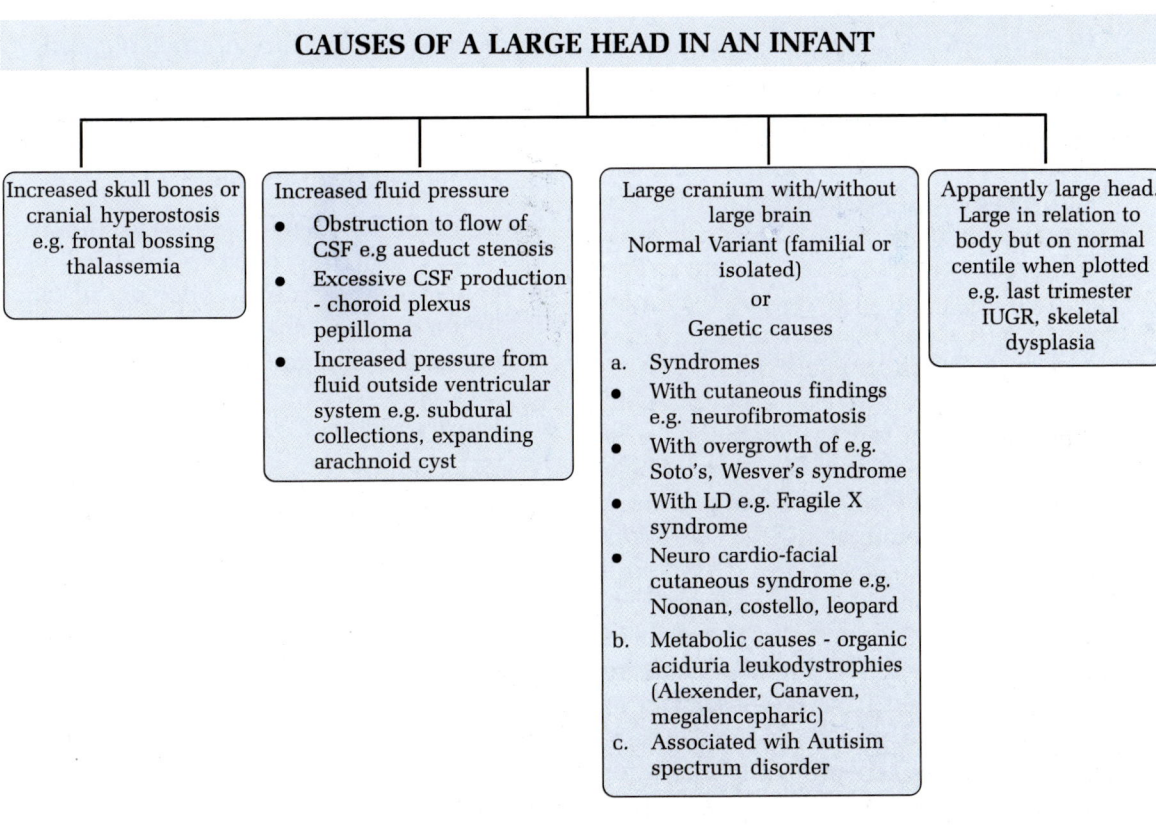

CAUSES OF A LARGE HEAD IN AN INFANT

Increased skull bones or cranial hyperostosis e.g. frontal bossing thalassemia	Increased fluid pressure	Large cranium with/without large brain	Apparently large head. Large in relation to body but on normal centile when plotted e.g. last trimester IUGR, skeletal dysplasia

Increased fluid pressure
- Obstruction to flow of CSF e.g aueduct stenosis
- Excessive CSF production - choroid plexus pepilloma
- Increased pressure from fluid outside ventricular system e.g. subdural collections, expanding arachnoid cyst

Large cranium with/without large brain
Normal Variant (familial or isolated)
or
Genetic causes
a. Syndromes
- With cutaneous findings e.g. neurofibromatosis
- With overgrowth of e.g. Soto's, Wesver's syndrome
- With LD e.g. Fragile X syndrome
- Neuro cardio-facial cutaneous syndrome e.g. Noonan, costello, leopard
b. Metabolic causes - organic aciduria leukodystrophies (Alexander, Canaven, megalencepharic)
c. Associated wih Autisim spectrum disorder

CLINICAL APPROACH

A. History

While eliciting the history in a child with a large head thefollowingconsiderations are useful.

> **Points in history**
>
> - Is the head large since birth or developed later?
> - Any history of preceding meningitis
> - Birth history
> - Family history of large head
> - Developmental history
> - Symptoms of raised intracranial tension
> - History of seizures

- **Is the head large since birth?**

  When did the parents notice that the head is large? Since birth or developed later?

  Children with anatomical megalencephaly are macrocephalic since birth, while those with metabolic megalencephaly usually have normal head circumference at birth and develop megalencephaly later. The head enlargement in these cases parallel neurological regression and clinical evidence of increased intracranial pressure. The ventricles are often small. Conditions with increased thickness of the skull bones do not have macrocephaly at birth, it only develops during infancy. Congenital aqueductal stenosis presents with a large head at birth, while in Dandy-Walker malformation macrocephaly is present in only 25 percent of the affected newborns at birth and in 75 percent by the age of 1 year. It is also essential to enquire whether the head size is still increasing or has become static. The latter points towards arrested hydrocephalus.

- **Preceding central nervous system illness:**

  Did the child suffer from meningitis in the past?

  Hydrocephalus is a commonsequelae of meningitis. It is specially seen with tubercular meningitis. Subdural empyema can develop as a complication of pyogenic meningitis in infants. It is common with H. influenzae meningitis. The effusion keeps increasing in size leading to increasing head circumference.

- **Birth history:**

  Did the baby sustain any trauma at birth? Did the baby deliver prematurely? Difficult labor can give rise to an intracranial bleed resulting in subdural collection of blood, which can keep increasing in size giving rise to macrocephaly. Intracranial bleeding is also common in preterm babies, who subsequently develop hydrocephalus.

- **History of head trauma:**

  In infants trivial fall can lead to rupture of blood vessels traversing the subdural space giving rise to gradual collection of blood in the subdural space leading to subdural hematoma and gradual macrocephaly.

- **Family history:**

  Head size of other family members must be enquired. Asymptomatic macrocephaly in immediate family members is a common cause of large head.

  Enquire about family history of genetic syndromes associated with macrocephaly especially neurofibromatosis developmental problems e.g. autism or learning disability.

- **Developmental history:**

  Did the child attain all the milestones at normal age? Has there been regression of milestones?

  Regression of milestones would suggest neurometabolic disease.

  Congenital hydrocephalus and anatomical megancephaly can give rise to delayed development.

  Rickets can give rise to delayed walking.

- **Symptoms of raised intracranial tension:**

  Enquire about symptoms of raised intracranial tension viz. irritability, high pitched cry, poor feeding, decreased alertness, headache, vomiting and seizures.

B. Examination

The following considerations are helpful.

> **Clinical signs**
>
> - Anthropometric measurements
> - Examination of head
> - Look for facial dysmorphism
> - Skeletal system
> - Assessment of mental function
> - Examination of eyes
> - Examination of nervous system

Anthropometric measurements:

It is essential to record the anthropometric measurements viz. Occipitofrontal circumference, height and weight. Early recognition of abnormal head size requires accurate serial measurements of the occipitofrontal circumference. Any orbitofrontal cortex (OFC) more than 2 SD from the mean raises a strong suspicion of macrocephaly. An OFC more than ± 3 SD from the mean almost certainly indicates an abnormal head size. Always compare the patient's OFC with the OFC and body dimensions of siblings and other family members.Measuring the height is also important, short stature with macrocephaly would be a feature of achondroplasia and mucopolysaccharidosis. While tall stature would be seen in Soto syndrome. If the OFC is within normal centiles, but the head seems apparently large, then one must consider late IUGR, skeletal dysplasia, rickets, osteogenesis imperfecta.

- **Head:**

  In a child with macrocephaly one must look for the shape of the skull. In case of hydrocephalus there is frontal prominence with craniofacial disproportion. The head appears large as compared to the face. In subdural hygroma the prominence is in the parietal region. In case of rickets there is frontal and parietal bossing. The anterior fontanelle is wide open and non-pulsatile in case of hydrocephalus, also the scalp veins are dilated and prominent.

  In case of Dandy-Walker malformation bulging of the skull is more prominent in the occipital than in the frontal region. A positive Macewan sign after the sutures have closed indicates hydrocephalus. Open squamoparietal suture beyond the first month of life is an early sign of hydrocephalus.

- **Face:**

  The face should be carefully observed. Sunset appearance of eyes would suggest hydrocephalus. Small face with a disproportionately large head would suggest hydrocephalus and if associated with short stature is a feature of Russell-Silver dwarfism. In case of thalassemia apart from frontal prominence the facial bones will be prominent with hypertelorism and dental malocclusion. Coarse features with thick lips, enlarged tongue, widely spaced peg-like teeth and depressed bridge of the nose is suggestive of mucopolysaccharidosis. Frontal bossing with depressed nasal bridge, mid facial hypoplasia and short stature would point towards achondroplasia. Children with Soto syndrome in addition to tall stature and a prominent forehead also have high arched palate and hypertelorism a small number also have dysmorphic features. The presence of neurocutaneous markers such as cafe-au-lait spots, sebaceous adenomas, shagreen patches, would suggest neurocutaneous syndromes.

- **Eyes:**

Apart from sunset appearance of eyes, which is a feature of hydrocephalus, the eyes should be examined for corneal clouding, which is a feature of mucopolysaccharidosis. A fundus examination would reveal papilledema in case of raised intracranial pressure and presence of cherry red spot would suggest storage disorder.

- **Skeletalsystem:**

The spine should be examined for the presence of meningocele or at times there may be a tuft of hair indicating spina bifida occulta. Achondroplasia is characterized by rhizomelic shortening of the limbs (proximal portion of the limbs is shorter than the distal position). There is lumbar lordosis and limitation of elbow extension. Children with Klippel-Feil syndrome have a low posterior hairline, short neck, head asymmetry, facial asymmetry and scoliosis. In case of rickets apart from

frontal and parietal bossing of the skull there would be widening of wrists, genu valgum deformity, rachitic rosary and Harrison sulcus.

- **Nervous system:**

In neurological assessment, it is essential to first assess whether the child is normal or mentally challenged. Mental subnormality, would be seen in some cases of hydrocephalus, Soto syndrome, neuroectodermal dysplasias and metabolic megalencephaly. Cranial nerves should be examined for palsies. Look for signs of raised intracranial tension viz. bulging fontanelle, splayed sutures. OFC crossing centiles, sunsetting eyes, prominent scalp veins, recent onset squint, lower limb spasticity, hyperreflexia, papilloedema. Truncal ataxia and nystagmus is a feature of Dandy-Walker malformation.

c. **Investigations:**

Presence of hepatosplenomegaly would suggest storage disorders or hematological disorders e.g. thalassemia. Most children who are asymptomatic and otherwise normal except for a large head, which is familial need not be investigated. In cases, with pathological macrocephaly relevant investigations must be done.

Which investigations to be done?

- Cerebrospinal fluid analysis
- Transfontanellar ultrasonography
- Computed tomography scan of head
- Magnetic resonance imaging
- Skeletal radiographs
- Chromosomal analysis

Cerebrospinal fluid examination:

Cerebrospinal fluid examination is indicated in children with hydrocephalus due to pyogenic/tubercular meningitis.

Transfontanellarultrasonography:

Transfontanellar USG is done in infants with open fontanelle for diagnosis of hydrocephalus. This modality is used for serial monitoring of ventricular size.

Computed tomography of head:

In an older child with closed fontanelle it is used for diagnosing hydrocephalus. The earliest sign is dilatation of occipital horns and atria of lateral ventricles. In achondroplasia CT scan shows a small posterior fossa and enlargement of the sphenoid sinuses. It is also useful for detecting subdural fluid collection. CT brain is normal in Soto syndrome.

- **Magnetic Resonance Imaging:**

Indicated in Dandy-Walker malformation, which would show cystic dilatation of the posterior fossa and partial or complete agenesis of the cerebellar vermis. It is also indicated in metabolic megalencephaly.

- **Skeletal Radiographs:**

X-ray of the spine will reveal characteristic fusion and malformations of vertebrae in case of Klippel-Feil syndrome. X-ray hands would be useful in cases of achondroplasia and rickets. X-rays of long bones would show multiple fractures in case of osteogenesisimperfecta and a marble bone appearance in case of osteopetrosis.

- **Chromosomal Analysis:**

Chromosomal analysis is indicated where the cause of macrocephaly appears to be a chromosomal aberration such as Fragile X syndrome.

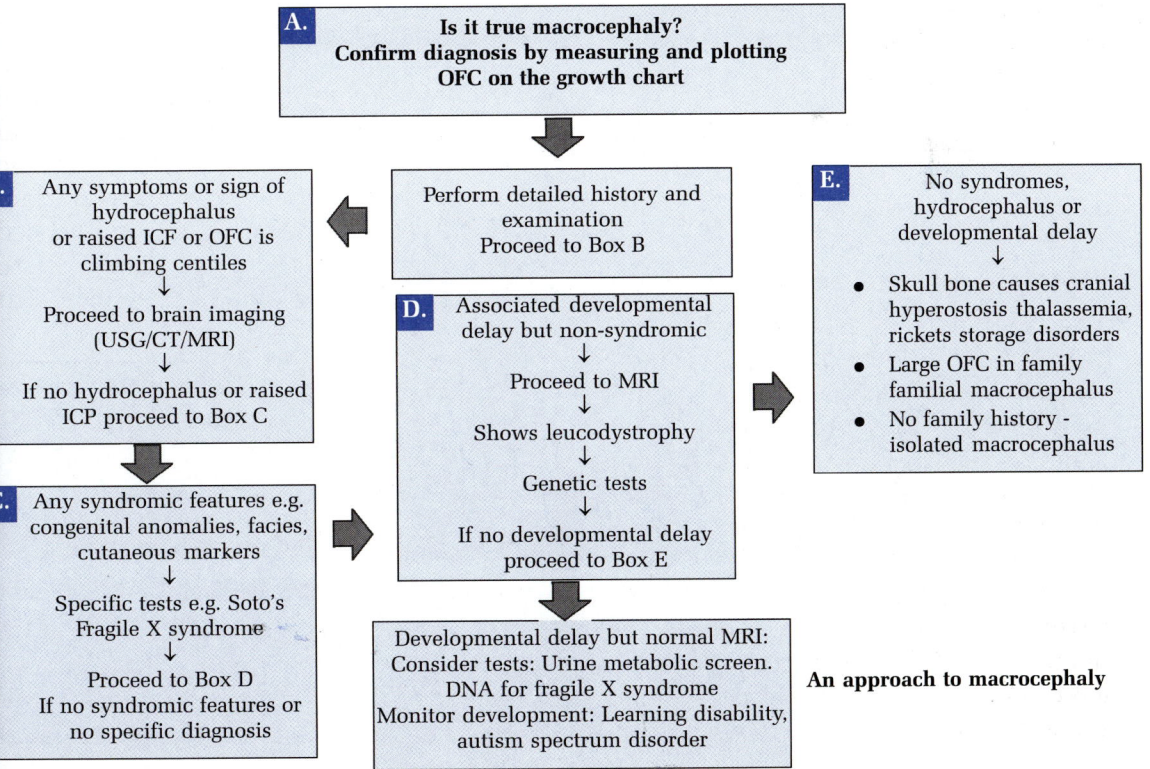

An approach to macrocephaly

SUMMARY

Before investigating any child with a large head one must rule out familial macrocephaly. The commonest cause of pathological macrocephaly is hydrocephalus usually following tubercular meningitis in this country. Serial measurements of he circumference, especially in the 1st year life will help in identifying ear hydrocephalus. This should particularly done in preterm babies as they can devel hydrocephalus due to intraventricular ble in the neonatal period.

SUGGESTED READING

1. Children with large head: Seal A. Arch Dis Child EducPract Ed 2013;98:122-125.

Age		Boys							Girls						
Years	Month	-35D	-25D	-15D	Median	+15D	+25D	+35D	-35D	-25D	-15D	Median	+15D	+25D	+35D
0	0	30.7	31.9	33.2	34.5	35.7	37.0	38.3	30.3	31.5	32.7	33.9	35.1	36.2	37.4
	1	33.8	34.9	36.1	37.3	38.4	39.6	40.8	33.0	34.2	35.4	36.5	37.7	38.9	40.1
	2	35.6	36.8	38.0	39.1	40.3	41.5	42.6	34.6	35.8	37.0	38.3	39.5	40.7	41.9
	3	37.0	38.1	39.3	40.5	41.7	42.9	44.1	35.8	37.1	38.3	39.5	40.8	42.0	43.3
	4	38.0	39.2	40.4	41.6	42.8	44.0	45.2	36.8	38.1	39.3	40.6	41.8	43.1	44.4
	5	39.9	40.1	41.4	42.6	43.8	45.0	46.2	37.6	38.9	40.2	41.5	42.7	44.0	45.3
	6	39.7	40.9	42.1	43.3	44.6	45.8	47.0	38.3	39.6	40.9	42.2	43.5	44.8	46.1
	7	40.3	41.5	42.7	44.0	45.2	46.4	47.7	38.9	40.2	41.5	42.8	44.1	45.5	46.8
	8	40.8	42.0	43.3	44.5	45.8	47.0	48.3	39.4	40.7	42.0	43.4	44.7	46.0	47.4
	9	41.2	42.5	43.7	45.0	46.3	47.5	48.8	39.8	41.2	42.5	43.8	45.2	46.5	47.8
	10	41.6	42.9	44.1	45.4	46.7	47.9	49.2	40.2	41.5	42.9	44.2	45.6	46.9	48.3
	11	41.9	43.2	44.5	45.8	47.0	48.3	49.6	40.5	41.9	43.2	44.6	45.9	47.3	48.6
1	0	42.2	43.5	44.8	46.1	47.4	48.6	49.9	40.8	42.2	43.5	44.9	46.3	47.6	49.0
	1	42.5	43.8	45.0	46.3	47.6	48.9	50.2	41.1	42.4	43.8	45.2	46.5	47.9	49.3
	2	42.7	44.0	45.3	46.6	47.9	49.2	50.5	41.3	42.7	44.1	45.4	46.8	48.2	49.5
	3	42.9	44.2	45.5	46.8	48.1	49.4	50.7	41.5	42.9	44.3	45.7	47.0	48.4	49.8
	4	43.1	44.0	45.7	47.0	48.3	49.6	51.0	41.7	43.1	44.5	45.9	47.2	48.6	50.0
	5	43.2	44.6	45.9	47.2	48.5	49.8	51.2	41.9	43.3	44.7	46.1	47.4	48.8	50.2
	6	43.4	44.7	46.0	47.4	48.7	50.0	51.4	42.1	43.5	44.9	46.2	47.6	49.0	50.4
	7	43.5	44.9	46.2	47.5	48.9	50.2	51.5	42.3	43.6	45.0	46.4	47.8	49.2	50.6
	8	43.7	45.0	46.4	47.7	49.0	50.4	51.7	42.4	43.8	45.2	46.6	48.0	49.4	50.7
	9	43.8	45.2	46.5	47.8	49.2	50.5	51.9	42.6	44.0	45.3	46.7	48.1	49.5	50.9
	10	43.9	45.3	46.6	48.0	49.3	50.7	52.0	42.7	44.1	45.5	46.9	48.3	49.7	51.1
	11	44.1	45.4	46.8	48.1	49.5	50.8	52.2	42.9	44.3	45.6	47.0	48.4	49.8	51.2

Year	Month														
2	0	44.2	45.5	46.9	48.3	49.6	51.0	52.3	43.0	44.4	45.8	47.2	48.6	50.0	51.4
	1	44.3	45.6	47.0	48.4	49.7	51.1	52.5	43.1	44.5	45.9	47.3	48.7	50.1	51.5
	2	44.4	45.8	47.1	48.5	49.9	51.2	52.6	43.3	44.7	46.1	47.5	48.9	50.3	51.7
	3	44.5	45.9	47.2	48.6	50.0	51.4	52.7	43.4	44.8	46.2	47.6	49.0	50.4	51.8
	4	44.6	46.0	47.3	48.7	50.1	51.5	52.9	43.5	44.9	46.3	47.7	49.1	50.5	51.9
	5	44.7	46.1	47.4	48.8	50.2	51.6	53.0	43.6	45.0	46.4	47.8	49.2	50.6	52.0
	6	44.8	46.1	47.5	48.9	50.3	51.7	53.1	43.7	45.1	46.5	47.9	49.3	50.7	52.2
	7	44.8	46.2	47.6	49.0	50.4	51.8	53.2	43.8	45.2	46.6	48.0	49.4	50.9	52.3
	8	44.9	46.3	47.7	49.1	50.5	51.9	53.3	43.9	45.3	46.7	48.1	49.6	51.0	52.4
	9	45.0	46.4	47.8	49.2	50.6	52.0	53.4	44.0	45.4	46.8	48.2	49.7	51.1	52.5
	10	45.1	46.5	47.9	49.3	50.7	52.1	53.5	44.1	45.5	46.9	48.3	49.7	51.2	52.6
	11	45.1	46.6	48.0	49.4	50.8	52.2	53.6	44.2	45.6	47.0	48.4	49.8	51.2	52.7
3	0	45.2	46.6	48.0	49.5	50.9	52.3	53.7	44.3	45.7	47.1	48.5	49.9	51.3	52.7
	1	45.3	46.7	48.1	49.5	51.0	52.4	53.8	44.4	45.8	47.2	48.6	50.0	51.4	52.8
	2	45.3	46.8	48.2	49.6	51.0	52.5	53.9	44.4	45.8	47.3	48.7	50.1	51.5	52.9
	3	45.4	46.8	48.2	49.7	51.1	52.5	54.0	44.5	45.9	47.3	48.7	50.2	51.6	53.0
	4	45.4	46.9	48.3	49.7	51.2	52.6	54.1	44.6	46.0	47.4	48.8	50.2	51.7	53.1
	5	45.5	46.9	48.4	49.8	51.3	52.7	54.1	44.6	46.1	47.5	48.9	50.3	51.7	53.1
	6	45.5	47.0	48.4	49.9	51.3	52.8	54.2	44.7	46.1	47.5	49.0	50.4	51.8	53.2
	7	45.6	47.0	48.5	49.9	51.4	52.8	54.3	44.8	46.2	47.6	49.0	50.4	51.9	53.3
	8	45.6	47.1	48.5	50.0	51.5	52.9	54.3	44.8	46.3	47.7	49.1	50.5	51.9	53.3
	9	45.7	47.1	48.6	50.1	51.6	53.0	54.4	44.9	46.3	47.7	49.2	50.6	52.0	53.4
	10	45.7	47.2	48.7	50.1	51.6	53.0	54.5	45.0	46.4	47.8	49.2	50.6	52.1	53.5
	11	45.8	47.2	48.7	50.2	51.7	53.1	54.5	45.0	46.4	47.9	49.3	50.7	52.1	53.5
4	0	45.8	47.3	48.7	50.2	51.7	53.2	54.6	45.1	46.5	47.9	49.3	50.8	52.2	53.6
	1	45.9	47.3	48.8	50.3	51.7	53.2	54.7	45.1	46.5	48.0	49.4	50.8	52.2	53.6
	2	45.9	47.4	48.8	50.3	51.8	53.2	54.7	45.2	46.6	48.0	49.4	50.9	52.3	53.7

3	45.9	47.4	48.9	50.4	51.8	53.3	54.8	45.2	46.7	48.1	49.5	50.9	52.3	53.8
4	46.0	47.5	48.9	50.4	51.9	53.4	54.8	45.3	46.7	48.1	49.5	51.0	52.4	53.8
5	46.0	47.5	49.0	50.4	51.9	53.4	54.9	45.3	46.8	48.2	49.6	51.0	52.4	53.9
6	46.1	47.5	49.0	50.5	52.0	53.5	54.9	45.4	46.8	48.2	49.6	51.1	52.5	53.9
7	46.1	47.6	49.1	50.5	52.0	53.5	55.0	45.4	46.9	48.3	49.7	51.1	52.5	54.0
8	46.1	47.6	49.1	50.6	52.1	53.5	55.0	45.5	46.9	48.3	49.7	51.2	52.6	54.0
9	46.2	47.6	49.1	50.6	52.1	53.6	55.1	45.5	46.9	48.4	49.8	51.2	52.6	54.1
10	46.2	47.7	49.2	50.6	52.1	53.6	55.1	45.6	46.9	48.4	49.8	51.2	52.6	54.1
11	46.2	47.7	49.2	50.7	52.2	53.7	55.2	45.6	47.0	48.5	49.9	51.3	52.7	54.1
0	46.3	47.7	49.2	50.7	52.2	53.7	55.2	45.7	47.1	48.5	49.9	51.3	52.8	54.2
5														

MICROCEPHALY

INTRODUCTION

A pediatrician usually comes across children with microcephaly in office practice. This condition is fairly common amongst children with developmental delay.

DEFINITION

Microcephaly can be defined as head circumference, which is three standard deviations below the mean for age and sex. Some authorities accept below two standard deviations as microcephaly. The former definition is more acceptable, reason being majority of the children with head circumference below two standard deviation develop normally without handicaps in contrast to majority of children with head circumference below three standard deviation, who have developmental handicaps.

Microcephaly can be primary or secondary. In case of primary microcephaly the brain inherently has a poor potential for growth. It may occur because of genetic or intrauterine disturbances in early gestation resulting in anomalous development of brain. Secondary microcephaly is due to the effect of environmental disturbances and noxious agents on the fetus in later pregnancy or in the postnatal period.

Microcephaly can be present at birth or it may develop in the first few years of life.

ETIOLOGY

Table: Causes of microcephaly

1. **Primary**

   - Genetic—Autosomal recessive autosomal dominant

   - Chromosomal—Down (21 trisomy) Edward (18 trisomy), Cri-du-chat (5 p-)

   - Dysmorphic syndromes—Cornelia de-Lange, Rubinstein- Taybi, Smith-Lemli-Opitz.

   - Exposure to teratogens% Familial

2. **Secondary**

   - Intrauterineinfections- cytomegalo-virus (CMV), rubella,toxoplasma human immunodeficiency virus (HIV).

   - Intrauterine toxins and drugs-alchohol, hydantoin, phenylketonuria etc.

   - Perinatal and postnatal insults to the brain, hypoxic ischemic encephalo-pathy, meningitis, encephalitis intracranial hemorrhage.

   - Craniostenosis.

CLINICAL EVALUATION

A. HISTORY

Before examining a child with microcephaly the following history must be elicited.

- **Family History**

  Do any sibling in the family have a small head? Is theirdevelopment normal or delayed? In familial asymptomatic microcephaly other members in the family may also have a small head, but are otherwise normal. The symptomatic or pathological microcephaly, which is associated with delayed development, can also have an autosomal dominant or recessive type of inheritance.

- **Gestational Age and Birth Weight**

  What was the gestational age of the baby at birth? Was he preterm or term? What was the birth weight?

  Intrauterine growth retardation is a feature of several chromosomal aberrations, dysmorphic syndromes and intrauterine infections.

  On the other hand infant of a diabetic mother is large for date.

- **History of Radiation During Pregnancy**

  Was the mother exposed to radiation during pregnancy? If yes, at what gestational period.

  Microcephaly and mental retardation are most severe, if exposure is before 15th week of gestation.

- History of Ingestion of Alcohol During Pregnancy Excessive intake of alcohol during pregnancy can damage the growing fetus giving rise to malformations.

  Anticonvulsants viz. phenytoin or sodium valproate, if taken during pregnancy can lead to fetalhydantoin syndrome.

- **History of Infections During Pregnancy**

  TORCH (T-toxoplasmosis, O-other infections, R-rubella, C-cytomegalovirus, H-herpes simplex virus) group of infections during pregnancy are known to give rise to growth retardation. Hence, an enquiry must be made whether the mother suffered from these infections during early pregnancy.

- **History of Diabetes in the Mother**

  Is the mother diabetic? If yes, was her blood sugar properly controlled during pregnancy?

  Uncontrolled diabetes in the mother during early pregnancy can give rise to microcephaly and other congenital malformations.

- **Hyperthermia During Pregnancy**

  High fever in the mother during early pregnancy, i.e. 4 to 6 weeks of gestation has been known to cause microcephaly.

- **Feeding Difficulty**

  Marked feeding problems in the neonatal period is a feature of Smith-Lemli-Opitz syndrome.

- **History of Perinatal Asphyxia**

  Was the baby asphyxiated at birth? How severe was the asphyxia? Did the baby develop hypoxic-ischemic encephalopathy?

  In a child who has sustained significant birth asphyxia with hypoxic-ischemic encephalopathy can have cerebral atrophy leading to microcephaly.

- **History of Postnatal Infections**

  If a child develops intracranial infections such as meningitis/ encephalitis particularly in the first 2 years of life when brain growth is rapid, the brain is likely to be damaged and loses its growth potential leading to microcephaly.

B. PHYSICAL EXAMINATION

Thorough examination of a child with microcephaly would help in arriving at a cause.

> **Signs to be looked for?**
> - Anthropometric measurements
> - Shape of the skull
> - Facial dysmorphism
> - Examination of the eyes
> - Any deafness
> - Presence of purpura/jaundice
> - Hepatosplenomegaly
> - Congenital heart disease

- **Anthropometric Measurements**

  Note the child's overall growth. Is he generally small or only head is small.

  The head circumference should be measured and plotted on the centile chart. If the measurement is below 3 SD, then the cause is definitely pathological. Severe microcephaly would suggest that the cause was in early embryonic life. Insult to the brain later in life usually beyond 2 years of life does not give rise to severe microcephaly. Serial measurement of head circumference are more meaningful than an isolated measurement.

  The head circumference of parents and other siblings should also be recorded. This would help in identifying familial microcephaly.

  Weight and height should be measured and recorded on the centile chart. If all the measurements are below the third centile, it indicates intrauterine growth retardation, which is a feature of chromosomal aberrations, dysmorphic syndromes and intrauterine infections.

- **Shape of the Skull**

  Look for craniosynostosis, which is due to premature fusion of cranial sutures even though the brain is growing normally. Look for early closure of fontanelle and palpable ridges of sutures. Examine the head for any scar marks (repair or closure of encephalocele).

Dysmorphism

The face should be carefully looked for dysmorphism. A set of dysmorphic features would suggest various genetic conditions.

Slanting forehead with prominent ears and nose with severe mental retardation would suggest familial microcephaly of autosomal recessive type. In autosomal dominant variety, there is upslanting palpebral fissures and prominent ears.

Trisomy 21 would have a typical mongoloid facies.

In trisomy 18 there is microstomia, micrognathia, low- set malformed ears and prominent occiput. Cri-du-chat is characterized by round facies, prominent epicanthic folds, low set ears, hypertelorism and characteristic cry. Rubinstein-Taybi syndrome is characterized by beaked nose, downward slanting of palpebral fissures, epicanthic folds with broad thumbs and toes.

Eyes

Look for ptosis. Presence of ptosis would suggest Smith-Lemli- Opitz syndrome. It is also a feature of fetal alcohol syndrome. Presence of cataract would suggest congenital rubella.

Look for chorioretinitis, which is a feature of intrauterine infections (CMV infection, rubella and toxoplasmosis).

Ears

Assessment of hearing must be done.

Deafness is a feature of CMV infection and rubella.

- **Purpuricspots**

  Presence of jaundice and purpuricspots would indicate intrauterine infections.

- **Hepatosplenomegaly**

  Hepatosplenomegaly is also seen in TORCH group of infections.

- **Examination of cardiovascular system**

  Look for evidence of congenital heart disease. It could be present in case of trisomy 21, trisomy 18, congenital rubella and infant of a diabetic mother.

- **Skeletalanomalies**

  Look for skeletal anomalies such as broad thumbs and toes, which is a feature of Rubeinstein-Tyabi syndrome. Rocker bottom feet in Trisomy 18, proximally placed thumb in cornelia de-dange. Hypoplastic distal phalanges in fetalhydantoin syndrome.

- **Central nervous system examination**

  Developmental assessment must be done. Mental subnormality can vary from mild to severe. The severity of mental retardation is related to the severity of microcephaly. Head circumference from 2-3 SD below the age has 13% risk of developing mental retardation while head circumference >3SD the incidence is 62%. Generalized hypotonia is a feature of several chromosomal anomalies and dysmorphic syndromes. Spasticdiplegia would be seen in cases of autosomal recessive type of microcephaly.

C. INVESTIGATIONS

Microcephaly can sometimes be diagnosed before birth by prenatal ultrasound. Most of the time, the diagnosis will not be made until birth or later in infancy.

Table: Investigations and probable diagnosis

	Investigations	Probable Diagnosis
1.	Neuroimaging of brain%	
	● CT scan – intracerebral calcification	Intrauterine infection
	● MRI useful in	Structural abnormalities of brain
2.	TORCH titres positive	Intrauterine infection
3.	Karyotyping	Chromosomal abnormalities
4.	Metabolic tests done in	Metabolic defects
5.	Urine culture for CMV positive	Cytomegalovirus infection

If cause of microcephaly is unknown, mother's serum phenylalanine levels should be done. High levels of phenylalanine in an asymptomatic mother can produce marked brain damage in an otherwise normal non-phenylketonuric infant.

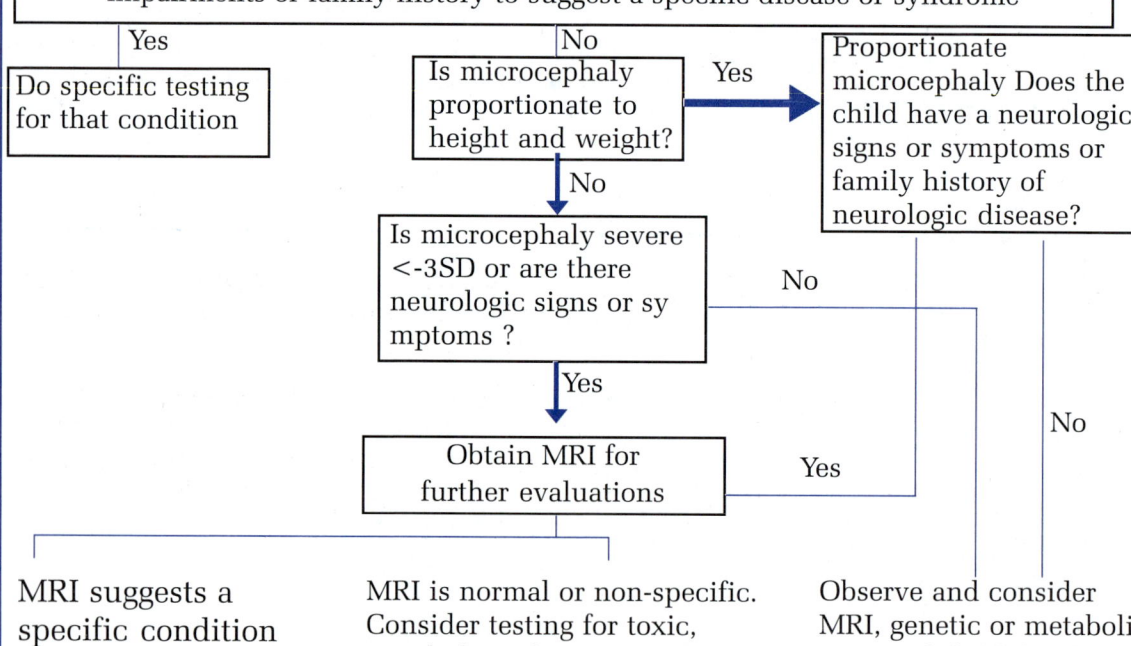

APPROACH TO POSTNATAL ONSET MICROCEPHALY

Does the child have clinical features, other organ involvement, vision / hearing impairments or family history to suggest a specific disease or syndrome

Yes → Do specific testing for that condition

No → Is microcephaly proportionate to height and weight?

Yes → Proportionate microcephaly Does the child have a neurologic signs or symptoms or family history of neurologic disease?

No → Is microcephaly severe <-3SD or are there neurologic signs or symptoms ?

Yes → Obtain MRI for further evaluations

MRI suggests a specific condition or pattern of injury. Do testing for that condition.

MRI is normal or non-specific. Consider testing for toxic, metabolic infectious, endocrine and genetic disorders. Consider testing for Rett syndrome in girls

Observe and consider MRI, genetic or metabolic testing if child develops neurologic signs or symptoms or worsening microcephaly

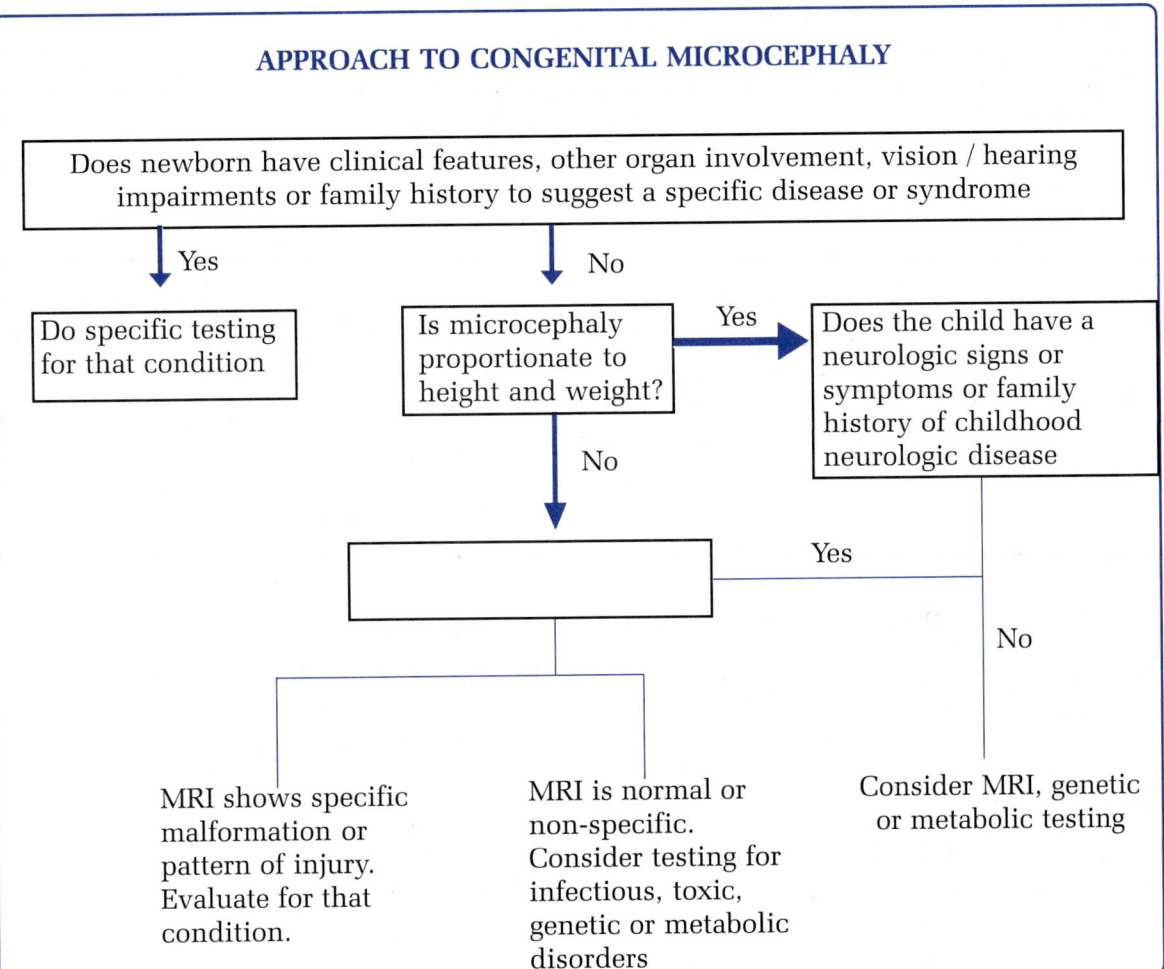

APPROACH TO CONGENITAL MICROCEPHALY

Does newborn have clinical features, other organ involvement, vision / hearing impairments or family history to suggest a specific disease or syndrome

Yes → Do specific testing for that condition

No → Is microcephaly proportionate to height and weight?

Yes → Does the child have a neurologic signs or symptoms or family history of childhood neurologic disease

No →

Yes →

No

MRI shows specific malformation or pattern of injury. Evaluate for that condition.

MRI is normal or non-specific. Consider testing for infectious, toxic, genetic or metabolic disorders

Consider MRI, genetic or metabolic testing

SUMMARY

Microcephaly is an important neurologic sign but there is non uniformity in the definition of microcephaly and inconsistency in the evaluation of affected children.

Children with head circumference three SD below the mean for age and sex have pathological microcephaly and need investigations.

Familial benign microcephaly must be ruled out. The child in this condition is neurologically normal.

Common cause of microcephaly in daily practice are secondary to birth asphyxia, intrauterine and postnatal infection.

SUGGESTED READING

1. Stephen Ashwel, David Michelson et al. Evaluation of the child with microcephaly. American Academy of Neurology.

6

FEVER

INTRODUCTION

Fever is the commonest symptom for which children are brought to the practitioner. Parents often get panic struck if fever is high grade and does not subside within a few hours of giving medication. The fear is much more among parents whose children keep getting febrile seizures. On the other hand some parents perceive fever if the forehead feels warm. In majority of cases fever is never documented. Hence, it becomes essential for the treating physician to ensure that the child is febrile before prescribing drugs.

DEFINITION

Fever is defined as elevation of body temperature in response to a pathological stimulus. It is important to understand the difference between core temperature and skin temperature. Core temperature: is the temperature of the deep tissue of the body, which remains almost constant within ± 1°F except when a person develops a febrile illness, while skin temperature: in contrast to core temperature rises and falls with the temperature of the surroundings. The average normal temperature is generally considered to be between 98°F and 98.6°F (36.7°C and 37°C) when measured orally and approximately 1°F higher when measured rectally.

When should the child be considered to have fever?
- If rectal temperature is above 38°C (100.4°F)

- If oral temperature is above 37.8°C (100.0°F)
- If axillary temperature is above 37.2°C (99°F)

TYPES OF FEVER

There are different patterns of temperature which help in determining the cause of fever

Continuous fever is one in which temperature never touches normal and fluctuation in temperature is less than 1°C.

Remittent fever also does not touch normal but fluctuation is more than 2°C.

Intermittent fever touches normal.

AETIOLOGY

Approach to a child with fever would depend upon the duration of fever with which he presents to the clinician.

Table : Causes of fever

I. **Fever of short duration (< 2 weeks)**
    Fever of short duration is almost always due to infection. At times heat stroke and Kawasaki disease do present with acute onset of fever.
    Depending upon the site of infection or focus of disease, generally there are localizing symptoms and signs due to underlying disease process. At times due to certain host characteristics and nature of the disease process, there may be no localizing features to suggest the site of

infection. Such a fever may be labeled as fever without focus (FWF).

Common causes of fever of short duration:

*Viral:*Coryza, tonsillitis, pharyngitis, pneumonia, measles, dengue, chickenpox, viral hepatitis.

Bacterial: Tonsillitis, otitis media, abscess, cellulitis, typhoid fever, gastroenteritis, pneumonia.

Protozoal: Malaria

II. Prolonged fever (> 2 weeks)

If fever persists beyond a fortnight it is known as PUO. Infections still continue to be the leading cause, but non-infectious causes should also be considered. Following are some of the conditions:

Infectious: Tuberculosis, typhoid, malaria, HIV, chronic fungal infections, occult abscess

Connective tissue disorders: Systemic lupus erythematosus, systemic onset rheumatoid arthritis, Kawasaki disease, periarteritisnodosa

Malignant disorders: Leukemia, lymphoma, neuroblastoma

Immune deficiency disorders: Sickle cell disease, agranulocytosis, child on steroids

Miscellaneous: Diabetes insipidus, thyrotoxicosis, factitious fever, anhidrotic ectodermal dysplasia

EVALUATION

In clinical practice no other symptom has such a large spectrum of diagnostic possibilities than fever. When fever presents with localizing symptoms and signs diagnosis becomes easy for e.g. tonsillitis, otitis media or cellulitis. Difficulty arises when there is no evident focus of infection. Either the focus

is clinically hidden or may evolve over time. A good history followed by meticulous examination to identify the focus of infection is essential to arrive at a diagnosis.

A. History

> **What to ask?**
> - Details of fever
> - Age of the child
> - Illness in other family members
> - Recent contact with infectious disease
> - Accompanying symptoms
> - Pre-disposing conditions
> - Immunization status
> - History of drug intake

Details of fever:

History should elicit the duration of fever, its onset and progress, type of fever. Is the fever associated with chills and rigors? Is the child normal in the interfebrile period? One must enquire whether fever has been documented. Many a times, in cases of undocumented fever the child may be afebrile but the mother may wrongly perceive fever due to warm forehead and palms as compared to rest of the body. It is often observed that parents cover infants excessively even during summer season. In such a situation the excess clothes should be removed and temperature recorded to ensure that the child is febrile.

Acute onset of fever usually denotes infection. Acute viral infection is the commonest infection and is characterized by fever at the onset which tends to subside over the next 3 to 4 days. Most viral fevers are self limiting but occasionally a child may develop complication which needs to be identified early. In case of dengue fever after fever subsides there is appearance of new symptoms which heralds onset of dengue shock syndrome. As against viral infection, fever in bacterial infections may not be high to begin with but peaks by 3-4 days and focus of infection starts getting localized. Malaria can also present with acute onset of fever, which is often intermittent. In viral infection and malaria the child appears normal between spikes of fever but not so in bacterial infection. Kawasaki disease also presents with high grade fever persisting beyond one week not responding to antibiotics.

If fever persists beyond the first week one must still consider infections. Most patients have already received antibiotics and hence the course of infection is 'likely' to be modified. Deep seated pyogenic abscesses in the liver or subphrenic space must be kept in mind.

When fever persists beyond two weeks, infection is still the main cause. It is better to think of uncommon presentation of common diseases rather than a rare disorder. Tuberculosis, resistant typhoid fever, resistant malaria, urinary tract infection, occult abscess, partially treated pneumonia are infections that should be ruled out. In malnourished children, those with sickle cell disease and other immunocompromised states common infections take long to respond. Systemic lupus erythematosus and systemic onset juvenile idiopathic arthritis can present as prolonged fever.

Age:

Febrile neonates and infants must be taken seriously. Fever could be due to a viral illness or severe fulminant bacterial sepsis.

Vaccination: Note the vaccines that the child has received.

Family history: Enquire if any member in the family is having fever or is there any recent contact with infectious disease.

Accompanying symptoms: Ask about accompanying symptoms which would give a clue to the cause of fever.

- Fever with chills and rigors: Malaria, viral fever, tonsillitis, acute otitis media, abscess, urinary tract infection
- Cough and cold: Viral fever
- Excessive crying: Acute otitis media, meningitis, pyogenic focus
- Diarrhoea, vomiting: Gastroenteritis
- Loss of appetite, nausea, pain in abdomen: Hepatitis
- Cough and fast breathing: Bronchiolitis, bronchopneumonia
- Burning in micturition, dysuria, crying during micturition: Urinary tract infection

Predisposing factors: Ascertain whether there are any conditions in the child which predispose to infection such as: vesicoureteric reflux, cardiac disease, ventricular shunt, immunodeficiency state.

History of drugs: Record the drugs the child has received and the response to treatment.

B. CLINICAL EXAMINATION

General appearance of the child, vital signs and alertness helps in assessing the seriousness of illness. A detail clinical examination from head to toe is important not only on the first day but also subsequently for appearance of new signs.

Physical signs to observe?
- General appearance
- Alertness
- Vital signs
- Examination of oral cavity
- Lymphadenopathy
- Rash

- Parotid swelling
- Pallor / icterus
- Joint swelling
- Bulging fontanelle
- Systemic examination

General appearance and alertness:

Is the child looking bright and playful or is he irritable, toxic and sick looking? Is the sensorium altered? The latter indicates meningoencephalitis, enteric encephalopathy, cerebral malaria.

Vital signs:

Check the pulse, respiratory rate and pattern of breathing. Record blood pressure and capillary refill time (CRT) in infants. Tachycardia, weak pulses, cold extremities and prolonged CRT would indicate fulminant sepsis with shock; also seen in dengue shock syndrome. Dyspnoea with cough seen in bronchiolitis and pneumonia.

Examination of oral cavity:

Oral cavity along with ear, eyes and nose must be examined for tonsillitis, diphtheritic membrane, pharyngitis, acute otitis media, Koplik spots in suspected measles. These appear as grey specks on a red base at the level of premolars. Fissured lips, strawberry tongue oropharyngeal congestion with non-purulent conjunctival injection is seen in Kawasaki disease.

Lymphadenopathy:

Lymph nodes in the neck, axillae and inguinal region should be examined. Any suppurative focus would lead to regional adenitis such as acute tonsillitis, abscess and dental infections. Other conditions which give rise to lymphadenopathy are tuberculosis, HIV infection, lymphoma, acute lymphoblastic leukemia, Kawasaki disease and inflammatory disorders such as systemic onset idiopathic rheumatoid arthritis. Matted lymph nodes with or without sinus is characteristic of tubercular lymphadenopathy. Epitrochlear lymph node enlargement is pathognomonic of infectious mononucleosis.

Rash:

Inspect for presence of rash. If present when did it appear? What is the distribution pattern? What type of rash is it?

Rash in measles appears on the 4th or 5th day of fever associated with running of nose and watering from eyes. It is maculopapular; first appears on the face and neck, near the hairline and subsequently spreads to the trunk, extremities, palms and soles.

In chicken pox the rash appears on the 1st or 2nd day of fever. It appears in crops. Initially, the rash is macular which evolves into papules and then vesicles which later become pustular. Lesions start from the face and trunk and spread over the whole body, palms and soles are spared.

Macular rash is also seen in infectious mononucleosis. Rash in case of Rubella is also macular which appears within 24 hours after onset of fever; begins from the face and spreads to involve the whole body. The rash lasts for 3 days. It is associated with suboccipital, posterior auricular and anterior cervical lymphadenopathy.

Rash in Kawasaki disease in polymorphous. Evanescent maculopapular rash with central clearing is seen in systemic JRA. Malar rash is characteristic of SLE. Presence of petechial rash purpura and ecchymosis suggests meningococcemia, dengue hemorrhagic fever or leukemia.

Parotid swelling:

Commonest cause of unilateral or bilateral parotid swelling is mumps. Suppurative parotitis is usually unilateral, extremely painful; there may be pus discharge from Stenson's duct.

Icterus / pallor:

Pallor in a child with high fever with chills consider malaria. Severe anaemia would also be present in acute lymphoblastic leukemia and sickle cell disease with aplastic crises due to infection.In viral hepatitis, dengue and leptospirosis icterus is present.

Arthritis:

When fever is associated with joint swelling is there involvement of single or multiple joints and which joints are affected. Usual causes are septic arthritis, rheumatic arthritis, tubercular arthritis, leukemia, systemic JRA and other inflammatory disorders. Bony tenderness in a child with fever consider acute leukemia.

Systemic examination:

All systems should be examined.

Abdomen: Palpate the abdomen for hepatosplenomegaly. Common causes of fever with hepatosplenomegaly are malaria, typhoid fever, viral hepatitis, infectious mononucleosis, dengue fever, septicemia and infective endocarditis. If fever is prolonged consider tuberculosis, leukemia lymphoma, chronic hepatitis, liver abscess and connective tissue diseases.

Apart from hepatosplenomegaly look for signs of acute peritonitis, acute appendicitis, any lump in abdomen which could be a malignant tumor. Look for tenderness in renal angles which is due to perinephric abscess.

Cardiovascular system: Auscultate the heart for presence of murmur. Changing murmur in a child with rheumatic fever could be due to active carditis. If a child with heart disease starts getting fever, he should be repeatedly examined for appearance of a new or changing murmur which would suggest bacterial endocarditis.

Respiratory system: Examine for signs of pneumonia, empyema.

Central nervous system: In an infant palpate the fontanelle. Tense bulging fontanelle would suggest meningitis. Look for signs of meningeal irritation.

General appearance of the febrile child

An alert and active child with a healthy appearance who is:

- Well hydrated
- Smiles
- Cries vigorously but is easily consoled
- Who watches the physician's movements
- Seeks his parents hand or soothing eyes and does not cause worry

These signs are reassuring and usually indicate a benign febrile state.

Red flags signs that demand urgent specific action in a febrile child

- Age below 3 months
- Behavioural abnormality – lethargy or extreme irritability
- Significant oliguria or anuria
- Tachycardia and tachyapnoea disproportionate to degree of fever
- Severe protein energy malnutrition
- Immunosuppressed state

FEVER WITHOUT FOCUS

So far we had seen how to approach a child with fever presenting with localizing symptomatology or developing signs over the next few days. However, due to certain host characteristics and nature of the disease process there may be no other symptom or sign in some children with fever. Unfortunately it is common to prescribe antibiotic without diagnosis and so partially treated bacterial infections may present without localization. In such a situation the term 'fever without focus' is used. Approach to such a child would be different.

Fever without focus can be:

1. Fever without localizing signs
2. Fever of unknown origin

Fever without localizing signs:

This group of children have acute onset of fever of short duration usually less than a week and there is no evidence in history or clinical examination of involvement of any system or organ. An older child can be observed and followed up for any evolving sign but febrile neonates and infants must be taken seriously because they are at risk of occult bacteremia. In a normal neonate especially during summer months dehydration fever must be excluded. Such neonates would respond to increased fluid intake and control of environmental temperature. It is suggested that all febrile neonates and infants from 0 to 36 months must be hospitalized for observation, investigation and treatment.

Pyrexia of unknown origin:

When fever (rectal temperature > 38°C) persists for more than 3 weeks duration and no cause is identified, despite carefully conducted observations and laboratory investigations for another one week it is labeled as PUO.

Common conditions responsible for PUO are infections, autoimmune diseases, malignancies and drug fever. Infections must be considered first. Tuberculosis, kalaazar, urinary tract infection, occult abscess, bacterial endocarditis, fungal infection also result in prolonged undiagnosed fever. Rickettesial infections, brucellosis, should also be considered.

Autoimmune disease such as systemic onset juvenile idiopathic arthritis, systemic lupus erythematosus, mixed connective tissue disorders, drug fever, can present as PUO.

Malignancies leukemia, lymphomas, neuroblastoma may result in PUO.

If fever persists for more than 6 months without diagnosis, it could be factitious fever.

Apart from a detail history and physical examination what is required in a case of PUO is repeated clinical examination for evolving clinical signs. In such cases, enquire whether there is history of exposure to animals, heavy metals and travel to an endemic area.

Fever in the infant and toddler

Approach to an infant and toddler with fever is very different hence is being discussed separately.

Neonates (<28 days) with fever may have few clues on history and clinical examination, however, 3% have a serious bacterial infection. In these cases one has to take history pertaining to pregnancy, delivery and early neonatal life. Infections that occur in the first 7 days of life are secondary to vertical transmission and those occurring after the first week are usually community acquired or hospital acquired.

Definitive identification of a serious bacterial infection requires laboratory investigation, full sepsis screen and a positive result in blood culture, CSF and/or urine. 5 to 10% of neonates with early onset group B streptococcal sepsis have concurrent meningitis.

Young infants: The general approach to fever in a febrile infant aged 28-60 days includes maintaining a high index of suspicion, because these patients often lack clues on physical examination. The prevalence of a serious bacterial infection in an infant below 3 months is approximately 6-10% mostly urinary tract infections.

Children aged 3 months to 3 years: Children aged 3 months to 3 years have a risk for occult bacteremia. The leading cause of blood stream infection is streptococcus pneumoniae, followed by H. influenza type b. S. pneumoniaeand E. coli are the most common pathogens.

Children with pneumococcal bacteremia may present with acute otitis media, pneumonia, sinusitis, cellulitis or non-specific febrile illness.

E. coli bacteremia is most common in children below 1 year of age and is usually with urinary tract infection. S. aureus is associated with skin, soft tissue, or musculoskeletal infections.

Approach to a febrile child age 3 months to 3 years consists of a targeted medical history, complete physical examination and judicious use of the laboratory tests.

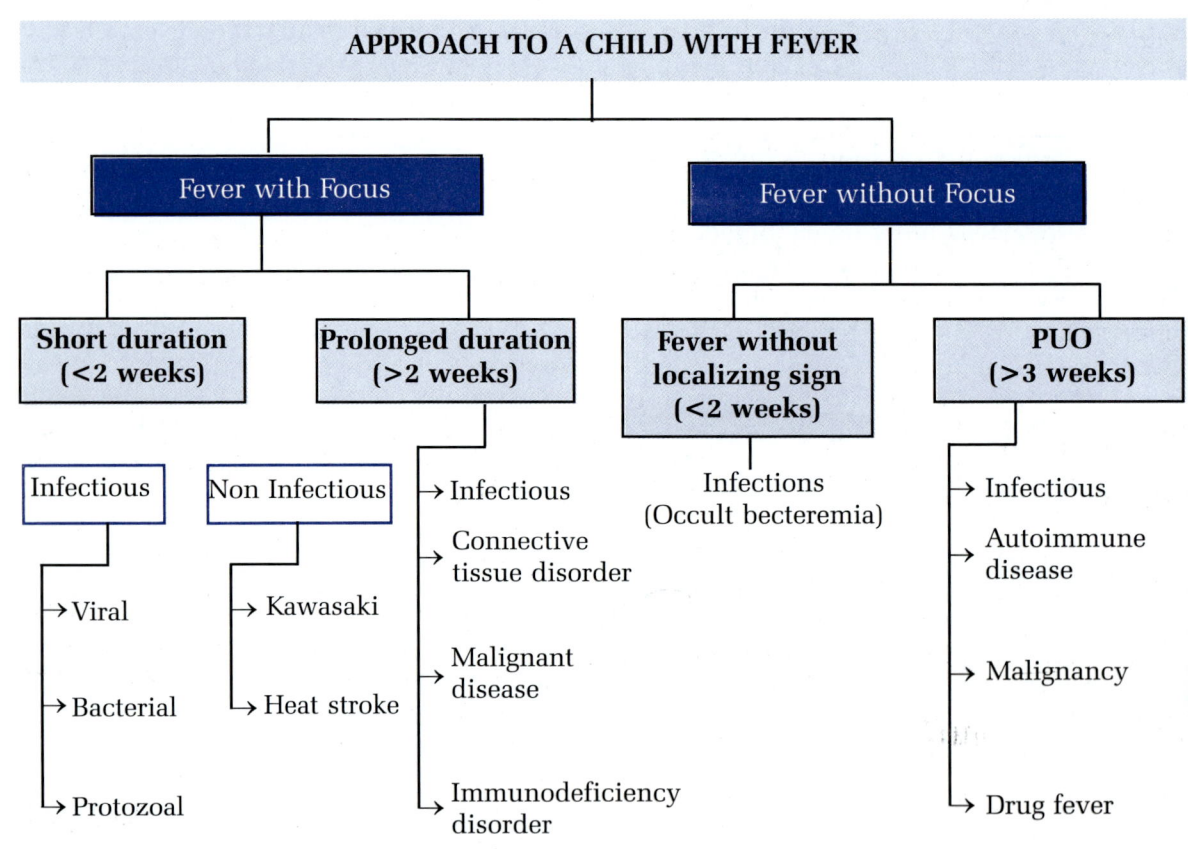

APPROACH TO A CHILD WITH FEVER

C. INVESTIGATIONS

Investigations are not needed in all children with fever. Majority of them in office practice come with simple viral fever of the upper respiratory tract which subsides in a few days. All they need is symptomatic treatment. Investigations are indicated in children presenting with high fever, fever lasting for a week, if there is a focus of pyogenic infection, child appearing toxic, history of recurrent fever and fever without focus.

Children presenting with fever of less than 2 weeks routine investigations and some serological tests would be required. In fever without focus more diagnostic tests would be necessary and in cases of PUO repeated tests may have to be conducted depending upon evolving signs. List of investigations are shown in box.

Which investigations to be done?

- Complete haemogram
- Urine analysis
- Blood culture
- X-ray chest
- Mantoux test
- Serological tests
- Erythrocyte sedimentation rate (ESR)% Liver function tests
- Viral markers
- C-reactive protein
- Bone marrow examination
- Abdominal ultrasonography
- Computed tomography (CT) scan
- Magnetic resonance imaging (MRI)

Complete blood count:

A lot of information can be obtained from simple blood count. Leucocytosis (TLC > 15000 / cumm) with raised neutrophils (> 10000/cumm) and thrombocytopenia (platelets < 100000/cumm) suggests bacterial sepsis. Leukopenia with lymphocytosis and eosinophilia suggests typhoid fever. Peripheral smear examination can reveal malarial parasite and immature cells in suspected leukemias. Atypical large lymphocytes in the peripheral smear is hallmark of infectious mononucleosis. Raised hematocrit and thrombocytopenia are seen in dengue fever. Thrombocytosis suggests collagen disease.

Urine examination:

Urine examination must be done in all cases of fever especially if fever is without a focus. Presence of pus cells and/or bacteriuria would suggest urinary tract infection. However, it needs confirmation by doing a urine culture.

C-reactive protein:

Quantitative CRP concentration is a valuable laboratory test in the evaluation of febrile young children who are at risk for occult bacteremia and severe bacterial infection with a better predictive value than WBC or ANC.

Blood culture:

It is indicated in typhoid fever and septicemia.

Serological tests:

Widal test is done in cases of typhoid fever. A rising titre is more suggestive. Serological tests are also indicated in cases of suspected Brucellosis and infectious mononucleosis.

Erythrocyte sedimentation rate:

Raised in cases of bacterial infection and collagen diseases.

Cerebrospinal fluid examination:

It is essential in cases of suspected meningitis and also in neonates and infants with bacterial sepsis or fever without focus.

Mantoux test:

A positive Mantoux would point towards tuberculosis.

X-ray chest:

Detects pneumonias and tuberculosis.

Liver function tests and viral markers:

Indicated in cases of viral hepatitis.

Bone marrow examination:

Essential for the diagnosis of aleukemic leukemia.

Ultrasonography/CT scan/MRI:

Imaging is indicated in cases of suspected abscess, lymphoreticular malignancies tubercular abdomen and tumors.

Seroimmunological tests:

Can be used in suspected autoimmune disorders for detection of autoantibodies.

Molecular diagnostic techniques:

Polymerase chain reaction (PCR) is now available for diagnosis of several infectious agents.

SUMMARY

Fever is the most common symptom for which a physician is consulted. Documentation of fever is almost always lacking even among educated parents. A large number of causes are responsible for fever. Once fever is confirmed, it is essential to identify any serious illness responsible for the fever. Most forms of pediatric infections are much more likely to be viral. In most cases of fever, bacterial infection gets localized in 3 to 4 days. If fever persists beyond 4 days without localizing signs, appropriate laboratory tests should be carried out. Clinicians must maintain a high index of suspicion for serious bacterial and /or viral infections in febrile infants and toddlers. The diagnostic approach in these cases consists of a targeted medical history, a complete physical examination and judicious use of laboratory tests.

SUGGESTED READING

1. Baker MD. Evaluation and management of infants with fever.Pediatr Clin North Am 1999;46:1061-72.

2. Ishimine P. Fever without source in children 0-36 months of age. Pediatr Clin North Am 2006;53:167-194.

3. Parekh P, Kaul K K. Fever. In: Manual of Pediatric Differential Diagnosis. 1st Ed. 2013. Jaypee Publishers, 47-59.

4. Gould J, Steele RW, et al. Fever in the infant and toddler. emedicine.medscape.com.

Chapter
7
LYMPHADENOPATHY

INTRODUCTION

Lymphadenopathy is defined as enlargement of lymph nodes due to inflammatory or non-inflammatory causes. There are about 500-600 lymph nodes in the human beings. These are distributed throughout the body and are found in clusters in underarms, groin, neck, chest and abdomen. The internal lymph nodes cannot be palpated easily and are present in thoracic and abdominal cavities. Evaluation of lymph nodes is an important part of general examination of every child. Lymph node enlargement is a very common clinical finding. Challenge to the pediatrician is to differentiate pathologic from non-pathologic lymphadenopathy.

Terminologies used:

1. Generalized lymphadenopathy: Involvement of more than two non-contiguous lymph node areas due to a systemic disease.

2. Localized lynphadenopathy: Involvement of one lymph node area.

3. Persistent lymphadenopathy: Persistence of lymphadenopathy for 3 months or more.

4. Significant lymphadenopathy: The lymph node enlargement is considered significant if any of the following factors are present:

- Size:
  - Inguinal nodes > 1.5 cm diameter
  - Cervical & axillary nodes > 1 cm in diameter
  - Epitrochlear nodes – any size
- Site: Multiple sites
- Matted nodes
- Red, tender, ulcerated nodes
- Associated with systemic signs and symptoms

Lymphatic Drainage

Head and Neck

Nodes	Drainage Area
Occipital	Back of scalp
Preauricular	Eyelids, conjunctiva, pinna and temporal region
Postauricular	External auditory meatus, pinna, scalp above the ear
Anterior cervical	Skin and superficial tissues of front of neck
Superficial cervical	Angle of jaw, skin over the lower part of the parotid gland and lobe of ear
Deep cervical	Oral cavity and neck
Posterior cervical	Scalp and neck, skin of arms

Submandibular	Mid face, buccal mucosa, tongue and submandibular region
Submental	Lower lip and floor of mouth
Right supraclavicular	Mediastinum and lungs
Left supraclavicular	Abdomen

Upper Limbs

Nodes	Drainage Area
Axillary	
Lateral (brachial)	Upper limb
Central	Receives afferents from lateral, anterior and posterior nodes
Medial	Superior breast, thoracic wall
Anterior (pectoral)	Anterior chest wall, breast
Posterior (subscapular)	Posterior chest wall, upper arm, lower post neck
Epitrochlear	Ulnar aspect of forearm and hand
Infraclavicular	Receives lymph from superficial vessels around the cephalic vein

Lower Limbs

Nodes	Drainage Area
Inguinal	Penis, scrotum, vulva, vagina, perineum, gluteal region, lower abdominal wall & lower anal canal
Femoral (upper innner thigh)	Foot, leg, groin and genitals
Popliteal	Legs and feet

ETIOLOGY

1. Infections:
   a. Viral:
   - Infectious mononucleosis
   - Human Immunodeficiency Virus (HIV)
   - Measles
   - Rubella
   b. Bacterial:
   - Streptococcal pyogens
   - Staphylococcal aureus
   - Cat scratch disease
   - Salmonella typhi
   - Tularemia
   - Brucellosis
   - M. tuberculosis
   - Atypical mycobacteria
   c. Spirochetal:
     - Syphilis
     - Lyme disease
     - Leptospirosis
   d. Protozoan:
     - Toxoplasmsosis
     - Malaria

e. Fungal:
  - Histoplasmosis
  - Coccidiomycosis
  - Tinea capitis

2. Malignancy:
  - Leukemia
  - Lymphoma-Non-Hodgkin lymphoma
  - Hodgkin lymphoma
  - Lymphosarcoma
  - Histiocytic lymphoma
  - Neuroblastoma
  - Rhabdomyosarcoma

3. Connective tissue disorders:
  - Juvenile rheumatoid arthritis
  - Systemic lupus erythematosus (SLE)
  - Serum sickness

4. Immunodeficiency syndromes:
  - Chronic granulomatous disease
  - AIDS
  - Hyper IgE syndrome
  - Hemophagocytic syndrome

5. Drugs:
  - Phenytoin
  - Allopurinol

6. Metabolic & storage diseases:
  - Gaucher disease
  - Niemann pick disease

7. Others:
  - BCG adenitis
  - Chronic reactive lymphadenopathy
  - Pediculosis
  - Kawasaki disease
  - Hyperthyroidism
  - Addison's disease

EVALUATION

Lymphadenopathy in children commonly arises from benign etiologies. A thorough history usually points the clinician in this direction. Furthermore, the physical examination guides the physician to the correct aetiology by focusing on the distribution of the enlarged nodes (i.e. regional or systemic), the exact characteristics of the involved nodes, and any other suspicious feelings.

It is important to remember that lymph nodes are not palpable in newborns and that the lymph node volume increases with antigenic exposure. Normal shotty lymph nodes are common in early childhood. One of the commonest cause of posterior cervical lymphadenopathy in our country is pediculosis and boils over the scalp. Chronic reactive cervical lymphadenopathy seen in young children is often due to recurrent upper respiratory infection.

Nodes smaller than 1 cm are often found in the cervical chain and in the femoral areas. They are somewhat larger in the inguinal areas. Similarly nodes smaller than 0.5 cm may be palpated in the occipital, postauricular and axillary chains. Small occipital and post-auricular nodes are common in infants, whereas cervical and inguinal nodes are common after age 2 years. However, finding lymph nodes of any size in the supraclavicular or epitrochlear areas is unusual. Thus, lymph nodes of the same size observed in two different regions may have markedly different implications. For example, a 1 cm node in cervical region is very likely benign, whereas a 1 cm supraclavicular node requires a biopsy and may reflect intrathoracic or intraabdominal malignancy. Non-inflammatory nodes greater than 2 to 2.5 cms deserve biopsy.

It is also important to remember that there are certain conditions, which mimic lymphadenopathy and need to be distinguished from lymph nodes viz. cystic hygroma in which transillumination test is positive. Branchial cleft cysts, which has a sinus also thyroglossal duct cyst. These cysts, when infected become tense and hard and tend to appear as lymph nodes. A firm fixed node should always raise the suspicion of malignancy.

For a rational approach to the cause of lymphadenopathy a meticulous history and clinical examination is essential.

A. History

> **Points in history**
>
> **What to ask?**
> - Age of the patient
> - Onset and duration
> - Progression
> - History of anorexia and weight loss
> - History of fever and night sweats
> - History of contact with tuberculosis
> - H/O Pain
> - H/O Drug intake
> - H/O Bleeding
> - H/O Bony tenderness
> - H/O Joint pain

Age of the Patient

While evaluating a child with lymphadenopathy the age of the patient is important. In a normal newborn, lymph nodes are not palpable. The lymphoid tissue increases with age and in young children small lymph nodes are normally palpable in the cervical region. Chronic reactive lymphadenopathy is common between the ages of 3 to 5 years.

In older children tuberculosis and lymphomas are common.

Onset and Duration

One must enquire since when have the parents noticed lymph node enlargement?

Whether the enlargement is of acute or subacute onset?

Acute onset lymphadenopathy usually starts with fever and is commonly due to viral or bacterial infections. Sometimes it can be seen in leukemis, Kawasaki disease and serum sickness.

A subacute onset in which the lymphadenopathy develops over 3 to 4 weeks is commonly seen in leukemia, lymphoma and autoimmune disease.

Progression

The progression of lymphadenopathy should be elicited. How rapidly the lymph nodes increased in size? Where the cause of lymphadenopathy is infection response to antibiotic treatment must be looked into. Normally, the lymph nodes regress after 2 weeks of good antibiotic therapy. In some cases, it may take 4 to 6 weeks. But by 4 weeks if the nodes do not subside one must consider other possibilities. In case of tubercular lymphadenopathy, if the lymph nodes do not show any regression in 4 to 6 weeks it should be considered as unresponsive. In some cases of Hodgkin lymphoma, there is fluctuating lymphadenopathy at times the lymph nodes regress and after sometimes may again appear.

Contact with Tuberculosis

If there is a history of contact with tuberculosis in a child who presents with lymphadenopathy, a serious effort should be made to look for tuberculosis.

History of Fever

History of fever should be elicited in all cases of lymphadenopathy.

Usually, in acute lymphadenitis due to viral or bacterial cause fever is high at the onset. In cases of tubercular lymphadenopathy there may be history of irregular fever over several days or weeks. In cases of leukemia fever may be variable in some cases low grade, in others high grade. In Hodgkin disease there may be Pelebstein type of fever with night sweats.

Anorexia and Weight Loss

Weight loss may not be a feature of acute lymphadenitis but in all chronic illnesses and malignancies anorexia and weight loss would be present.

History of Pain

Pain and signs of inflammation surrounding a group of enlarged nodes are helpful in reaching a diagnosis, particularly if an infectious source is found distal to the node area. These findings strongly suggest an infectious primarily bacterial cause.

Drug Intake

Enlargement of lymph nodes, most commonly in the cervical region may occur as a complication of phenytoin or carbamazepine therapy.

History of Bleeding

One should suspect leukemia if patient is bleeding from any site.

History of Bony Tenderness

This points towards leukemia.

History of Joint Pain

Presence of joint pain indicates collagen vascular diseases like SLE, JIA and leukemia.

B. Clinical Examination

> **Points on physical examination**
> - Lymph node size
> - Localized or generalized
> - Which group of lymph nodes are affected
> - Consistency of lymph nodes
> - Oral cavity ears, especially tonsils
> - Pallor, rash, purpuric spots
> - Joint involvement
> - Hepatosplenomegaly

Lymph Node Size

Lymph node size should be assessed in all cases because size of normal lymph nodes vary with age. In the normal newborn lymph nodes are not palpable and in case they are it suggests congenital infection such as cytomegalovirus. As age increases the lymphoid tissue increases in size upto the age of 8 years and then regresses. Cervical and axillary lymph nodes are considered pathological when the size is more than 1 cm. Inguinal lymph nodes are significant if the size is more than 1.5 cm. In general, in young children a lymph node size more than 2 cm is taken as significant.

Is there Localized or Generalized Lymphadenopathy?

Localized lymphadenopathy is more common than generalized lymphadenopathy. Generalized adenopathy is defined as enlargement of more than two non-contiguous node regions and indicates systemic disease and is often accompanied by abnormal physical findings in other systems.

Localized lymphadenopathy is usually due to infection in the involved node and or its drainage area.

Location

The affected group of lymph nodes must be thoroughly examined and a search for focus of infection in the drainage areas must be made, for, e.g. the commonest lymphadenopathy for which children are brought in offie practice is posterior cervical and suboccipital lymph nodes. This lymphadenopathy is usually due to pediculosis or pyoderma of the scalp and one can easily miss it if the drainage area is not looked for. Often they are misdiagnosed as tubercular and the patient receives a course of antitubercular treatment.

SUBMANDIBULAR

Submaxillary adenopathy may develop secondary to stomatitis tonsillitis periapical dental abscess. Axillary lymphadenopathy may occur from infections on the arms whereas inguinal and femoral adenopathy may be secondary to infections on the in lower extremities. Preauricular adenopathy may be caused by cat scratch disease, chlamydial conjunctivitis, listeriosis or tuberculosis.

Mediastinal or hilar adenopathy of an infectious etiology may occur in patients with tuberculosis, chronic sinusitis, histoplasmosis and infectious mononucleosis. Bilateral involvement is the rule and pulmonary disease is common in tuberculosis.

Enlargement of supraclavicular lymph nodes are always pathological. Right supraclavicular lymph nodes enlargement suggests pathology in the mediastinum and lungs, while left supraclavicular lymph nodes indicates lesion in the abdomen. If an infant has a left supraclavicular lymph node, one must consider BCG adenitis. This occurs if BCG is injected above the insertion of the deltoid muscle or a larger dose is given subcutaneously.

Enlargement and tenderness of posterior auricular, posterior cervical and occipital lymph nodes indicate rubella infection. Generalized superficial lymphadenopathy may occur in patients with measles, chickenpox, mumps or other viral diseases.

Infectious mononucleosis is accompanied by lymphadenopathy that is symmetric with involvement of the posterior cervical nodes. Histoplasmosis with the exception of mediastinal lymphadenopathy is an uncommon cause of lymph node enlargement.

Generalized adenopathy may be noted after typhoid immunization. Regional adenitis may follow pertusis vaccine, diphtheria toxoid and tetanus toxoid immunization.

Lyme disease may be characterised by generalised lymphadenopathy.

Juvenile rheumatoid arthritis is a diagnostic consideration in children with unexplained fever and persistent lymphadenopathy.

Rapidly enlarging, confluent or fixed nodes and supraclavicular lymphadenopathy may be malignant.

Lymphosarcoma commonly involves the cervical and mediastinal lymph nodes. Hodgkin disease is usually characterised by an insidious, painless, unilateral enlargement of regional lymph nodes, most frequently cervical. Right supraclavicular node may enlarge secondary to mediastinal disease, whereas left supraclavicular adenopathy may occur with abdominal involvement. Non-Hogkin's lymphoma may present as rapidly enlarging peripheral or mediastinal lymphadenopathy.

It is therefore important to know the drainage area of various lymph nodes.

Consistency of Lymph Nodes

Most lymph nodes are benign soft easily compressible and mobile.

Nodes that are warm, tender and fluctuant indicate infection and inflammation.

Hard nodes usually due to fibrosis of surrounding area are due to malignancy, firm and rubbery nodes are seen in Hodgkin lymphoma. Matting of lymph nodes are seen in tuberculosis and invasive malignancy.

Consistency	Conditions
Soft	Infections / inflammatory conditions
Firm	Hodgkin's lymphoma, SLE
Hard	Malignancy, lymphoma
Stony hard	Malignancy, metastasis
Firm, rubbery	Hodgkin's lymphoma
Fluctuant	Suppurative infection
Shotty (Resembling lead pellets)	Viral infections

Examination of Oral Cavity and Ears

One must carefully look for any focus of infection in the throat and ears. Also look for enlargement of tonsils, any presence of exudates or follicles. Infection in the tooth and nose can also give rise to regional lymphadenopathy.

Examination of Skin

Presence of severe pallor would indicate leukemia. Anemia is also a feature of collagen vascular disease. Purpuric spots would suggest leukemia, infectious mononucleosis. Rash is a feature of collagen disease.

Joint Involvement

Joint swelling and pain is seen in leukemias and collagen vascular disease.

Bony tenderness is a feature of leukemia.

Hepatomegaly

Hepatosplenomegaly if associated with lymphadenopathy is a feature of leukemias, lymphomas, Hodgkin disease infectious mononucleosis, collagen vascular disease, disseminated tuberculosis and storage disorders.

Most lymphadenopathy in children is due to benign self limited disease such as viral infections and hence extensive investigations are not needed. However, some preliminary tests are required in all cases with significant lymphadenopathy.

C. Investigations

In most patients, only the history and physical examination are needed to establish the likely diagnosis. However, if the diagnosis must be further refined, several tests can be performed. Generally, clinician should perform the least invasive test that provides the most information. Furthermore, clinicians should tailor testing to the most likely diagnosis instead of performing a battery of tests on all patients with lymphadenopathy.

> **Which investigations to be done?**
> - Complete blood count
> - Mantoux test
> - X-ray chest
> - Bone marrow examination
> - Lymph node biopsy
> - X-ray chest
> - Imaging studies – USG, CT

Complete Blood Count

The test would reveal the presence and degree of anemia.

The complete blood count may reveal the reactive lymphocytes of infectious mononucleosis or a granulocytosis suggesting bacterial infection. Bicytopenia would be a red flag sign of hematologic malignancy such as leukemia or lymphoma or metastatic disease like neuroblastoma. Isolated leukopenia and neutropenia may also be seen with viral infections.

C-reactive protein or raised ESR would suggest collagen vascular disease.

Platelet count is essential for diagnosis of thrombocytopenia seen in viral infections and leukemia.

Mantoux Test

Should be done in persistent signifiant lymphadenopathy. A positive mantoux test suggests tuberculosis.

X-ray Chest

Useful for detection of mediastinal glands and parenchymal lung involvement.
Presence of mediastinal glands require prompt assessment of neoplastic or granulomatous causes.

Anatomic location of mediastinal masses	
Anterior mediastinum	Lymphoma
	Thymoma
	Benign teratoma
	Substernal goiter
	Thymic cyst
Middle mediastinum	Lymphoma
	Tuberculosis
	Sarcoidosis
	Histoplasmosis
	Sarcoma
Posterior mediastinum	Neuroblastoma
	Ganglioneuroma
	Neurofibroma
	Sarcoma
	Germ cell tumour

Bone Marrow Examination

It is indicated in suspected leukemias and storage disorders.

Lactate Dehydrogenase

Lactate dehydrogenase (LDH) is useful as a screening test for lymphoma.

Fine Needle Aspiration Cytology

Although fie needle aspiration cytology (FNAC) is recommended for the diagnosis of lymphadenopathy it has several drawbacks. Firstly, it has a high false negative rate, architecture of the lymph node is not preserved and is not useful for immunohistochemistry.

If tuberculosis is thought to be present, then the needle aspiration should be avoided to prevent the spread of infection.

Lymph Node Biopsy

Lymph node biopsy should be considered in situations where there is massive lymphadenopathy. It is also indicated if lymphadenopathy is not clearing within 4 to 6 weeks of proper antibiotic therapy or if the child has associated cytopenias, hepatosplenomegaly, bony tenderness, persistent or unexplained fever, weight loss or hard nodes.

Ultrasonography and computed tomography scan of chest and abdomen

Ultrasonography and computed tomography scan of chest and abdomen are indicated in cases of abdominal and mediastinal lymphadenopathy.

SUMMARY

Lymphadenopathy is most common in young children whose naïve immune systems respond more frequently to newly encountered infections. There are many different causes. Children are often with posterior cervical lymphadenopathy, the commonest cause for which is pediculosis and boils over scalp. Most of these children are wrongly treated for tuberculosis. History, examination and a few routine tests will help in arriving at a diagnosis in most cases. However, some may need lymph node biopsy.

SUGGESTED READING

1. Evaluation and management of lymphadenopathy in children, Alison M. Friedman, Pediatrics in Review, Feb 2008, Vol. 29, Issue 2.

2. Childhood Cervical Lymphadenopathy. Alexander K.C. Leung, W. Lane, M. Robson. J Pediatr Healthcare 2004;18(1).

3. Aruchamy Lakshamnswamy. Clinical Pediatrics, History Taking and Case Discussion. 3rd Ed.

4. Green, Pediatric Diagnosis, Interpretation of Symptoms and Signs in Children & Adolescent. 6th Ed.

Chapter

8

PALLOR

INTRODUCTION

Pallor generally indicates anemia, but it can also be seen in poor peripheral circulation, i.e. shock and severe edema as in nephrotic syndrome. Severe anemia often imparts a yellowish hue to the skin and hence may be mistaken for jaundice. Some children may have a pale complexion without having anemia and in those with a dark skin, pallor cannot be recognized by skin color.

Anemia is common in children especially in India and identifying the cause is important. Even though anemia in childhood has many causes, the correct diagnosis can usually be established with relatively little laboratory cost.

DEFINITION

A child is considered anemic if the hemoglobin is less than normal for his age. Hemoglobin values change with age.

ETIOLOGY

Anemia can be classified in 2 ways. Firstly, according to morphology of red blood cells and secondly on the basis of aetiological factors responsible for anemia. The latter appears to be more convenient in daily clinical practice.

Table: Causes of anaemia

- Nutritional: Deficiency of iron, folate, vitamin B12, protein.

- Hemolytic
  Congenital:
  - Hemoglobinopathies - Thalassemia, sickle cell anemia
  - Enzyme deficiency - Glucose-6-phosphate dehydrogenase (G6PD) deficiency, pyruvate kinase deficiency
  - Membrane defects - Spherocytosis, elliptocytosis

  Acquired: Autoimmune hemolytic anemia: Hypersplenism, malaria, hemolytic uremic syndrome.

- Hemorrhagic (Blood Loss)
  - Obvious or concealed hemorrhage: Purpura, coagulopathies, trauma.

- Hypoplastic/Aplastic (Bone Marrow Suppression)
  - Congenital: Fanconi anemia, Diamond Blackfan, osteopetrosis.
  - Acquired: Drugs, viruses, leukemia.

- Mixed etiology:
  - Infections and inflammation: Intestinal malabsorption, tuberculosis, collagen disease
  - Chronic renal failure.

EVALUATION

A. HISTORY

A detail history on the following points must be taken before proceeding for examination.

Points in history

- Age of the child
- Onset of anaemia
- Ethnic background
- Family history and consanguinity
- H/O breathlessness, fatigue
- Dietary history
- Chronic infections or disease
- Passage of blood from any site
- Color of stools and urine
- Repeated blood transfusions
- H/O pica and worm infestation
- Environmental exposure to lead
- Is the child receiving any medications

Age of the child:

Age at which child presents with anemia is important. In the newborn period, baby can be anemic either due to twin-to-twin transfusion, hemolytic disease of the newborn, spherocytosis or G6PD deficiency. The latter two conditions present more as pathological jaundice. In a child with thalassemia, anemia is not present at birth. It manifests by the age of 3 to 6 months. In children between the age of 6 months to 3 years, iron deficiency anemia is common especially in our country, due to poor dietary habits. Again, in the adolescent period, anemia could be due to poor diet and in girls due to menorrhagia.

Dietary history:

Nutritional anemia is the most common cause of anemia in childhood. Enquire about the child's diet. Is the baby breast fed or top fed? If top fed, which milk is the baby taking? Is it diluted? How much milk does the babyconsume? Is the infant receiving solid food?Infants receiving only whole cow's milk develop anemia, because of poor iron content of cow's milk and also because it results in occult gastrointestinal bleeding. Exclusive breast feeding beyond 6 months of age results in iron deficiency anemia due to lack of iron content in milk. Infants receiving goat's milk develop folic acid deficiency. A vegan mother's breastfed child is prone to develop megaloblastic anemia due to vitamin B12 deficiency in the mother.

It is commonly observed in our country that toddlers are given only milk and very little solid food by parents, as they believe that milk is very nutritious. Such children though plump are anemic.

Similarly, grown up children and adolescents can develop anemia as they consume food lacking micronutrients. Consumption of fast food in this age group is common leading to deficiency anemia.

Ethnicity:

The child's ethnic background would suggest certain hemoglobinopathies, e.g. sickle cell anemia is seen in certain tribals of Madhya Pradesh, Chhattisgarh, Maharashtra and Orissa. The prevalence of thalassemia gene is high among Kuthis, Kathiawadi Punjabis, Sindhies, Lohanas. G6PD deficiency is common amongst Punjabi, Sindhi and Parsi communities.

Family history:

A similar type of anaemia in other family member would suggest a genetic cause for anemia. A history of neonatal hyperbilirubinemia, anemia, jaundice, splenomegaly, gallstones or splenectomy in family members would point towards congenital hemolytic anemia. History of consanguineous marriage among parents should also be enquired. Beta thalassemia and sickle cell disease are inherited as autosomal recessive conditions. Hereditary spherocytosis demonstrate an autosomal dominant inheritance pattern. G6PD deficiency is inherited as an X-linked recessive trait.

History of chronic infections or disease:

Anemia is a common manifestation of many chronic illnessesin children such as tuberculosis, chronic urinary tract infection, intestinalmalabsorption. The anemia in such cases has a mixedetiology viz. marrow suppression, nutritional deficiencies andhemolysis.

History of medications:

Is the child receiving any drugs, which could give rise to anemia? Anticonvulsant drugs, e.g. phenytoin and phenobarbitone and cytotoxic drugs such as methotrexate have been associated with folate deficiency. Prolonged use of drugs such as non-steroidal anti-inflammatory drugs (NSAIDs) can cause anemia by producing long-standing blood loss from the gastric mucosa. Certain drugs viz. primaquine, nalidixic acid, nitrofurantoin can precipitate hemolysis in children with G6PD deficiency.

History of passage of blood from any site:

Anaemia can result from either moderate to severe acute blood loss or chronic loss of blood in small quantities. Enquire whether child is passing blood from any site viz. epistaxis, hematuria, melena or episodes of hematochezia. Hence, color of stool and urine would be important. If there is a history of passing cola-colored urine with sudden onset of pallor and jaundice, it points towards an acute hemolytic crisis usually due to G6PD deficiency.

Onset of anemia:

A sudden onset of anemia is often due to hemorrhage either obvious or hidden. It is also seen in children with acute hemolysis. Gradual onset is a feature of dietary deficiencies, hypoplastic anemia,chronic hemolysis, anemia of chronic diseases or occult blood loss as in hookworm infestation.

History of joint swelling and pain:

Is the child suffering from pain or swelling of any joints? Such a history would suggest leukemias or collagen diseases. In coagulation disorders, there could be a history of joint swelling and pain due to hemarthrosis. Episodic painful crisis are typical of sickle cell disease.

History of jaundice:

Does the child get recurrent jaundice? Recurrent jaundice with anemia points towards a hemolytic process. History of hyperbilirubinemia with anemia in the neonatal period may indicate congenital spherocytosis or G6PD deficiency. In childhood, mild jaundice (lemon yellow) is often seen in cases of spherocytosis and sickle cell anemia. In sickle cell disease, jaundice becomes deep, whenever there is a crisis. Jaundice is uncommon in thalassemia.

History of fever:

The most common cause of fever with anemia in our country is malaria. Fever can also be present in cases of leukemia, aplastic anemia and in chronic infections.

repeated blood transfusion:

History of repeated blood transfusions in a child usually points towards the presence of inherited hemolytic anemia such as thalassemia and sickle cell disease. Children with hypoplastic anemia, osteopetrosis and various leukemias would also need repeated transfusions.

Environmental exposure:

One must enquire about occupation of parents especially any exposure to lead. Chronic exposure to environmental lead exacerbates iron deficiency.

General symptoms:

Listlessness, loss of appetite, irritability, poor concentration and easy fatiguability are common symptoms associated with anemias. One must also enquire for history of pica.

Was the baby born premature?

Intrauterine transfer of iron from mother to baby occurs chiefly in the last trimester of pregnancy. Therefore preterm babies have poor iron stores and hence are predisposed to develop an early and exaggerated physiological anaemia of infancy.

EXAMINATION

After having taken a detail history it is essential to carry out a careful examination. During a general and systemic examination the following signs should be looked for:

Signs on examination

- Anthropometry
- Vital signs
- Facies
- Eyes
- Skin
- Lymphadenopathy
- Tongue and nails
- Pigmentation of knuckles
- Bony tenderness
- Joint swelling
- Congenital anomalies
- Signs of systemic illness
- Systemic examination

Facies:

A typical hemolytic facies is seen in cases of thalassemia. It resembles mongoloid facies characterized by prominent frontal and parietal eminences, depressed bridge of nose, malar prominences, crowding of teeth and upturning of vermilion border of the upper lip. In case of systemic lupus erythematosus, a butterfly rash is characteristic.

Anthropometry:

Weight, height and head circumference should be noted. Poor growth may suggest malnutrition or chronic disease such as chronic renal failure or hypothyroidism that are responsible for anemia. Any long-standing anemia would hamper growth.

Pallor:

Pallor should be looked for in the oral mucous membrane, nails, tongue, conjunctiva, palms and soles. Waxy pallor of generalized edema may mimic anemia, while severe anemia may present a yellowish hue to the skin.

Jaundice:

One must examine the sclera for jaundice. Presence of jaundice would suggest hemolytic anemia. The pallor is out of proportion to the jaundice, which often has lemon-yellow hue. In case of sickle cell anemia jaundice can be dark yellow.

Bleeding and bruising:

It is essential to look for petechiae, purpura or ecchymotic patches. Presence of bleeding will suggest either a bleeding disorder, aplastic or hypoplastic anemia or leukemias.

Lymphadenopathy:

Presence of lymphadenopathy would suggest either a malignant process such as leukemias and lymphomas or chronic infection such as tuberculosis.

Tongue:

Apart from tongue appearing pale in cases of iron deficiency anemia, the papillae are atrophied. Mouth ulcers are noted in children with neutropenia. Presence of oral thrush may indicate immunodeficiency or poor feeding practices.

Nails:

Pallor can be appreciated on nails. It should be kept in mind that sometimes the nails may appear pale due to their excessive thickness. In such cases presence of anaemia should be confirmed by looking at other sites. In case of iron deficiency anemia, the normal convexity of nails becomes attenuated and they start appearing flat. In severe cases they may become concave or spoon shaped (koilonychia). In fact, koilonychia is a very specific sign of iron deficiency anaemia. Nails may become thin and brittle and longitudinal ridges appear on them. Clubbing of fingers and toes due to chronic hypoxia can be seen in case of sickle cell disease.

Bony tenderness:

In a case of anemia one must elicit sternal tenderness. Presence of bony tenderness would indicate infiltrative disorders of the marrow such as leukemia.

Pigmentation of knuckles:

It is a classical sign of megaloblastic anem due to vitamin B12 deficiency.

Examination of joints:

It is essential to examine the joints in a chi with anemia. Dactilytis of hands and fe (hand foot syndrome) when present indicat sickle cell disease. Vascular necrosis of lar joints (hip knee, etc.) due to microinfarc leading to joint swelling. Pain is also a featu of sickle cell disease. Features of rickets wou be seen in cases of chronic renal failure.

Congenital anomalies:

Features of congenital anomalies in a chil with anemia points towards constitution aplastic anemia. Apart from dysmorphicfaci microcephaly, polydactyly, squint, cafe-au-la spots, hypogonadism and skeletal anomali especially absence of thumb, is a feature Fanconi's anemia, while eye anomalies vi glaucoma, cataract, strabismus and upper lim anomalies are seen in Diamond-Blackfa Syndrome.

Vital signs:

Vital signs viz. pulse rate, respiratory rate an blood pressure should be recorded. Marke tachycardia and respiratory distress in a anaemic child indicates heart failure an would need urgent blood transfusion.

Edema:

Edema is seen in protein caloric malnutritio and in cardiac failure due to severe anemia

Examination of abdomen:

Hepatosplenomegaly in a child with anemi points towards hemolytic process, marro infiltrative diseases viz. leukemias osteopetrosis and myelofibrosis. Spleen ca so be palpable in 15 percent cases of iron deficiency anemia. Presence of hepatosplenomegaly almost excludes aplastic anemia.

Cardiovascular system:

The cardiovascular system must be carefully examined for cardiomegaly, which may indicate long-standing anemia and also for the presence of hemic murmur.

INVESTIGATIONS

Before discussing the various investigations that can be done in a child with anemia it is important to remember that the normal range for peripheral blood counts vary significantly with age. Newborns have large red cells as compared to children and adults, with higher MCV at birth. Subsequently, MCV falls and reaches the lowest at around 6 months of age. Thereafter MCV increases gradually until it reaches adult values after puberty.

Table: Following are the normal hemoglobin levels at different ages

Age	Hb (g/dL)	
	Mean	2 SD
Birth (cord blood)	16.5	13.5
1-3 days	18.5	14.5
7 days	17.5	13.5
14 days	16.5	12.5
1 month	14.0	10.0
2 months	11.5	9.0
6 months	11.5	9.5
1 year	12.0	10.5
2-6 years	12.5	11.5
6-12 years	13.5	11.5
12-18 years Girls	14.0	12.0
Boys	14.0	13.0

The normal number of white cells is higher in infancy and early childhood than later in life. Neutrophils predominate in the differential white cell count at birth and in the older child. There is a predominance of lymphocytes (upto 80%) between ages 1 month and 6 years. Normal values for platelet count vary little with age.

The initial laboratory evaluation of a child with anemia should consists of a complete blood count, with differential and platelet count, a reticulocyte count and a detailed review of the peripheral smear. Then based on clinical examination and Complete Blood Count (CBC) report, the patient is subjected to further investigations if required. All the investigations listed below are not essential in every case.

First line investigations:

Interpretation of the hemoglobin and hematocrit base levels is done on the reference range for the specific age group. Hemoglobin and hematocrit levels can be used interchangeably. Essentially, the hematocrit level is 3 times the hemoglobin value. If the patient is anaemic, look for the following red cell indices:

- Mean corpuscular volume (MCV)
- Mean corpuscular hemoglobin (MCH)
- Mean corpuscular hemoglobin concentration (MCHC)

Reference ranges for these parameter also vary with age. Of these MCV is particularly helpful in classifying anaemia. Microcytic anaemia suggests iron deficiency, lead poisoning, or thalassemia. Macrocytosis suggests folate / B12 deficiency or reactive reticulocytosis. Another valuable parameter in classifying anaemia is the RBC distribution width (RDW). This is the statistical description of the heterogenecity of the RBC sizes. It is increased in anisocytosis (variable sizes of red cells).

Selective rise in white blood cell counts (leukocytosis) is seen in infections and leukemias. Falsely elevated leukocyte count is seen in thalassemia. This rise in count is because of normoblasts, which are not destroyed by the WBC fluid.

Pancytopenia is a feature of depressed bone marrow activity seen in cases of hypoplastic anemia and in hemolytic anemia with aplastic crisis due to parvovirus infection. Low platelet count is seen in hypoplastic anemia, leukemias and immune thrombocytopenic purpura. Thrombocytosis (increase in platelet count) is a feature of iron deficiency anemia and collagen diseases.

Reticulocyte count:

Reticulocyte count indicates active erythropoiesis. Elevated reticulocyte count is observed in cases of hemolysis or blood loss and patients responding to hematinic therapy. In some autoimmune hemolytic anaemias, reticulocytopenia is present due to lysis of reticulocytes by the same antibiotics. It is also decreased in anaemias of chronic disorders, bone marrow failure or megaloblasticanaemia.

Peripheral smear:

Examination of peripheral smear helps to identify the cause of the anaemia through recognition of abnormal cell morphology.

- Schistocytes or fragmented cells (microangiopathic hemolytic anaemia)
- Spherocytes (hereditary spherocytosis, autoimmune hemolytic anaemia)
- Ghost, helmet, blister or bite cells (G6PD deficiency)
- Sickle cells (sickle cell disease)
- Target cells (hemoglobin C) also seen in thalassemia, other hemoglobinopathies
- Stippled red cells (suggests lead poisoning)
- Increased polychromasia (reticulocytosis)

It is important to remember that normal RB morphology does not rule out hemolysis.

Second line investigations:

Depending on the clinical diagnosis an result of first line (routine) tests shou additional laboratory tests should be done

- Bilirubin level, lactate dehydrogena (hemolytic anemia)
- Coomb's test (autoimmune hemolyt anaemia)
- Hemoglobin electrophores (hemoglobinopathies)
- Red cell enzyme studies e.g. G6PI pyruvate kinase
- Osmotic fragility
- Serum iron, total iron binding capacit ferritin (iron deficiency anemia)
- Folate, Vitamin B12 levels (macrocytic megaloblasticanaemia)
- Blood typing and cross matchir (isoimmuneanaemia in neonate)
- Bone marrow aspiration and biops (myeloproliferative disease, leukemia and hypoplasticanaemia)
- Viral titers (e.g. EB virus, CMV)
- BUN and creatinine levels (assess ren function)
- T4 / TSH (rule out hypothyroidism)
- Stool for occult blood (multiple specimen

Radiology:

- *Chest X-ray:* May show cardiomegaly cases of chronic anemia.
- *Skull X-ray:* Hair on end appearance see in congenital hemolytic anemia specially thalassemia.
- *Long bones X-ray:* Indicated i osteopetrosis in which the appearance very characteristic. These bones sho increased density masking the distinctio between the cortex and the medullar cavity. (Marble bone appearance).

Ultrasonography of abdomen:

In older children with spherocytosis and sickle cell USG abdomenis indicated if gallstones are suspected.

Karyotyping:

In children with Fanconi'sanaemia karyotyping may revealchromosomal breaks.

SUMMARY

Anemia is common in children. Normal color of the skin in Indian children varies from dark to fair. Some normal children have a complexion that appears pale. Hemoglobin values change with age.

Clinically there are four major causes of anemia viz. nutritional deficiencies, hemolytic anemia, hypoplasia/aplasia of the marrow and hemorrhage. Proper history and examination would help in arriving at a clinical diagnosis, which can be confirmed by appropriate investigations.

SUGGESTED READING

1. Pediatric acute anaemia workup (2015). Emedicine.medscape.com.
2. A practical approach to the child with anaemia. www.ncbi.nim.nih.gov.pubmed.

9 JAUNDICE IN AN OLDER CHILD

INTRODUCTION

Jaundice can result from a variety of disorders hence approach to a child with jaundice is one of the most challenging problems encountered in clinical practice. The differential diagnosis in older children and adolescents is very different from infants and neonates, hence it will be discussed separately.

DEFINITION

Jaundice also known as icterus is defined as a condition characterized by yellowish discoloration of tissues and body fluids, due to an increase in the circulating bilirubin. It is clinically detected by presence of varying coloration from yellowish to deep yellow or yellowish green of skin mucous membrane and scleras. In normal children the total serum bilirubin is less than 1 mg%. Jaundice can be detected clinically when the total serum bilirubin exceeds 5 mg% in neonates and 2 mg% in older children. One should look for jaundice only in natural light. It is very hard to detect jaundice in artificial light especially in fluorescent light.

Bilirubin has a high affinity for elastic fibers, hence jaundice becomes manifest first in the sclera, which is very rich in elastic fibers followed by hard palate, face and abdominal wall. Regression occurs in the reverse order and jaundice disappears last from the sclera. Because jaundice may be the presenting feature of life threatening conditions such as fulminant liver failure, a prompt and logical evaluation is necessary to identify the more serious disorders that require urgent management.

ETIOLOGY

The causes of jaundice in a child can be broadly classified into three categories:

Table: Causes of jaundice

A. **Pre-hepatic jaundice**

It is characterized by unconjugated hyperbilirubinemia.

a. Hemolytic anemia: Thalassemia, sickle cell anemia, hereditary spherocytosis, glucose-6-phosphatase dehydrogenase (G6PD) deficiency, autoimmune anemia

b. Familial jaundice: Gilbert's syndrome, Criggler-Najjar syndrome.

B. **Hepatocellular Jaundice**

1. Infections

   a. Viral

   Hepatotropic virus: A, B, C, D, E, F and G

   Non-hepatotropic virus: Mumps, measles, rubella, cox sackie, Epstein barr virus

   b. Bacterial: Typhoid, brucellosis, disseminated tuberculosis, E. coli, septicemia

   c. Spirochetal: Weil's disease

   d. Protozoal: Malaria, toxoplasmosis, Kala-azar.

2. Drugs:
   a. All antitubercular drugs except streptomycin
   b. Paracetamol
   c. Non-steroidal anti-inflammatory drugs (NSAIDs)
   d. Anticonvulsants: Valparin, carbamazepine
   e. Antibiotics: Erythromycin.
3. Toxins
   a. Alfatoxins produced by fungus aspergillusflavus, which contaminates cereals and nuts
   b. Poisonous mushroom.
4. Metabolic disorders
   Wilson's disease, Galactosemia, a1 antitrypsin deficiency, cystic fibrosis, hereditary tyrosinemia, hereditary fructose intolerance
5. Autoimmune hepatitis.
   Type 1 and 2

C. **Cholestatic Jaundice**
   1. Extrahepatic cholestasisCholedochal cyst, gallstones, glands in the portahepatis.
   2. Intrahepatic cholestasisViral hepatitis, galactosemia, Watson-Alagille syndrome, Byler syndrome, Budd chiari syndrome
   3. FamilialDubin Johnson syndrome

EVALUATION

Evaluation of child with jaundice involves an appropriate and accurate history, a carefully performed physical examination and skilled interpretation of signs and symptoms. Further evaluation is aided by judicious selection of diagnostic tests.

A. HISTORY

Points in history
- History of fever
- Prodromal symptoms
- Onset and duration of jaundice
- Pain in abdomen
- Color of urine and stool
- History of contact
- Transfusion history
- History of recurrent jaundice
- Family history of jaundice
- History of drug ingestion
- History of pruritis
- Vaccines that the child has received
- Clustering of cases
- History of hematemesis

History of fever:

Enquire whether the child has fever. Fever at the onset of illness is seen in acute hepatitis. History of fever with chills suggests viral hepatitis, malarial hepatitis, liver abscess, leptospirosis or cholangitis. In case of viral hepatitis, fever tends to subside with onset of jaundice. If fever persists beyond the onset of jaundice it is likely to be malaria or Salmonella infection.

Prodromal symptoms:

It is important to find out whether the illness was preceded by any prodromal symptom such as malaise, anorexia, nausea and abdominal discomfort, which would indicate viral hepatitis.

Onset and duration of jaundice:

How long has the child been suffering from jaundice? Was the onset acute, subacute or chronic? An acute onset is seen in acute viral hepatitis, while subacute or chronic onset suggests chronic hepatitis or metabolic disease.

Autoimmune hepatitis though mostly associated with chronic liver disease, 25-30% of children may mimic acute viral hepatitis. Wilson disease may present as acute self-limited hepatitis or as fulminant hepatic failure, a1 antitrypsin deficiency may rarely present as acute hepatitis.

Pain in abdomen:

Does the child complaint of pain in abdomen? Pain in the right hypochondrium is seen in hepatitis, liver abscess and cholecystitis.

Color of urine and stool:

Whenever the child presents with jaundice, it is essential to enquire about the color of urine and stool. If the color of urine is normal it indicates unconjugated hyperbiliribinemia, as seen in hemolytic anemia and Gilbert disease. In hepatocellular and cholestatic jaundice the urine is high colored. In hemolytic anemia the color of stools is normal, while it is pale or clay colored in cholestatic jaundice.

Transfusion history:

If there is a history of receiving blood transfusion or blood products, one must consider hepatitis B or C, 6 months prior to presentation.

History of recurrent jaundice:

Is this the first episode of jaundice or does the child get recurrent jaundice? The latter would suggest congenital hemolytic anemia,such as spherocytosis, sickle cell anemia etc. or familial jaundice such as Gilbert disease or Dubin Johnson syndrome.

Family history of jaundice:

Is there a history of recurrent or persistent jaundice in any members of the family? Such a history would suggest congenital hemolytic anemias such as spherocytosis and sickle cell anemia or metabolic disease viz Wilson disease, galactosemia, tyrosenemia, Gilbert disease and Dubin Johnson syndrome. Mode of inheritance in these metabolic disorders is autosomal recessive.

Has any family member suffered from jaundice in the recent past?

If such a contact has occurred especially with siblings and other family members, the possibility of hepatitis A and E must be considered. These are transmitted by oro-fecal route.

History of drug ingestion:

Is the child receiving any drugs? Antitubercular drugs and anticonvulsants are known to give rise to drug hepatitis. In children with G6PD deficiency ingestion of certain drugs such as primaquin, nalidixic acid sulfas, etc. can give rise to severe hemolysis and the child suffers from severe anemia and mild jaundice.

History of pruritis:

Itching points towards cholestatic jaundice.

Immunization status of the child:

Has the child received vaccines against hepatitis A, B and typhoid? Such a history will help in identifying those protected from these vaccine preventable causes.

Clustering of cases:

Clustering of cases is seen in epidemics of hepatitis E.

History of hematemesis:

If a child with jaundice develops hematemesis the cause is portal hypertension. In case of acute viral hepatitis, hematemesis is due to liver cell failure (hypoprothrombinemia) and indicates a bad prognosis.

Pain in hands and feet:

Recurrent pain and swelling over the dorsum of hands and feet would suggest sickle cell disease (hand foot syndrome).

3. EXAMINATION

A carefully conducted examination can help to arrive at a definite diagnosis regarding the cause of jaundice in the child.

Points on examination

- Anthropometry
- Examination of eyes
- Clubbing
- Signs of liver cell failure
- Leg ulcers
- Systemic examination

Anthropometry:

Growth parameters to be recorded to assess growth failure, which would indicate chronic liver disease.

Examination of eyes:

The color of jaundice should be looked for. Lemon yellow color suggests hemolytic jaundice, deep yellow seen in hepatocellular jaundice, while orange/green hue is seen in cholestatic jaundice.

Presence of pallor associated with jaundice indicates hemolytic jaundice. It is also seen following hemetemesis in liver cell failure.

The eyes should be carefully examined for presence of Kayser-Fleischer (KF) ring, presence of which would indicate Wilson disease. Cataract in a child with jaundice would suggest galactosemia or Wilson disease. Presence of Bitot spots would indicate cholestatic jaundice as absorption of fat soluble vitamins is impaired in cholestasis.

High grade fever, pallor, icterus and splenomegaly suggests malaria.

Clubbing:

Clubbing of finger nails is seen in chronic liver disease.

Signs of liver cell failure:

In any child presenting with jaundice, one must look for signs of liver cell failure viz Spider naevi, palmar erythema, ecchymosis and rapidly developing edema.

Leg ulcers:

Leg ulcers are seen in congenital hemolytic anemias.

Systemic Examination:

- Abdominal distension – ascitis.
- Liver should be carefully palpated and percussed to assess texture and size.
- Nodular shrunken liver suggests cirrhosis.
- Tender, hepatomegaly suggests acute hepatitis.
- Splenomegaly would suggest hemolytic anemia and portal hypertension.
- Neurologic: Confusion, asterixis, heperreflexia may all be feature of hepatic encephalopathy.

C. INVESTIGATIONS

- Bilirubin fractionation:
  - Unconjugated hyperbilirubinemiais often due to hemolytic disease.
  - In case of unconjugated hyperbilirubinemia the following tests should be done viz. CBC, reticulocytes, direct and indirect. Coomb's test, haptoglobin and Hb electrophoresis if suspecting hemoglobinopathy.
  - Conjugated hyperbilirubinemia suggests hepatobiliary disease.
  - In such a case the following tests are indicated.
  - Liver enzymes:
    Alanine aminotransferase (ALT, SGPT) typically shows a mild rise (2 to 5 fold increase) in chronic liver disease as against 20-100 fold rise usually seen with acute viral hepatitis. Alkaline phosphatase may also be raised. It is less than 3 times elevated in hepatoceuar jaundice and more than 3 times in cholestatic jaundice. Levels are normal in hemolytic jaundice. Thus predominant elevation of ALT / AST suggests hepatocellular injury, whereas predominant elevation of ALP / GGT suggests biliary tract disease.
  - Coagulation profile:
    PT, aPTT, INR. Prothrombin time is most sensitive indicator of liver function. It is raised because of impairment of synthesis of coagulation factors by liver or because of cholestasis associated Vitamin K deficiency. In the latter case, the correction of PT occurs following Vitamin K administration whereas in the former, PT does not normalize after Vitamin K therapy.

- Other laboratory investigations:
  - Abdominal USG to establish hepati architecture and rule out biliary trac disease.Useful in choledochal cysts portal hypertension and cirrhosi liver.
  - Hepatitis serology.Viral markers fo acute viral hepatitis.These serologica tests should only be done if on suspects viral hepatitis as the caus of jaundice. Elevated immunoglobulir M (IgM) antibody to hepatitis A viru (anti-HAV) is observed in hepatiti A.Elevated IgMAnti HBc along witl HBsAg positivity seen in acut hepatitis B.
  - Serum ceruloplasmin, 24 hou urinary copper excretion – Wilson' disease.

SUMMARY

Jaundice is yellowish discoloration of the skin, sclera and mucous membranes due to elevated bilirubin as a result of abnorma bilirubin metabolism and/or excretion. The bilirubin can either be unconjugated (indirec bilirubin) or conjugated (direct bilirubin). Jaundice is best observed in daylight. The firs step in diagnosing the cause of jaundice is to determine if it is direct (obstructive hepatobiliary) or indirect (hemolytic jaundice). Clinically deep jaundice, acholic (pale clay colored) stools and yellow urine favor obstructive jaundice. Lemon tinge ol skin and absence of change in color of urine and stool favor hemolytic jaundice. Confirmation is obtained by estimating serum bilirubin. Raised direct bilirubin confirms obstructive and raised indirect variety points to hemolytic jaundice. Hemolysis causes rec cell breakdown, which is reflected in hyperbilirubinemia of indirect type, raised urine urobilinogen and increased reticulocyte count in the peripheral blood. Further search or a diagnosis within the two types ofjaundice is then made on the basis of history, clinical examination and more elaborate laboratory investigations.

SUGGESTED READING

1. Pashankar D, Schneiber RA. Jaundice in older children and adolescents. Pediatrics in Review 2001;22(7):219-226.

2. Non-Neonatal Jaundice. Learn Pediatrics.ubc.ca.

Chapter

JAUNDICE IN NEONATE

INTRODUCTION

Hyperbilirubinemia is a common problem in the neonatal period. Nearly two-thirds of full term and three-fourths of preterm babies develop jaundice, most of which is physiological. At no other time in life is jaundice physiological. It is challenging at times for a treating physician to distinguish physiological from pathological jaundice. In 3 to 5% of newborns, serum bilirubin levels can exceed physiological limits, raising concerns of brain damage.

DEFINITION

What is physiological jaundice?

Most term newborns develop jaundice on 2nd or 3rd day of life, which rises to a maximum of 8 mg% by day 4 and almost disappears by end of 1st week. A rise upto 12 mg% is considered to be within physiological limits. In preterm infants, the rise may start a day or two later and reaches its peak by 7th day and disappears by the end of 2nd week.

What are the criteria for diagnosis of pathological jaundice?

Pathological jaundice is diagnosed if:

1. Jaundice appears within 24 hours of birth.
2. Serum bilirubin rises by 5mg/day or 0.5 mg/h.
3. If jaundice persists beyond 2 weeks in term and 3 weeks in a preterm infant.

4. Whenever direct bilirubin component i more than 2 mg% or more than 10% t 15% of total bilirubin.
5. If there are signs of underlying illness in any infant such as vomiting, lethargy poor feeding, excessive weight loss apnea, tachypnea or temperature instability.

ETIOLOGY

Common causes of pathological jaundice in our country are blood group incompatibilities, infections, idiopathic jaundice (breast milk jaundice), G6PD deficiency, bruising and cephalhematoma.

Table: Causes of neonatal jaundice

A. Unconjugated Hyperbilirubinemia

- Exaggerated physiological jaundice, e.g. prematurity, birth asphyxia hypothyroidism
- Hemolytic anemia: blood group incompatibilities—Rh, ABO, hereditary spherocytosis, G6PD deficiency, pyruvate kinase deficiency, alpha thalassemia
- Extravascular blood: large cephalhematoma, bruises, hematomas, etc.
- Polycythemia
- Metabolic causes: galactosemia, maternal diabetes
- Hypothyroidism

- Genetic disorders: gilbert disease, Crigler-Najjar syndrome
- Infections: sepsis, intrauterine infections - TORCH stands for toxoplasmosis, other (syphilis, varicella-zoster, parvovirus B19), rubella, cytomegalovirus and herpes.
- Increased enterohepatic circulation: Intestinal atresia,Hirschsprung disease, meconium ileus, swallowed blood, meconium ileus and/or meconium plug syndrome.

B. Conjugated Hyperbilirubinemia

- Biliary atresia
- Choledochal cyst
- Neonatal hepatitis
- Infections: viral, bacterial
- Inspissated bile syndrome
- Alagille syndrome
- Genetic disorders: Dubin-Johnson syndrome, Rotor syndrome, galactosemia, tyrosinemia, alpha 1-antitrypsin deficiency
- Total parenteral nutrition induced cholestasis.

EVALUATION

In order to arrive at a definitive diagnosis to the cause of jaundice in the neonate, it is essential to take a detailed history followed by examination and on the basis of a working diagnosis investigations have to be carried out to arrive at a final diagnosis.

A. History

It is essential to take a detail history.

Points in history

- Presentation and duration of jaundice
- Family history
- History of pregnancy and delivery
- Postnatal history

Table: Causes of neonatal jaundice based on day of appearance

1. Jaundice appearing within 24 hours of age
   - Hemolytic disease of newborn: Rh, ABO and minor group incompatibility
   - Intrauterine infections
   - G6PD deficiency
   - Hereditary spherocytosis
   - Crigler-Najjar syndrome
   - Alpha-thalassemia
2. Jaundice appearing between 24 and 72 hours of life
   - Physiological
   - Septicemia
   - Polycythemia
   - Concealed hemorrhages: Cephalhematoma subarachnoid bleed, intraventricular hemorrhage
3. Jaundice appearing after 72 hours of life
   - Septicemia
   - Idiopathic jaundice
   - Hypothyroidism
   - Metabolic disorders

Presentation and duration of neonatal jaundice:

Typically physiological jaundice appears on the second or third day of life. Jaundice if visible during first 24 hours of life is likely to be pathological and needs investigation. Jaundice presenting after 3 to 4 days needs close monitoring. Infants with severe jaundice or if icterus continues beyond the first 2 weeks need to be screened for metabolic disease such as galactosemia and hypothyroidism. Adequacy of breast milk and stool color should be assessed.

Family history:

Has any member of the family or sibling suffered from jaundice in the neonatal period particularly if it needed treatment. A history of jaundice and anemia in the newborn period would suggest blood group incompatibility, congenital spherocytosis and G6PD deficiency.

If any member in the family has undergone splenectomy for jaundice or had gallstones, one must consider spherocytosis.

History of liver disease in early infancy in the family points towards galactosemia, alpha 1-antitrypsin deficiency,

Gilbert disease, Crigler-Najjar syndrome, Tyrosinosis. History of consanguinity would suggest metabolic diseases such as galactosemia, tyrosenemia and cystic fibrosis inherited as autosomal recessive.

Maternal illness during pregnancy:

Did the mother suffer from fever during pregnancy? If she did have fever consider TORCH group of infections in the newborn or congenital malaria. Infants of diabetic mother tend to develop hyperbilirubinemia. Drugs such as sulfas, nitrofurantoin and antimalarials if consumed by the mother may cause hemolysis in G6PD deficient infant. Also enquire whether she took any herbal remedies.

Details of labour:

History of labor should be enquired because certain conditions during labor can lead to hyperbilirubinemia in the newborn.

Prolonged labor or premature rupture of membranes can lead to jaundice due to sepsis.

Traumatic delivery can lead to large extravascular bleeding and hemolysis leading to jaundice.

Birth asphyxia can lead to hyperbilirubinemia.

Oxytocin administered to the mother during labor can also lead to hyperbilirubinemia in the newborn, so also delayed cord clamping by causing polycythemia.

Postnatal history:

History of the newborn is essential to determine the cause of jaundice. Was there any delay in the passage of meconium? Is the neonate persistently vomiting? Is the baby breastfed? Is there adequate secretion of milk? Is there excessive somnolence in the baby? Does he get choked during feeds? What is the color of urine and stool? Any exposure to total parental nutrition.

Delayed passage of stool or infrequent stooling will suggest intestinal obstruction or hypothyroidism as a cause of hyperbilirubinemia. If there is a history of persistent vomiting one should suspect sepsis, pyloric stenosis or galactosemia.

Breast milk jaundice manifests as persistence of physiological jaundice beyond the first week. Its maximum intensity is between 10 to 14 days and jaundice can persistsupto 4 to 8 weeks. It is due to inhibitory factors such as 3-alpha-20-beta-pregnendiol present in breast milk, but lactation is adequate.

On the other hand, breastfeeding jaundice is due to inadequate lactation during first few days leading to relative dehydration, hemoconcentration, delayed colonization of gut and enhanced enterohepatic circulation.

If there is history of excessive somnolence in the baby along with choking during feeds and delayed passage of stools one must consider congenital hypothyroidism.

Pale stools after 48 to 72 hours of birth would suggest biliary atresia.

B. Examination

> **Points on examination**
> - Assessment of weight and gestational age
> - Examination of hand
> - Examination of skin
> - Examination of eyes
> - Signs of sepsis
> - Systemic examination

Assessment of weight and gestational age:

The weight and gestational age of the neonate should be assessed because both the preterm and small-for-date baby has an increased risk of developing hyperbilirubinemia. Preterm due to immaturity of liver enzymes and small-for-date due to polycythemia and infections.

Assess for presence of jaundice:

Neonatal jaundice first becomes visible in the face and forehead. Identification is aided by pressure on the skin, since blanching reveals the underlying color. Jaundice then gradually becomes visible on the trunk and extremities. Jaundice disappears in the opposite direction.

Examination of head:

The head should be examined for presence of cephalhematoma. It would give rise to hyperbilirubinemia. Measure the head circumference. Microcephaly would indicate intrauterine infection. Macrocephaly is often seen in congenital toxoplasmosis.

Examination of skin:

Presence of pallor is often associated with hemolytic anemia and extravascular blood loss.

One should carefully look for the presence of petechiae and bruising. Presence of petechiae would indicate congenital infections, sepsis and erythroblastosis.

Examination of eyes:

The eyes should be examined for presence of cataract, which would indicate a metabolic disease such as galactosemia or an intrauterine infection. Presence of congenital anomalies such as microphthalmia, coloboma of iris, etc. would suggest intrauterine infection. The fundus must be carefully examined for chorioretinitis, which is a feature of rubella and cytomegaloviral infections.

Signs of sepsis:

The neonate should be evaluated carefully for signs of sepsis such as off feeds, dullness, hypothermia and poor cry.

Systemic examination:

The abdomen should be palpated for the presence of hepatosplenomegaly seen in intrauterine infections, congenital malaria, hemolytic anemia, neonatal hepatitis and congenital tuberculosis.

Altered sensorium, shrill cry with tense bulging fontanelle would suggest meningitis. Overt neurological findings such as changes in muscle tone, seizures or altered cry in a significantly jaundiced neonate are danger signs indicating development of kernicterus.

C. Investigations

Depending upon the clinical suspicion investigations must be planned. In a newborn, one must first get a serum bilirubin estimation done and assess whether it is an unconjugated or conjugated hyperbilirubinemia. Based on the result, further investigations should be planned.

Estimation of serum bilirubin:

Usually a total serum bilirubin level is the only test required in an infant with moderate jaundice who presents on the second or third day of life. However, in infants who have hepatosplenomegaly, pallor, petechiae, thrombocytopenia or findings suggestive of hepatobiliary disease, metabolic disorder, or congenital infection, early measurement of bilirubin fractions is suggested. The same also applies to infants who remain jaundiced beyond the first 7-10 days of life.

- If there is **indirect hyperbilirubinemia** then blood type and Rh determination in mother and infant along with hemoglobin and hematocrit values and DCT (Direct Coomb's Test), peripheral smear for normoblasts, RBC morphology, evidence of hemolysis and reticulocyte count must be done. If the peripheral smear shows spherocytes and other features of hemolysis then osmotic fragility and G6PD estimation is indicated. If there is no evidence of hemolysis then a sepsis screen, thyroid profile and TORCH titres must be done.

- If there is **direct hyperbilirubinemia** i.e. when serum direct bilirubin is >2 mg% of total bilirubin or >2% of total bilirubin, then liver function tests should be done. SGOT and SGPT levels are raised in hepatocellular disease. Alkaline phosphatase and g-glutamyltransferase (GGT) levels are often elevated in cholestatic disease. Also PT and PTT should be done.

- Tests for viral infection are indicated in infants with hepatosplenomegaly, petechiaeand other evidence of hepatocellular disease.

- Reducing substance in urine. This is useful screening test for galactosemia.

Imaging studies:

- Ultrasonography of liver and bile ducts is warranted in infants with laboratory or clinical signs of cholestatic disease.

- Radionuclide scanning: A radionuclide liver scan for uptake of hepatoiminodiacetic acid (HIDA) is indicated if extrahepatic biliary atresia is suspected. Patients are pretreated with phenobarbital 5 mg/kg/day for 3-4 days before performing the scan.

APPROACH TO NEONATAL JAUNDICE

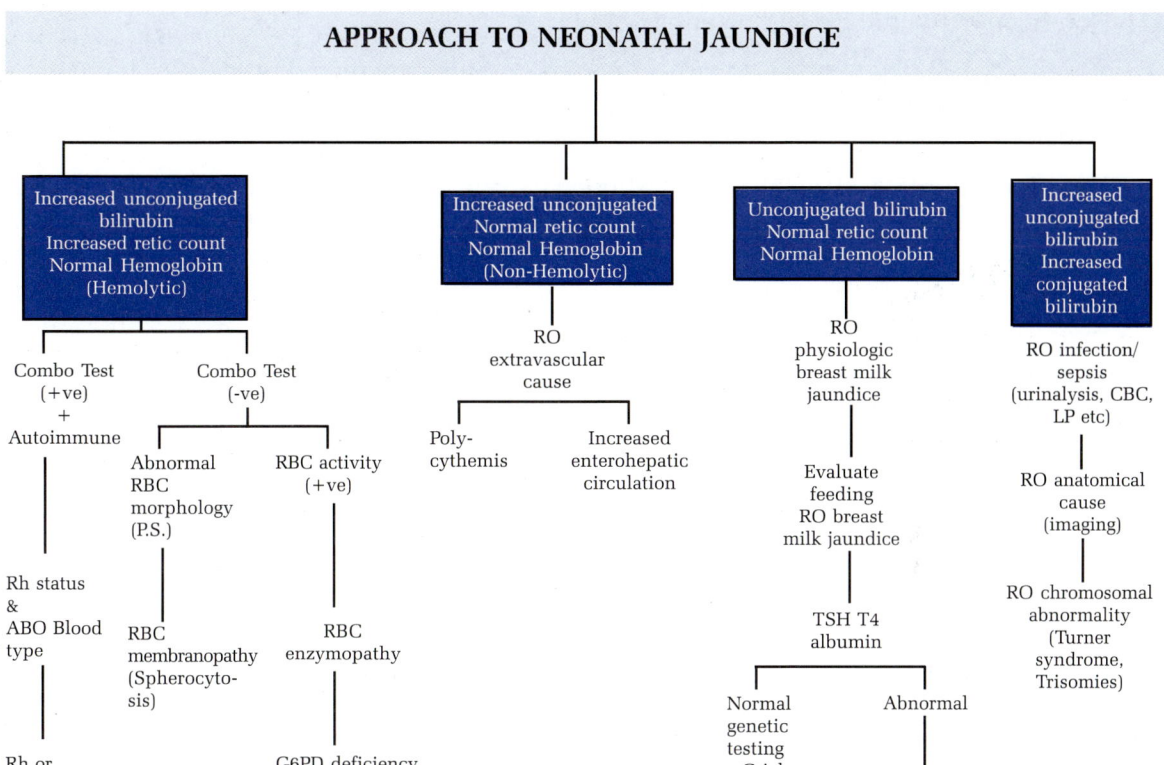

SUMMARY

Jaundice is frequently encountered in neonates. In the neonatal period most newborns have physiological jaundice. At the same time, it is very important to differentiate it from pathological jaundice as unconjugated hyperbilirubinemia in the newborn can lead to kernicterus, subsequently resulting in permanent brain damage. On the basis of history and clinical examination one must decide whether the jaundice is hemolytic, hepatocellular or obstructive. The diagnosis can be finally confirmed by relevant investigations.

SUGGESTED READING

1. Non-neonatal jaundice: learn.pediatrics.ubc.ca.

2. Friedman, LS "Chapter 16. Liver, biliary tract, and pancreas disorders". McPhee, SJ, Papadakis MR. Current Medical Diagnosis and Treatment 2011: http://www.accessmedicine.com/content.aspx2alb=7993.

3. Neonatal jaundice clinical presentation. History, physical examination. Emedicine. medscape.com.

4. Neonatal jaundice. learn.pediatrics.ubc.ca.

5. Neonatal jaundice. Diagnosis - approach. Best practice.bmj.com.

11 BLEEDING DISORDER

INTRODUCTION

A practicing physician often faces the challenge of evaluating a child with a potential bleeding disorder. Bleeding or bruising can occur spontaneously or following trauma. Whenever it occurs spontaneously or after a trivial injury, it is significant and needs investigation as to its cause.

Blood keeps flowing through the smallest capillaries throughout the life without clotting and yet when there is an injury it clots effectively and rapidly to prevent major blood loss followed by timely dissolution of the clot formed. This delicate balance is achieved through vascular factors, platelets and plasma proteins like coagulation factors their inhibitors and fibrinolytic factors working synchronously.

Bleeding disorders may occur as a result of:

- Quantitative and qualitative abnormalities of platelets
- Vascular abnormalities
- Quantitative and qualitative abnormalities in plasma coagulation factors
- Accelerated fibrinolysis.

ETIOLOGY

Table: Causes of bleeding disorders

I. Platelet Disorders

   a. Decreased platelet number

      i. Increased destruction of platelets:

- Idiopathic thrombocytopenic purpura, disseminated intravascular coagulation (DIC), necrotizing enterocolitis (NEC), hemolytic uremic syndrome, hypersplenism, thrombotic thrombocytopenic purpura, sepsis.

      ii. Decreased production of platelets:

- Fanconi anemia, Wiskott-Aldrich syndrome, osteopetrosis, acquired aplastic anemia, leukemia, folate and vitamin B12 deficiency

   b. Platelet Dysfunctions:

      i. Congenital: Bernard-Soulier syndrome, Glanzmann thrombasthenia, Scott syndrome.

      ii. Acquired: Uremia, cirrhosis, sepsis, viral infections, myeloproliferative disorders.

II. Vascular Disorders

Henoch-Schonlein purpura, Ehlers-Danlos syndrome, meningo-coccemia, scurvy.

III Coagulation Disorders

- Hereditary disorders: Hemophilia a factor VIII deficiency, hemophilia B factor IX deficiency, Von Willebrand disease factor VIII and vascular factor, hemophilia C factor XI deficiency, parahemophilia factor V deficiency, factor VII, X, XII, XIII deficiency.

- Acquired disorders: Deficiency of vitamin K dependent factors, liver disorders, hemorrhagic disease of newborn, malabsorption, acquired hemophilia, DIC.

EVALUATION

While approaching a child with bleeding, systematic approach starting with clinical history, detailed examination, screening laboratory tests and at the end confirmatory test is essential.

Important questions that one should address while faced with a bleeding child are

- Is the bleeding significant?
- Is it a local or a systemic cause?
- Is it inherited or acquired in nature?
- Is it due to vascular or platelets or coagulation abnormality.
- Or is it multifactorial?

- **Is the bleeding significant?**

  Bleeding follows trauma but generally stops in 1-3 minutes with pressure. One should suspect a bleeding disorder when bleeding occurs spontaneously, does not stop on pressure, recurs, leads to significant blood loss or there are systemic clues or positive family history.

- **Is it a local or a systemic cause?**

  Bleed due to local cause is from one site and recurs from same site without systemic clues. Some of the common local causes of bleeding are epistaxis due to nose picking, bleeding from little's area, nasal foreign body, vigorous blowing of nose during rhinitis and dry nasal mucosa, lower GI bleed due to polyps, rectal fissure, umbilical bleeding due to slipped ligature, umbilical granuloma, oral bleeding due to poor dental hygiene, tongue bite, etc.

- **Is it inherited or acquired in nature?**

  Inherited bleeding disorders start very early in life (mild hemophilia is an exception) and there is history of bleeding from umbilical cord, huge cephalhematoma, excessive bleeding when primary teeth fall, bleeding after minor surgery like circumcision or joint bleeds, etc. Often there is positive family of similar bleeding. Hemophilia A, B and Wiskott Aldrich syndrome are X-linked recessive disorders with history of bleeding in males on maternal side. Other coagulation factors deficiency are autosomal recessive disorders with history of bleeding in both the sexes, in siblings or cousins and consanguinity in family. Qualitative platelet defects, dysfibrinogenemia are hereditary hemorrhagic telangiectasis are examples of autosomal dominant conditions with history of bleeding in parents and grand parents suggesting vertical transmission.

Acquired disorders start late in life (Vitamin K deficiency associated hemorrhagic disease of newborn is an exception). There would be no evidence of bleeding in the past even with some surgeries and no family history of similar bleeding. There must be some systemic illness like liver, renal disease or history of intake of drugs such as NSAIDs, malabsorption syndromes, SLE, leukemias, bone marrow diseases.

B. Physical Examination

Before proceeding for examination it is important to understand that the term 'purpura' is used to denote leakage of blood in the skin. When the size of this bleed is pinpoint (< 2 mm) it is known as petechiae. When the size is between 3 to 10 mm, it is known as purpura. Ecchymosis are large areas of extravasation of blood in the skin exceeding 10 mm. They may be flat or raised above the surface. It cannot be blanched by pressure with a finger or glass slide.

Signs to be looked for?
• Confirm whether there is true bleeding
• Site of bleeding
• Assess growth
• Look for jaundice and pallor, eczema
• Look for lymphadenopathy and hepatosplenomegaly
• Are the gums bleeding?
• Any skin rash or gangrenous patches
• Does the child look ill?
• Any involvement of joints

Confirm whether there is true bleeding:

Firstly, it is essential to confirm whether there is true bleeding or is it some other lesion resembling bleeding, e.g. drug eruption and erythema nodosum, which appear like ecchymosis. Drug eruptions do not change color over time. Erythema nodosum appear over extensor surfaces and are red and tender. Viral exanthematous illness and mosquito bites may be confused with petechieal rash. The latter does not blanch on pressure.

- **Appearance of the child:**

  If the child looks acutely ill and toxic with massive skin hemorrhages one must consider septicemia or meningococcemia.

- **Site of bleeding:**

  Presence of petechiae and bleeding into the mucous membrane indicate platelet abnormality. Either there is thrombocytopenia or platelet dysfunction. Hematomas in the deep tissues, subcutaneous or intramuscular bleeds and hemarthrosis suggests coagulopathy.

- **Assessment of growth:**

  Short stature with absent radii, pigmentation and purpura would suggest Fanconi's anemia.

- **Look for pallor, jaundice and eczema:**

  Presence of pallor, purpura and mild icterus would suggest hemolytic uremic syndrome, while eczema, purpura and recurrent infections will favor Wiskott-Aldrich syndrome.

- **Lymphadenopathy and hepato-splenomegaly:**

  In a child with purpura one must carefully look for presence of lymphadenopathy and hepato-splenomegaly. In case of leukemia apart from purpura there would be pallor, lymphadenopathy, splenomegaly and bony tenderness. In osteopetrosis there will be pallor purpura and hepatosplenomegaly. Bleeding, deep icterus, hepatosplenomegaly would suggest a liver disease.

- **Are there bleeding gums?**

  Bleeding gums, pseudoparalysis of lower limbs, scorbutic beading and limb pains are features of scurvy.

- **Skin rash:**

  In case of Henoch-Schonlein purpura there is initially urticarial rash occurring in crops particularly over buttocks, arms and legs. Later on the rash becomes hemorrhagic.

- **Involvement of joints:**

  Hemarthrosis is seen in coagulopathies. Joint involvement is also seen in Henoch-Schonlein purpura, leukemias and scurvy.

  Hyperextensibility of joints and skin hyperclasticity is a feature of Ehlers-Danlos syndrome.

Table: Signs and conditions

	Signs	Conditions
1.	Joint bleeding, muscle bleeding, deep seated ecchymosis	Hemophilia, Von Wille-Brand disease
2.	Telangiectasia in oral or nasal mucosa with local bleeding	Hereditary telangiectasia
3.	Pigment disorder with partial albinism	Hermansky Pudlak syndrome
4.	Thrombocytopenia with absent radius	TAR syndrome
5.	Syndactyly	Factor V deficiency
6.	Keloids	Factor XIII deficiency
7.	Recurrent ecchymosis, poor scars, hyperextensible joints and cutis elastica	Ehler Danlos syndrome
8.	Recurrent infections eczema, bleeding	Wiskott Aldrich syndrome
9.	Giant hemangioma bleeding, localized DIC	Kasabach Merritt syndrome

LABORATORY INVESTIGATIONS

In a suspected bleeding disorder the following screening tests must be done. Based on the clinical evaluation and the results of these tests subsequent studies can be considered to confirm the diagnosis.

Screening tests

- Complete blood count (CBC)
- Review of peripheral smear
- Prothrombin time (PT)
- Activated partial thromboplastin time (aPTT)

Complete blood count:

- If epistaxis is associated with severe anemia it points to an underlying bleeding disorder. Microcytic anemia indicates prolonged blood loss.
- Normocytic anemia is seen in case of recent hemorrhage with significant amount of blood loss.
- Thrombocytopenia along with anemia and leukocyte abnormality indicate leukemia, lymphomas, etc.
- Pancytopenia would indicate hypoplastic/aplastic anemia.

● **Peripheral smear:**

- In the peripheral smear one must look for clumping of platelets, platelet morphology and leukocyte morphology, immature cells, burr cells.
- Low platelet count must be confirmed by review of the smear because clumping of platelets can cause falsely low automated count.
- Study of platelet morphology: In case of giant platelet disorders, e.g. Bernard-Soulier or May-Hegglin anomaly majority of platelets will be of size similar to or larger than erythrocyte.
- In immune thrombocytopenic purpura both normal and large platelets are seen.
- Wiskott-Aldrich syndrome: Smaller than normal size of platelets are seen.
- Presence of blast cells in the peripheral smear suggest leukemia.

● **Prothrombin Time and Activated Partial Thromboplastin:**

Time Prothrombin time and activated partial thromboplastin time are screening tests for coagulopathy.

- PT evaluates the intrinsic pathways of the coagulation cascade.
- aPTT evaluates the extrinsic pathways of the coagulation cascade. aPTT is normally ± 10 sec of control. PT is normally ± 3 seconds of control. PT is better interpreted as INR which should be below 1.2. Both these tests are highly sensitive to temperature and hence should be performed as soon as possible after sample collection. If there is going to be a delay in performing the tests, it is better to extract plasma and keep it in fridge till tests are performed. PT alone is prolonged in factor VII deficiency. aPTT alone is prolonged in factor VIII, IX or XI deficiency.

● **Thrombin clotting time (TCT):**

TCT measures thrombin induced conversion of fibrinogen to fibrin. Normal TCT is ±3 seconds over control. Prolonged TCT will suggest either a hypo/dys-fibrinogenemia. Simultaneous estimation of fibrinogen level by chemical methods will help to further differentiate these conditions as prolonged TCT with absent or low fibrinogen levels will suggest a hypo-fibrinogenemia respectively while normal fibrinogen level will suggest dysfibrinogenemia.

● **Coagulation factor assay:**

When a factor deficiency is suggested by mixing studies specific coagulation factor assay is indicated.

● **Thrombin time:**

When it is prolonged it signifies low fibrinogen activity.

- **Platelet aggregation studies:**

  These studies are done in those children where one suspects platelet function disorders such as Bernard-Soulier syndrome or Glanzman thromboasthenia.

- **Bone marrow studies:**

  Bone marrow studies are indicated where one suspects bone marrow suppression such as aplastic anemia or bone marrow infiltration as in leukemia and lymphomas. However, bone marrow examination is contraindicated in coagulopathies.

- **X-rays of long bones:**

  X-rays of long bones are done in cases of scurvy, osteopetrosis and leukemias.

  - Peniciling of cortex, signet ring appearance of epiphysis, rarefaction of bones, subperiosteal hematoma seen in scurvy.
  - Increased bone density, distinction between cortex and medullary cavity is lost (marble-like appearance) is diagnostic of osteopetrosis.

- **Immunoglobulin M Level**

  In suspected Wiskott-Aldrich syndrome, IgM level can be markedly reduced.

SUMMARY

Apart from bleeding occurring in surgical trauma resulting from accident or surgery, there are non-surgical causes of bleeding where bruising and bleeding can occur spontaneously or after a trauma, which is too trivial to explain the extent of bleeding.

Platelets, capillary integrity and normal coagulation process prevent any spontaneous bleeding in normal individuals. Therefore spontaneous bleeding can result from three basic types of abnormalities. First platelet deficiency in number (thrombocytopenia) or in quality (thrombasthenia). Secondly, capillary dysfunction (vascular causes) and thirdly defects of coagulation mechanism. Each of these can be from a hereditaryor acquired cause.

Therefore in a child with bleeding problem, a careful history including family history, past history, detailed clinical examination, important screening tests and then appropriate specialized tests will help in diagnosis and better management.

SUGGESTED READING

1. Nitin Shah: Approach to a bleeding child. Indian Journal of Practical Pediatrics, Vol. 18, 2016.

12   HEPATOMEGALY

INTRODUCTION

Hepatomegaly is frequently observed in clinical practice. Either it is observed alone or in association with splenomegaly.

Hepatomegaly means enlargement of liver resulting from an increase in the number or size of cells and structures within the liver. The total span of the liver is increased. Before labeling a child to have hepatomegaly, one has to ensure that it is not simply a pushed down liver due to pathology in the lung, pleural space or subdiaphragmatic region, in which case the liver may be palpable more than 2 cm below the right costal margin.

Liver is normally palpable upto 3 cm below the right costal margin in the newborn and upto 2 cm throughout childhood. It is normally soft in consistency and has rounded margin.

The normal liver span varies with age. Average span being 5 to 6 cm in a healthy term infant; 6 to 7 cm between 1 to 5 years; 7 to 9 cm between 5 to 10 years and 10 to 12 cm between 10 to 16 years of age.

ETIOLOGY

Hepatomegaly can represent intrinsic liver disease or may be the presenting physical finding of a generalized disorder. Early diagnosis and treatment of children who have liver disease is important because specific treatments are available for some diseases that can prevent progression or hepatic failure.

Table: Causes of hepatomegaly

1. Infections:
   a. Viral-hepatitis, mumps, measles, rubella, acquired immunodeficiency syndrome (AIDS)
   b. Bacterial-typhoid, tuberculosis, brucellosis
   c. Protozoal-malaria, toxoplasmosis, amoebiasis, kala-azar
   d. Fungal-histoplasmosis
   e. Intrauterine infections-toxoplasmosis, rubella, cytomegalovirus and herpes (TORCH) infections.

2. Hematological conditions:
   Anemias-thalassemia, sickle cell disease, congenital spherocytosis, iron deficiency anemia

3. Neoplasms:
   Leukemias, lymphomas, hepatoma, hepatoblastoma, Wilm's tumor, neuroblastoma

4. Passive congestion of liver:
   Congestive cardiac failure, Constrictive pericarditis, Budd-chiari syndrome.

5. Chronic liver disease:
   Cirrhosis, chronic hepatitis.

6. Collagen diseases:
   Systemic lupus erythematosus, juvenile idiopathic arthritis, polyarteritisnodosa.

7. Neoplasms:
   Hepatoma, hepatoblastoma, metastatic liver disease.

8. Space occupying lesions:
    Hydatid cyst, liver abscess, hemangioma.
9. Metabolic diseases:
    Wilson disease, galactosemia, cystic fibrosis, alpha-1-antitrypsin deficiency, mucopolysaccharidosis, glycogen storage disease and lipidosis.
10. Miscellaneous:
    Congenital hepatic fibrosis, osteopetrosis, Reye syndrome.

EVALUATION

While recording the history the following questions should be specifically asked.

A. History

> **Point in history**
>
> - Is there any history of recent infection? e.g. rash, pharyngitis, cough, fever, poor feeding
> - Has the child consumed any contaminated food suffered from diarrhea and/or vomiting
> - Any history of loss of consciousness or seizures?
> - Any preexisting liver diseases, lung diseases, or congenital heart disease
> - Any complications during pregnancy and perinatal period. Any growth and developmental delay
> - Maternal history of hepatitis B, C, CMV, EBV or HIV
> - Family history of cystic fibrosis, alpha-1-antitrypsin deficiency, storage diseases, heart diseases, autoimmune diseases
> - Change in stool color
> - History of drug or toxin ingestion
> - Is the child receiving any medications
> - History of recent travel

Age at Presentation

In the neonatal period and first 3 months of life the common causes of hepatomegaly are neonatal hepatitis, congenital biliary atresia, intrauterine infections, galactosemia and erythroblastosisfetalis, also conditions such as alpha-1-antitrypsin deficiency and gangliosidosis can present from birth to 3 months of age with hepatosplenomegaly. In later infancy and childhood infections are a common cause. Wilson disease does not generally manifest until after 5 years of age. Hepatomegaly due to chronic liver disease and portal hypertension are seen in older children.

Onset of Illness

One must enquire whether the illness is of an acute onset, which would indicate an acute infection, while a gradual onset would suggest a chronic illness. Sometimes viral hepatitis may be fulminant in onset.

Fever

Does the child have fever? Is the fever high grade? Is it associated with chills and rigors.

Fever would be an important symptom in cases of hepatitis, malaria and other infections. High grade continuous fever with tender hepatomegaly would suggest a liver abscess.

Fever is also present in collagen diseases.

Jaundice

Does the child have jaundice? Did he have jaundice in the past? Does he get recurrent jaundice?

Presence of jaundice is a symptom of liver disease. Recurrent jaundice is seen in congenital spherocytosis, sickle cell disease. Jaundice is also seen in cases of galactosemia.

Color of Stool and Urine

What is the color of urine and stools?

Passage of dark colored stools and urine would suggest a liver disease. Acholic stools is a feature of cholestasis.

Family History

Family history of liver disease would be present in hereditary conditions such as Wilson disease and storage disorders. A family history of anemia and hepatomegaly would be obtained in cases of thalassemia. H/O consanguinity would be present in thalassemia, SCA and metabolic diseases.

History of Injections

Did the child in the past receive any injections, blood transfusion, or vaccines? Such a history may be obtained in cases of serum hepatitis.

Gastrointestinal Hemorrhage

Did the child have hematemesis or melena? Gastrointestinal bleeding could be due to rupture of esophageal varices in case of portal hypertension or due to hypopro-thrombinemia in cases of advanced liver disease.

Vomiting

Does the child vomit?

Vomiting from neonatal period with failure to thrive is a feature of galactosemia. Acute onset of vomiting, altered sensorium and hepatomegaly are features of Reye syndrome.

Convulsions

Does the child get seizures?

Recurrent convulsions do occur in cases of galactosemia and glycogen storage disease.

Joint Involvement

Any history of joint pain or swelling would indicate a collagen disease.

History of Infection During Pregnancy A history of TORCH group of infections in the mother during pregnancy should be enquired. Intrauterine infections could present with hepatomegaly.

History of Death in Siblings

It is important to enquire whether there have been deaths in previous siblings and at what age. Death in the neonatal period could be due to erythroblastosis, while in later infancy could be due to biliary atresia or neonatal hepatitis or metabolic disease.

History of blood transfusion

History of frequent blood transfusion would be present in thalassemia major. History of exchange blood transfusion in neonatal period would be present in G6PD deficiency and hereditary spherocytosis.

Pain in Abdomen

If the child complaints of pain in abdomen, the cause of hepatomegaly could be hepatitis, congestive hepatomegaly or liver abscess. If a child has massive hepatomegaly with no other symptoms, the likely cause is a storage disorder.

History of cough and dyspnea

Chest pain and dyspnea are signs of cardiac decompensation and indicate presence of congestive cardiac failure.

B. Physical Examination

After recording a detail history one must do a thorough general and systemic examination. Efforts should be made to especially look for the following.

Points on Examination

- Facies
- Anthropometry
- Eyes
- Jaundice/pallor
- Vital signs
- Lymphadenopathy
- Edema
- Spider nevi
- Palmar erythema
- Xanthomas
- Focus of infection
- Skeletal system
- Skin ulceration
- Systemic examination

Facies

Hemolytic facies associated with hepatomegaly and anemia would suggest hemoglobinopathy especially thalassemia. Doll-like face is typical of glycogen storage disorders.

Coarse facies is seen in cases of mucopolysaccharidosis. Butterfly rash over the face suggests lupus.

Anthropometry

Anthropometry is important to assess the growth of a child presenting with hepatomegaly.

In case of galactosemia there would be failure to thrive. Stunting is seen in cases of glycogen storage disorder and lysosomal storage disorder. Intrauterine growth retardation is also seen in cases of intrauterine infections.

Microcephaly is often associated with intrauterine infections.

Head

Microcephaly is common in CMV infection and congenital rubella syndrome while hydrocephalus is seen in toxoplasmosis.

Eyes

A lot of information can be gathered from examination of the eyes. Congenital anomalies such as microphthalmia, cataract are seen in congenital rubella syndrome. Kayser-Fleischer ring (KF ring) is diagnostic of Wilson disease. Corneal clouding is seen in Hurler syndrome. Presence of jaundice would suggest liver disease, while pallor would indicate anemia. Cherry red spot would be present in Gaucher and Niemann-Pick disease.

Vital Signs

Vital signs is important to record the pulse, blood pressure and respiration. Presence of dyspnea with tender hepatomegaly is a feature of congestive cardiac failure.

Neck

Engorged neck veins and raised jugular venous pulse is seen in constrictive pericarditis and CCF.

Lymphadenopathy

Significant lymphadenopathy associated with hepatomegaly is seen in leukemias, lymphomas and disseminated tuberculosis. Generalized lymphadenopathy can also be seen in cases of intrauterine infections and systemic lupus erythematosus.

Skin Ulcerations

If in early infancy a child has snuffles, rhagades, ulcerations and fissures in the mouth and anus along with hepatosplenomegaly and pseudoparalysis the cause is congenital syphilis.

Edema

Presence of pitting edema would indicate liver cell failure. It is also a feature of congestive cardiac failure.

Spider Nevi and Palmar Erythema

Presence of spider nevi and palmar erythema suggests chronic liver disease. Spider naevi are prominent over face and chest. Palmar erythema is also a feature of chronic liver disease. It is a blotchy erythema most noticeable over the thorax and hypothenar eminences and tips of fingers.

Focus of Infection

In suspected cases of liver abscess one must look for focus of infection elsewhere such as pyoderma, osteomyelitis, etc.

Skeletal System

Joints including the spine must be examined.

Swelling and tenderness of joints is present in systemic lupus erythematosus.

Gibus is often present in cases of mucopolysaccharidosis.

Systemic Examination

One must carefully examine the abdomen. Measure the span of the liver to decide about hepatomegaly. Feel for the consistency of liver and whether it is tender.

Soft tender hepatomegaly is seen in cases of inflammatory disease. It is also seen in congestive cardiac failure. Firm hepatomegaly indicates chronic liver disease, infiltrative disease or neoplasia. In case of liver abscess not only is there a tender hepatomegaly, but there is also intercostal tenderness.

Table: Consistency of liver

Soft	CCF, Acute infective hepatitis, fatty liver, other infections
Firm	Chronic active hepatitis, cirrhosis, chronic malaria, kala-azar, metabolic conditions, neonatal hepatitis, lymphoma
Hard	Congenital hepatic fibrosis, macronodular cirrhosis, CML, hepatoma, hepatoblastoma
Cystic	Hemangioma
Pleomorphic	Abscess

Next one must feel for enlargement of spleen. In several conditions, hepatomegaly is associated with splenomegaly such as in typhoid fever, malaria, miliary tuberculosis, thalassemia, storage disorders, cirrhosis of liver leading to portal hypertension, leukemias, intrauterine infections (TORCH) and osteopetrosis.

Examine the abdomen for the presence of fluid. Ascitis is seen in chronic liver disease, portal hypertension and tuberculosis. In cases of constrictive pericarditis the child will have ascitis with tender hepatomegaly and distended jugular venous pressure (JVP).

In the cardiovascular system look for raised JVP, cardiomegaly, presence of murmur and gallop rhythm. Raised JVP with cardiomegaly would suggest cardiac failure. In suspected rubella syndrome, look carefully for patent ductusarteriosus (PDA) and pulmonary stenosis.

Generalized hypotonia and loss of developmental milestones with hepatomegaly is a feature of lysosomal storage disorder. Presence of tremors and choreform movements is seen in Wilson disease.

The fundus must be examined. Cherry red spot in the macula suggests Niemann-Pick disease and gangliosidosis.

Clues from physical examination

Skin: Petechiae and purpura (malignancy), pruritus / jaundice (liver disease and rashes (infection))

Eyes: Icterus, cherry red spots or cloudy cornea (lipid storage disease). Kayser-Fleischer ring (Wilson's disease)

CNS: Decreased level of consciousness, seizures (hypoglycemia due to storage disease)

CVS/Respiratory: Murmur, abnormal heart sounds (S3S4) (congenital heart disease) abnormal breath sounds (alpha-1 antitrypsin deficiency)

GI: Tenderness, distension, ascitis, hepatomegaly (liver disease, gall stones), splenomegaly (hemolytic anemia)

MSK: Joint tenderness (hepatitis), bone pain (malignancy)

C. Investigations

Hepatomegaly may be a transient finding during systemic viral illness, which may need just a few routine investigations, but persistent hepatomegaly is an indication for further evaluation.

Which investigations to be done?
- Complete blood count
- Liver function test
- Viral markers
- Ultrasonography of abdomen
- Hemoglobin electrophoresis
- Blood sugar levels
- Serum ceruloplasmin levels
- X-ray chest
- Bone marrow examination
- Liver biopsy
- Antinuclear antibody (ANA) estimation
- X-ray long bones

Table: Probable cause based on investigations

	Investigations	Probable Cause
1.	Complete blood count	
	• Leucocytosis	Infection, inflammation, leukemia
	• Normoblasts and increased retic count	Hemolytic anemia
	• Malarial parasite	Malaria
2.	Liver function tests	
	• Serum bilirubin raised	Liver disease
	• Elevated transaminases (SGOT, SGPT)	Hepatocellular injury from inflammation
	• Low serum albumin	Deteriorating hepatic function
	• Prothrombin time prolonged	Reye's syndrome, deteriorating hepatic function
3.	Australia antigen positive	Hepatitis B
	• Viral markers for A, E & B	Hepatitis
4.	Ultrasonography of abdomen	Organomegaly, abscess, cyst
5.	Haemoglobin electrophoresis	Haemoglobinopathies
6.	Blood sugar levels	
	• Hypoglycemia	Galactosemia, glycogen, storage disorder, Reye's syndrome

7. Serum ceruloplasmin levels low	Wilson's disease
8. X-ray chestMiliary shadows	Miliary tuberculosis
9. Bone marrow examination • Immature cells • Typical cells	LeukemiaLipidosis
10. Liver biopsy useful in	Chronic liver disease, Wilson's disease
11. ANA estimation – positive	Systemic lupus erythematosus
12. X-ray long bones – typical findings	Osteopetrosis, mucopolysaccharides

Complete Blood Count

Total leukocyte count would be raised in cases of infection and inflammation and also in leukemias. Peripheral smear examination would be helpful in cases of malaria and also in hemolytic anemia. In case of malaria the parasite may be found and in hemolytic anemia, there would be normoblasts in the peripheral smear with increased reticulocyte count.

Liver Function Tests

a. **Serum bilirubin:** Rise in serum bilirubin would indicate liver disease.

b. **Serum glutamic oxaloacetic transaminase (SGOT)/serum glutamic pyruvic transaminase (SGPT):** Elevated transaminases is most commonly caused by hepatocellular injury from inflammation.

c. **Serum albumin and prothrombin time:** Low serum albumin levels and increased prothrombin time indicates deteriorating hepatic function. In Reye syndrome prothrombin time is prolonged.

Australia Antigen and Viral Markers for Hepatitis

These are indicated where the cause of hepatomegaly is viralhepatitis.

Ultrasonography of the Abdomen

Ultrasonography of the abdomen would help in confirming organomegaly. It is very useful in cases of liver abscess, cysts, tumors, liver metastasis and portal hypertension.

Hemoglobin Electrophoresis

Hemoglobin electrophoresis is indicated where the cause of hepatomegaly clinically appears to be thalassemia.

Blood Sugar Levels

Blood sugar levels suspected cases of galactosemia and glycogen storage disorder it must be done. Hypoglycemia is observed in these conditions. In Reye syndrome blood and CSF sugars are consistently low, while SGOT, SGPT and lactate dehydrogenase (LDH) are significantly raised.

Serum Ceruloplasmin Levels

Estimation of serum ceruloplasmin level is indicated in suspected cases of Wilson disease, in which the levels are low.

X-ray Chest

Skiagram of the chest is done for evidence of tuberculosis. It is especially useful in miliary tuberculosis, which can present as hepatosplenomegaly. It is also helpful for detection of cardiomegaly.

Bone Marrow Aspiration

Indicated in cases of leukemia, Gaucher and Niemann-Pick disease. In leukemias the marrow would be packed with immature cells. In case of lipidosis typical cells will be present.

Liver Biopsy

Liver biopsy should be done in cases of chronic liver disease. In case of glycogen storage disease type-1 liver cells will show increased fat and glycogen and absence of glucose-6-phosphate enzyme. Liver biopsy is also useful in Wilson disease.

Electrocardiography and Echocardiography

If the liver is enlarged and tender and the cause appears to be congestive cardiac failure then an electrocardiography (ECG) and echocardiography is helpful in arriving at a diagnosis.

Antinuclear Antibody Estimation

Antinuclear antibody estimation is done in suspected cases of systemic lupus erythematosis, in which it is positive.

X-ray Long Bones

In a child having hepatosplenomegaly with anemia suspected clinically to be suffering from osteopetrosis. X-ray long bones would reveal marble bone appearance, which is diagnostic. In case of mucopolysaccharidosis also skeletal X-rays are diagnostic.

CT scan abdomen

Liver masses detected on ultrasonography may be defined further by CT scan. Hepatic angiography is indicated in the evaluation of suspected vascular tumors.

SUMMARY

Hepatomegaly is a sign that can be caused by a variety of conditions that affect different organ systems. When evaluating a child with hepatomegaly it is very important to identify conditions in which immediate intervention is needed and provide appropriate treatment options. The liver is normally palpable in children. Total liver span varies with age. Liver is considered pathological, if the size is more than normal for the age of the child or it is tender or the consistency is firm. Common causes for hepatomegaly in routine practice are infections. If a child presents with massive hepatomegaly, which is firm in consistency one must consider storage disorder. Investigations should be planned based on clinical diagnosis.

HEPATOMEGALY

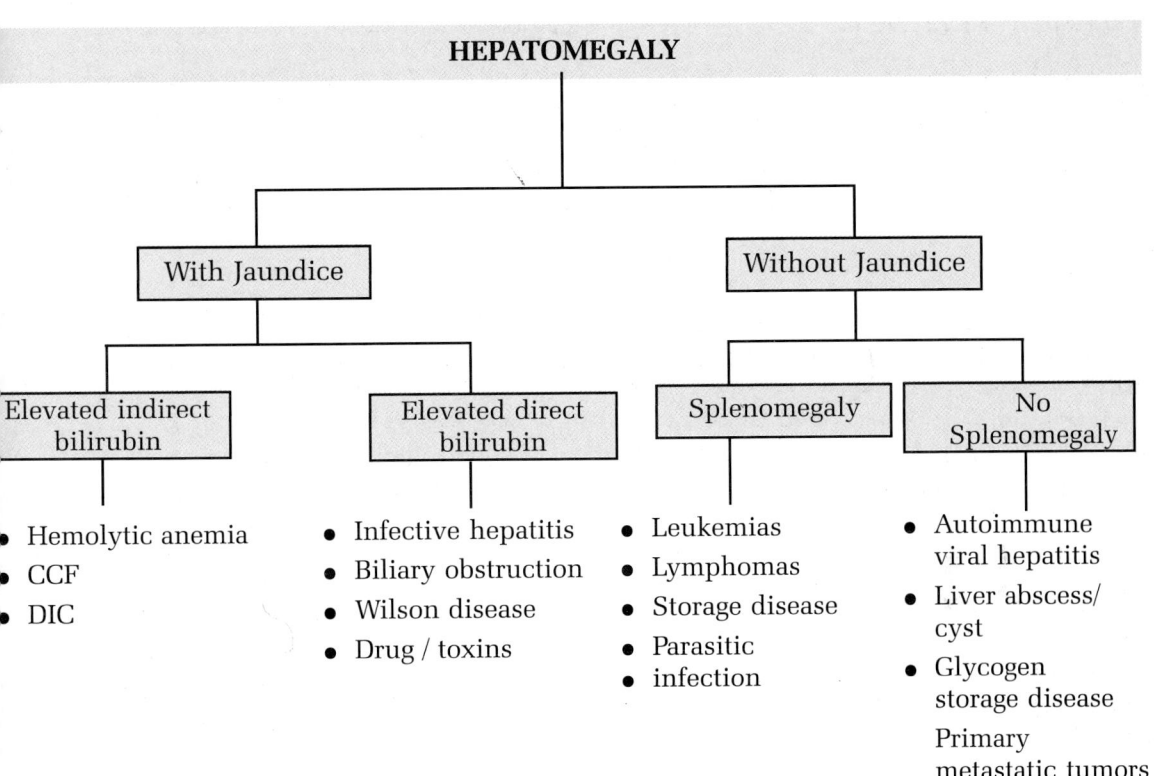

With Jaundice

- **Elevated indirect bilirubin**
  - Hemolytic anemia
  - CCF
  - DIC

- **Elevated direct bilirubin**
  - Infective hepatitis
  - Biliary obstruction
  - Wilson disease
  - Drug / toxins

Without Jaundice

- **Splenomegaly**
  - Leukemias
  - Lymphomas
  - Storage disease
  - Parasitic
  - infection

- **No Splenomegaly**
  - Autoimmune viral hepatitis
  - Liver abscess/ cyst
  - Glycogen storage disease
  - Primary metastatic tumors

SPLENOMEGALY

INTRODUCTION

Splenomegaly in childhood is generally first detected upon physical examination. One third of newborns and 10 percent of children may normally have a palpable spleen. The tip of the normal, palpable spleen is soft, smooth, non-tender and less than 1 to 2 cm below the left costal margin. A pathologically enlarged spleen is often firm, may have an abnormal surface and is frequently associated with signs and symptoms of the underlying disease.

In infants, spleen enlarges vertically downward while in children, it enlarges diagonally downward. By the time spleen becomes palpable, it has already enlarged by 2 to 3 times its normal size.

ETIOLOGY

Table: Causes of splenomegaly

1. **Infections:** Malaria, enteric fever, tuberculosis, septicemia, infective endocarditis, kala-azar, infectious mononucleosis, intrauterine infections, acquired immunodeficiency syndrome (AIDS), Brucellosis.

2. **Anemias:** Thalassemia, sickle cell anemia, spherocytosis. Iron deficiency anemia.

3. **Congestive splenomegaly:** Portal vein thrombosis, cirrhosis of liver, neonatal hepatitis, extrahepatic biliary atresia, non-cirrhotic portal hypertension, congestive cardiac failure.

4. **Collagen vascular disease:** Juvenile idiopathic arthritis, systemic lupus erythematosis.

5. **Neoplasia:** Leukemia, lymphomas.

6. **Storage disorders:** Gaucher, Niemann Pick disease, mucopolysaccharidosis.

7. **Miscellaneous:** Histiocytosis, immune thrombocytopenic purpura, congenital splenic cyst, hydatid cyst, osteopetrosis, myelofibrosis.

EVALUATION

When assessing a child with splenomegaly, the major splenic functions should be kept in mind: its hematopoietic phagocytic and immunologic roles and its role as a reservoir for blood borne elements. The spleen is a major hematopoietic organ during fetal life. However, it is capable of resuming extramedullary hematopoiesis in children and adults with bone marrow failure. The spleen removes the senescent and abnormal RBCs, as well as the particulate material from the blood. It is a major lymphoreticular organ that acts as a filter for infectious organisms and also acts as a site of immunoglobulin M and properdin production. Finally it acts as a reservoir for platelets, reticulocytes and plasma proteins, especially factor VIII. Because the spleen has so many functions, splenomegaly may be caused by a wide variety of disorders.

The cause of splenomegaly can often be ascertained by history and physical

...xamination combined with relatively inexpensive and readily available laboratory tests.

HISTORY

Points in history

- Age of the child
- Onset of illness - acute or chronic
- Caste of the patient
- Any history of fever and night sweats
- Has the child lost weight?
- Is there a history of abdominal trauma?
- Any history of illness in the neonatal period
- History of jaundice
- History of having received a blood transfusion
- Family history of anemia
- Has anybody in the family undergone cholecystectomy or splenectomy?
- History of heart disease
- History of past surgeries
- History of hematemesis and melena.

Age of the Child

Etiology of splenomegaly varies with age. In the newborn the commonest cause could be intrauterine infections, congenital malaria, hemolytic disease of the newborn.

In infancy neonatal hepatitis, extrahepatic biliary atresia are common causes of splenomegaly.

Splenic sequestration in sickle cell disease occurs early in life usually below the age of 6 years, before splenic involution that ultimately occurs in most patients with sickle cell disease.

Onset of Illness

Was the onset of illness acute or did the symptoms appeared over a period of time?

Acute splenomegaly occurs due to sequestration crisis in cases of sickle cell disease. Apart from splenomegaly the child appears pale, is in shock and has acute pain in abdomen.

Chronic liver disease, extrahepatic portal hypertension, storage disorders have a gradual onset.

Caste of Patient

Hemoglobinopathies are common in various ethnic groups. Thalassemia is prevalent amongst Gujaratis, Punjabis and Sindhis, while sickle cell is common in certain tribes of Central India.

History of Fever

Does the child get fever? If yes since how long? Is it high grade with chills and rigors?

Fever with splenomegaly indicates infection.

Prolonged fever is also observed in cases of malignancies and collagen vascular disease.

Fever with night sweats is a feature of Hodgkin disease.

Fever with chills and rigors is common in malaria and viral infections.

History of Weight Loss

If the child is losing weight over the past several months, it points towards a chronic infection such as tuberculosis or malignancies.

History of Abdominal Trauma

Enquire whether the child in the past sustained an abdominal injury. Trauma can lead to subcapsular hematoma, which may eventually develop into a pseudocyst in the spleen.

History of Illness in the Neonatal Period A detail history of illness in the neonatal period should be enquired. Did the child suffer from sepsis or shock? Any history of omphalitis? Was the umbilical cord catheterized? All these would lead to portal vein thrombosis and subsequently portal hypertension.

History of Jaundice and Anemia

A past history of hyperbilirubinemia and anemia would suggest spherocytosis as the cause of splenomegaly.

History of Receiving Blood Transfusion

Is the child receiving repeated blood transfusions? In such a situation the cause of splenomegaly could be hemoglobinopathy. Blood transfusion can also lead to hepatitis B.

Family History

Has any member in the family suffered from a similar illness? Has any family member undergone cholecystectomy or splenectomy?

Family history of similar illness could point towards a hereditary condition such as hemoglobinopathies, spherocytosis or storage disorder and if any family member has undergone cholecystecomy or splenectomy it would indicate hereditary hemolytic anemia.

Hematemesis or Melena

History of hematemsis or melena associated with splenomegaly would indicate portal hypertension or liver disease.

History of Heart Disease

One must enquire whether the child gets palpitation, dyspnea or in an infant history of feeding difficulty, excessive sweating. All these symptoms would indicate cardiac failure leading to congestive splenomegal If a known case of heart disease develop fever and pallor and the spleen is palpab the cause is bacterial endocarditis.

History of Abdominal Surgery

Any history of abdominal surgery should b enquired as it could lead to infectio thrombosis and portal hypertension.

Loss of Developmental Milestones

In a child with splenomegaly if there is history of regression of milestones one mu consider storage disorders.

B. Physical Examination

Physical examination will determine wheth the splenomegaly is isolated or part of generalized hyperplasia of lymphoid an reticuloendothelial tissues.

Points on examination
- General appearance
- Pallor
- Petechiae, purpura
- Jaundice
- Pruritus
- Rashes
- Eyes
- Lymphadenopathy
- Clubbing
- Joints
- Bony tenderness
- Systemic examination

General Appearance

If the child appears ill and there is failure to thrive, one must consider chronic infections like tuberculosis, chronic hemolysis, metabolic disease, malignancy or collagen vascular disease. Coarse facies is a feature of mucopolysaccharidosis.

Pallor

Presence of pallor would suggest hemolysis, marrow infiltration, hypersplenism, bacterial endocarditis.

Petechiae/Purpura

One should carefully look for the presence of petechial and purpuric spots, which would indicate thrombocytopenia. Presence of thrombocytopenia with splenomegaly will suggest hypersplenism, autoimmune disorder or leukemia.

Jaundice

Presence of jaundice will point towards hemolytic anemia and liver disease.

Pruritus

Itching is seen in cases of liver dysfunction and sometimes in Hodgkin lymphoma.

Rashes

Malar rash is pathognomonic of systemic lupus erythematosus (SLE). It involves the cheek, bridge of nose and lower eyelids, but spares the nasiolabial folds.

Evanescent maculopapular rash with central clearing prominent on the trunk is seen in juvenile idiopathic arthritis.

Eczematous rash is seen in Langerhan cell histiocytosis and immunodeficiency syndrome.

Eyes

Cloudy cornea is seen in mucopoly-saccharidosis,microphthalmia, cataract and microcornea would suggest congenital rubella. Presence of uveitis and iritis is seen in rheumatoid arthritis.

Lymphadenopathy

Presence of lymphadenopathy with splenomegaly would be seen in disseminated tuberculosis, infectious mononucleosis, histiocytosis and collagen disease.

Clubbing

Presence of clubbing is seen in bacterial endocarditis and biliary cirrhosis.

Joints

Joint involvement both pain and swelling would suggest systemic lupus erythematosus, idiopathic arthritis or autoimmune disease.

Bony Tenderness

Bony tenderness is a feature of leukemia.

Systemic Examination

Splenomegaly is also graded according to the size of spleen palpable below the left costal margin.

Grading	Palpable below left costal margin
Mild	< 3 cms
Moderate	4 to 7 cms
Massive	> 7 cms

Distension of abdomen with prominent veins and ascitis would suggest liver disease.

Enlarged firm liver in addition to splenomegaly would point towards cirrhosis of liver and also storage disorders. Abdominal tenderness could be elicited in gallstones and hepatitis.

Presence of dyspnea would indicate congestive cardiac failure due to anemia or heart disease.

Infective endocarditis should be considered in the presence of murmur.

Examination of the Nervous System

Loss of developmental milestones would suggest storage disease, chronic infection or immunodeficiency disorder.

Poor vision would suggest osteopetrosis.

The fundus should be carefully examined for cherry red spots, which are present in lipid storage disorders.

Splenomegaly is usually due to systemic disease and not the result of primary splenic disease. Therefore, diagnostic studies are not directed at the spleen itself. Instead, they are orientedat diagnosing disease states that result in splenomegaly. Themostusefulinitial laboratory tests include the complete blood count (CBC) with differential peripheral blood smears and liver function tests.

Table: Which investigations to be done ?

Sr. No.	Investigations	Probable Cause
1.	Complete blood count	
	• Pancytopenia	Hypersplenism, bone marrow infiltration Infection, leukemia
	• Increased WBC count	Leukemias
	• Immature WBCs	Hemolytic anemia
	• Normoblasts	Infectious mononucleosis
	• Atypical lymphocytes	Malaria
	• Peripheral smear for malarial parasite	Hemolytic anemia
	• Reticulocytosis	
2.	Liver function tests	
	• Hypoalbuminemia	Liver disease
	• Prolonged prothrombin time	
	• Indirect and direct hyperbilirubinemia	
	• Isolated indirect hyperbilirubinemia	Hemolysis
	• Raised alkaline phosphatase	Biliary obstruction
3.	ANA titre estimation – elevated	Systemic lupus erythematosus
4.	Specific antibody titre – raised	Infectious mononucleosis, CMV, HIV, toxoplasma
5.	Bone marrow examination diagnosis in	Leukemias, storage disorders, lymphomas
6.	USG abdomen in	Splenic cyst, portal hypertension
7.	Splenic biopsy in	Storage disorders, histiocytosis

Complete Blood Count

Presence of pancytopenia is seen in hypersplenism and bone marrow infiltration. Increased white blood cell (WBC) count is seen in infection and leukemia. Immature WBCs in leukemias and normoblasts in hemolytic anemia. Atypical lymphocytes in infectious mononucleosis. Peripheral smear could also reveal the presence of malarial parasite. Hemoglobin concentration and red blood cell (RBC) smear may reveal anemia. Reticulocytosis is seen in hemolytic anemia. Platelet count-presence of thrombocytopenia could be due to decreased production suggesting bone marrow infiltration, increased destruction as in case of viral infection or hypersplenism.

Liver Function Tests

Hypoalbuminemia prolonged prothrombin time, indirect and direct hyperbilirubinemia indicate liver dysfunction.

Isolated indirect hyperbilirubinemia indicates hemolysis.

Elevated SGOT and SGPT indicates liver damage seen in cases of hepatitis.

Raised alkaline phosphatase suggests biliary obstruction.

Antinuclear Antibody Titer Estimation

In suspected case of SLE it is indicated. Positive ANA isdiagnostic of SLE.

Specific Antibody Titer

Specific antibody titer in infectious mononucleosis, cytomegalovirus (CMV), toxoplasma and human immunodeficiency virus (HIV).

Blood Culture

Blood culture in suspected septicemia.

Bone Marrow

Examination is indicated in suspected cases of leukemia, lymphoma and storage diseases.

Ultrasonography

Ultrasonography abdomen will help in confirming splenomegaly.

It will also help in cases of splenic cyst.

In cases of portal hypertension, doppler USG will demonstrate collateral blood vessels and reversal of portal vein blood flow.

Histology

Splenic biopsy is rarely indicated.

Some of the conditions where it is done is in cases of Gaucher disease, Niemann-Pick disease, glycogen storage disease and histiocytosis.

Imaging studies

Computed tomographic scanning is used to evaluate splenic trauma and focal splenic pathology. MRI of the spleen can further clarify abnormalities in size and shape and can define parenchymal disease. Technetium 99m sulfur colloid scan is used to assess splenic function.

SUMMARY

Spleen is normally palpable in a sizeable number of neonates and children. Infections are the commonest cause of splenomegaly and need routine investigations. Massive splenomegaly can be due to thalassemia major, portal hypertension and storage disorder. The diagnosis in such cases is based on relevant investigations.

14

EDEMA

INTRODUCTION

Children with edema are often brought by parents with the complaints of swelling over body or puffiness of face.

DEFINITION

The term 'edema' refers to the accumulation of abnormal and excessive amount of fluid in the intercellular tissue spaces, or body cavities. It may be generalized or localized. The term 'anasarca' denotes edema, which is severe and generalized producing marked swelling of the subcutaneous tissue. More localized interstitial fluid collections include ascites and pleural effusions.

Edema may be pitting or non-pitting depending upon whether a pit can be produced over the part after sustained pressure is applied to skin over a bony surface such as the shin or ankle. Non-pitting edema is indicated by no pit formation after sustained pressure over the skin. Obstruction of lymphatic flow in the lymphatic channels causes non-pitting edema as in hypothyroidism and filariasis.

Inflammatory swellings like that of an abscess, cellulitis, arthritis, etc. are not included under edema.

ETIOLOGY

Generalized edema is typically chronic and progressive. It may result from cardiac, renal, endocrine or hepatic disorders as well as from severe burns, malnutrition or the effects of certain drugs and treatment.

Common factors responsible for edema are hypoalbuminemia and excess sodium ingestion or retention, both of which influence plasma osmotic pressure.

Table: Causes in children and neonates

Generalized:

- Pitting:Cardiac - congestive cardiac failure, constrictive pericarditisRenal - nephritis, nephrotic syndromeNutrition - protein energy malnutrition, beri-beri, anemia, protein loosing enteropathy, severe burnsLiver - cirrhosis liver with portal hypertension.
- Non-pitting:Hypothyroidism.

Localized:

- PittingVeno-caval obstruction—superior venocaval obstruction results in edema of upper part of body; inferior vena caval obstruction causes edema of lower part of the bodyVenous thrombosis—insect bite.
- Non-pitting : Angioneurotic edema Filariasis Milroy's disease

Table: Causes in neonates

Generalized : Prematurity, hydropsfetalis and cardiac failure.

Localized : Edema of presenting part, Turner syndrome, Milroy's disease.

EVALUATION

Both history and clinical examination are important in evaluating a child with edema.

A. History

The following points should be specially noted, while eliciting the history in a child with edema.

Points in history

- Where did the swelling first appear?
- Any diurnal variation in the edema?
- History of preceding sore throat or boils?
- History of hematuria
- Any alteration in the amount of urine passed?
- Past history of jaundice?
- Symptoms of cardiac failure?
- Detailed nutritional history?
- Gestational age in case of newborn?

Where did the swelling first appear?

Did it appear over the face especially eyelids or on the dependent parts?

In case of renal disease, edema first appears over the eyelids, while in cardiac failure swelling first appears over the dependent parts. Does it come and go?

Any diurnal variation in the edema?

In case of renal disease puffiness of the face is there in the morning and as the day progresses the swelling becomes less.

Any history of hematuria?

Presence of hematuria would suggest nephritis.

Is the child passing adequate urine?

History of oliguria or anuria would point towards renal failure.

History of sore throat or boils:

Has the child suffered from sore throat or boils in the recent past? Presence of such a history would point towards acute post streptococcal glomerulonephritis.

History of jaundice:

If there is jaundice in a child with edema the cause could be hepatic illness with portal hypertension.

Symptoms of cardiac failure:

Is the child having breathlessness and palpitation? Such a history would suggest cardiac failure. In an infant ask whether there is feeding difficulty? Does the child have excessive sweating? Is there failure to thrive? In an infant feeding difficulty, excessive sweating and failure to thrive are features of cardiac failure.

Dietary history:

A detailed nutritional history should be taken in terms of total calories consumed and protein intake.

In protein energy malnutrition, the dietary recall will suggest low protein and calories intake.

Edema that appears after ingestion of a particular food or drug would suggest angioedema.

Is the edema recurrent?

Recurrent edema localized to an area such as lips, eyelids, scalp, etc. is seen in case of angioedema. If the edema is localized and congenital it would suggest Turner's syndrome or Milroy's disease. History of itching is a feature of allergic edema.

History of diarrhea:

Does the child get recurrent diarrhea? Recurrent or persistent diarrhea would suggest protein losing enteropathy or gluten sensitivity.

Gestational age:

In case of newborn with generalized edema enquire about the gestational age of the neonate. Is there any Rh incompatibility? Prematurity and hydropsfetalis will give rise to generalized edema.

Table: Symptoms and their significance

Symptoms	Significance
Mode of onset	Sudden (<72 hours), acute nephritis, allergic reactions
Site and evolution	Legs - face - ascitis → cardiac cause Face - legs - ascitis→ Renal Acute edema of face and neck, SVC obstruction
Timing	Increase in morning → Hypoproteinemia Increase in evening → Congestive cardiac failure
Exposure	Medications, food preservatives Danders → allergic reaction
Nutritional history	Low protein intake → PEM
Past history	Sore throat and joint pain → Rheumatic carditis Umbilical vein sepsis or umbilical vein catheterization → hepatic cause Chronic illness, persistent diarrhea → PEM, milk allergy, gluten sensitivity, protein losing enteropathy

Associated symptoms	Significance
Orthopnea, noisy breathing, poor weight gain, feeding difficulties, bluish episodes	Cardiac cause
Yellowish discoloration, dark urine, black tarry stool, itching, petechiae	Hepatic cause
Rash, joint pains	Connective tissue disorders
Nausea, vomiting, retarded growth	Uremia
Massive generalized edema	Nephrotic syndrome
Blood in urine and decreased urine	Acute nephritis
Anorexia, lethargy, diarrhea, vomiting, decreased growth and frequent infections	Malnutrition
Cow's milk intake, diarrhea,abdominal pain	Protein losing enteropathy

B. Clinical Examination

Points on examination

- Assessment of growth
- Extent of edema
- Record vital signs
- Signs of vitamin and mineral deficiency
- Look for icterus
- Examination of skin and hair
- Stigmata of Turner syndrome
- Systemic examination

Assessment of growth:

The child's growth should be assessed using various anthropometric measurements. Growth failure is a feature of protein energy malnutrition. It would also be seen in protein losing enteropathy and cardiac failure. If anthropometry reveals short stature in a female child with localized edema over dorsum of feet and hands, one must consider Turner syndrome.

Extent of edema:

Look whether edema is generalized, localized, massive or just puffiness of eyelids. Is it over the dependent parts, i.e. legs. In an infant or a child confined to bed, look whether there is pitting edema over the sacrum. Ensure whether the edema is pitting or non-pitting.

Generalized massive edema is a feature of nephrotic syndrome and Kwashiokor. Edema over dependent parts is usually seen in cardiac failure. Puffiness of eyelids, specially on getting up in the morning is seen in nephritis. Generalized non-pitting edema is a feature of myxedema. In Turner's syndrome, Milroy disease and filariasis, edema is localized and non-pitting. Recurrent edema over a localized area such as lip or eyelid suggest angioedema.

Vital signs:

Record the vital signs viz. pulse, respiration and blood pressure. Assess whether the child has tachypnea, tachycardia, dyspnea, cyanosis. In case of congestive cardiac failure, apart from edema, the child will have tachycardia, tachypnea, dyspnea, hepatomegaly and cardiomegaly. Presence of hypertension would suggest a renal cause such as nephritis and nephrotic syndrome.

Signs of vitamin and mineral deficiency:

The child should be examined for signs of vitamin A, B, C, iron and zinc deficiency. For vitamin A deficiency, examine the eyes for xerosis and skin for hyperkeratosis. For vitamin B deficiency, look for angular stomatitis, cheilosis. For vitamin C look for spongy or bleeding gums and scorbutic bleeding. Deficiency of vitamins and minerals would be a feature of malnutrition.

Icterus:

Presence of icterus would suggest a hepatic cause.

Examination of skin and hair:

Presence of boil marks would suggest a post streptococcal infection and is seen in post streptococcal glomerulonephritis. Presence of dermatosis (mosaic, flaky paint dermatosis, crazy pavement) is a feature of Kwashiokor. Similarly, the hair would be dry, lustreless and easily pluckable. Presence of palmar erythema and spider nevi would suggest portal hypertension.

Stigmata of Turner'ssyndrome:

In a female child, with short stature and localized non-pitting edema, look for webbing of neck, shield shape chest, increased carrying angle and presence of nevi.

Systemic examination:

A proper systemic examination should be done with following in mind. Presence of a firm hepatomegaly with jaundice, ascitis and signs of portal hypertension, would be seen in cirrhosis of liver. In edema due to cardiac failure, the heart should be examined for the cause of failure viz. signs of myocarditis, congenital heart or rheumatic heart disease. If the child with edema has encephalopathy and hypertension, the likely cause is acute nephritis with hypertensive encephalopathy.

C. Investigations

1. General Investigations:

- Urine examination routine and microscopy: Proteinuria, casts and hematuria are indicative of renal disease.

- Renal function tests and electrolytes:
  - Raised serum urea and creatinine indicate renal disease, hyperkalemia, hypokalemia, hyperphosphatemia, hypocalcemia

- CBC:
  - Microcytic hypochromic anemia: Iron deficiency from occult GI bleed (Cow's milk allergy)
  - Normocytic normochromic anemia: Chronic disease
  - Megaloblastic anemia: Vitamin B12 and folate deficiency from small bowel disease
  - Eosinophilia: Angioedema or protein losing enteropathy

- Liver function tests:
  - Hypoalbuminemia
  - Hyperbilirubinemia → liver disease

- Chest X-ray and electrocardiogram:
  - Cardiomegaly, prominent perihilar vascular markings left ventricular hypertrophy → intravascular fluid overload
  - ST elevation with T wave inversion – pericarditis
  - ECG can provide clue to other causes of heart failure

2. Specific Investigations:

These should be done depending upon th most likely cause.

- Cardiac cause: Echocardiography
- Nephrotic syndrome: 24 hour urin protein, urine protein to creatinine ratic fasting lipids, screen for secondar causes viz. SLE, hepatitis B
- Nephritic syndrome: Serum complements, screen for secondar causes e.g. streptococcal infection, SLE IgA nephropathy
- Chronic liver disease: Screen fo underlying cause, assess complication e.g. hyperammonemia, coagulopathy
- Gluten hypersensitivity: Anti gliadinIgG / IgA anti-endomysial IgA, jejunal biopsy
- Malnutrition: Blood glucose, sepsi screen, stool and urine for pus cells and parasites, electrolytes, calcium phosphorus, alkaline phosphatase serum proteins, X-ray and Mantoux test

SUMMARY

Edema also referred to as 'swelling' 'bogginess', 'puffiness','bloating', 'ballooning of skin' or 'pitting of skin' are expressions used by lay parents to express edema. There are several causes of edema. In clinical practice the common causes of edema in children are due to renal disease, cardiac failure malnutrition and liver disease. Nephrotic syndrome is characterized by massive edema massive albuminuria, hypercholesterolemia and hypoalbuminemia. The other common renal cause in children is acute pos streptococcal glomerular nephritis in which there is mainly puffiness of face, hematuria and often hypertension. In our country malnutrition continues to be an important cause of edema.

In congestive cardiac failure, apart from edema, there would be tachycardia, tachypnea, cardiomegaly and hepatomegaly.

History and clinical examination will help in arriving at a tentative diagnosis, which can be confirmed by a few investigations.

SUGGESTED READING

1. Approach to a child with edema. Epomedicine.com, 2014.

2. Dharel Dinesh. Approach to a child with edema. www.authorstream.com.

3. Evaluation and management of edema in children. www.uptodate.com.

VOMITING

INTRODUCTION

Vomiting is a common symptom in infants and children. The causes are numerous and diverse and can vary from faulty technique of feeding and parental anxiety, to serious organic disorders. If vomiting is severe or persistent it results in loss of fluid and electrolytes, leading to dehydration and dyselectrolytemia. Despite there being many complex tests available, diagnosis primarily relies on a thorough history and physical examination.

DEFINITION

Vomiting and associated terms:

1. Vomiting is forceful expulsion of gastric contents through the mouth and is usually accompanied by vigorous contractions of the abdominal muscles and descent of diaphragm.

2. Regurgitation: Is non-forceful, expulsion of food and secretions from the esophagus or stomach through the mouth not accompanied by nausea or forceful contractions of abdominal muscles. Regurgitated milk is usually unaltered.

3. Nausea: Is a feeling of inclination to vomit.

4. Retching: Is the effort to vomit, short of expulsion of gastric contents and may be considered an abortive attempt to vomit.

5. Rumination (or merycism) is the term used to describe a habit of bringing up semidigested food and chewing it again. This is usually done by cattle and is referred to as 'chewing the cud'. Some infants, who develop this habit are able to regurgitate the feed at will and then chew it. It can in some situations be a serious psychological disorder resulting in failure to thrive.

The causes of vomiting, in all age groups may be classified into three main groups:

I. **Mechanical:** Due to obstructive lesions of the gastrointestinal tract (GI), which can be complete or partial; congenital or acquired.

II. **Reflex vomiting:** Resulting from irritating afferent stimuli from the viscera, urinary tract, labyrinth, etc. or from certain drugs and metabolites through the chemoreceptor trigger zone.

III. **Central vomiting:** Through irritation or stimulation of the vomiting center, as in raised intracranial tension inflammatory lesions of central nervous system (CNS), e.g. meningitis, encephalitis, epilepsy and epileptic equivalents like migraine and cyclic vomiting.

At times the same etiologic factor may produce vomiting by two ways, e.g. a drug may act locally by irritating the stomach and also by afferent impulses to the vomiting center.

Causes and evaluation of vomiting will be discussed in relation to age, beginning with the newborn and going on to infancy and childhood. This age based approach is useful, since the causes and approach is different in different age groups and hence will help the clinician to easily arrive at a diagnosis.

VOMITING IN THE NEWBORN

ETIOLOGY

Table: Causes of vomiting in the newborn

1. Congenital anomalies of gastrointestinal tract:Esophageal atresia tracheoesophageal fistula, gastroesophageal reflux, duodenal stenosis, duodenal atresia, pyloric stenosis, small intestinal atresia, malrotation of gut, meconium ileus, necrotizing enterocolitis, diaphragmatic hernia.

2. Central nervous system causes: Intracranial bleed, Meningitis encephalitis, birth asphyxia.

3. Cardiac causes: Myocarditis.

4. Inborn errors of metabolism: Galactosemia.

5. Septicemia.

6. Endocrine disorders:Congenital adrenal hyperplasia-salt losing type.

7. Miscellaneous:Ingestion of amniotic fluid, maternal medication, aerophagy.

EVALUATION

A large number of normal neonates vomit on the first day of life due to gastritis, as a result of amniotic fluid ingestion. It responds to stomach wash and is never persistent. Regurgitation following feeds due to improper technique of feeding and aerophagy is also common. Persistent, projectile and bile-stained vomiting suggests intestinal obstruction. Early onset vomiting suggests high intestinal obstruction, while delayed onset suggests distal obstruction.

A. History

Points in history

- History of diabetes in the mother
- Polyhydramnios in mother
- Did the baby sustain birth asphyxia?
- What is the gestational age of the newborn?
- Day of onset of vomiting
- What is the color of vomitus?
- Relationship of vomiting with feeding
- Any history of choking during feeds
- Has the neonate passed meconium?
- Is the baby off feeds?
- History of seizures
- Passage of blood in stools
- Is the baby receiving top milk?

Following history must be taken before examining the neonate.

History of diabetes in the mother:

Is the mother diabetic? Was blood sugar well-controlled from early pregnancy? In infants of diabetic mothers, a cluster of anomalies are seen identified by the acronym VATER association (vertebral anomalies, anal anomalies, esophageal atresia with tracheoesophageal fistula, renal anomalies and radial limb dysplasia).

History of polyhydramnios in the mother:

Polyhydramnios in the mother is often associated with atresia ofupper gastrointestinal tract.

Did the baby sustain birth asphyxia?

What was the condition of baby at birth? Was he asphyxiated? Babies, who sustain birthasphyxia can vomit due to cerebral irritation.

Gestational age of the newborn?

Is the baby full term or preterm. Prematurity is the most consistent and important risk factor associated with neonatal necrotizing enterocolitis. It is extraordinarily infrequent among term infants and almost never diagnosed in older infants or children.

Day of onset of vomiting:

How soon after birth did the neonate start vomiting? Many neonates vomit on the first day itself, which is due to gastritis as a result of amniotic fluid ingestion. It responds to stomach wash with normal saline and is never persistent. Later on occasional regurgitation does occur often due to improper technique of feeding and aerophagy. Vomiting is early in onset in high intestinal obstruction and is delayed in distal obstruction. In hypertrophic pyloric stenosis and in cases of galactosemiavomiting, generally starts after 2 weeks of age.

Color of vomitus:

What is the color of vomitus? Is it clear or bile stained? Does it contain curdled or uncurdled milk? Pure mucus may indicate obstructive lesion proximal to the stomach such as in esophageal atresia, coagulated milk not stained with bile suggests obstruction proximal to ampula of vater. Bile stained vomit indicates obstruction beyond the ampulla of vater. Fecal vomiting occurs, when obstruction is in the lower gut. Blood mixed vomits, apart from indicating bleeding from the mucosa, may result fromswallowed maternal blood.

Relation of vomiting with feeding:

Is vomiting related to feeding? In case of gastroesophageal reflux the vomiting characteristically occurs, as soon as the baby is returned to the cot after the feed. When held upright the baby does not vomit. In cases of pyloric stenosis, the baby vomits even if held upright. It is large, non-bilious and projectile.

Choking during feeds:

Does the neonate get choked during feeds? In case of esophageal atresia, there would be a history that the baby regurgitates with the first feed and gets choked and cyanosed every time an attempt is made to feed the neonate. There would also be history of excessive drooling of saliva.

Passage of meconium:

In a newborn without an imperforate anus non-passage of meconium would point towards meconium ileus. While delayed passage of meconium in a full term baby indicates Hirschsprung disease.

Is the baby off feeds?

If the baby is dull and has stopped accepting feeds one must consider septicemia or galactosemia.

History of seizures:

Is the neonate getting seizures? If a neonate with vomiting gets seizures one must think of birth trauma, septicemia or galactosemia.

Passage of blood in stools:

Is the neonate passing blood in stools? It is usually seen in low birth weight neonate receiving top milk and also in cases of necrotizing enterocolitis.

Is the baby receiving top milk?

Vomiting is seen in neonates receiving top milk, which could be due to milk allergy.

B. Examination

> **Points on examination**
> - Growth assessment-Is there failure to thrive
> - Dysmorphicfacies
> - Sex of the neonate
> - General appearance
> - Bulging fontanelle
> - Jaundice
> - Cataract
> - Temperature
> - Umbilical cord
> - Examination of abdomen
> - Examination of genitalia
> - Per-rectal examination

The neonate should be carefully examined for the following.

Growth assessment:

Failure to thrive will be seen in neonates with persistent vomiting, especially in cases of pyloric stenosis and inborn errors of metabolism like galactosemia in which vomiting appears after 1 to 2 weeks of milk feeding. Congenital adrenal hyperplasia with salt losing syndrome also presents in the neonatal period with failure to thrive due to vomiting with or without diarrhea.

Dysmorphicfacies:

Congenital intestinal obstruction is often associated in neonates with chromosomal aberrations. Forty percent cases of duodenal atresia are seen in infants with Down syndrome.

Sex of the neonate:

Pyloric stenosis is common in first male child.

General appearance:

Baby with septicemia, necrotizing, enterocolitis may look very sick, lethargic, scleromatous and in shock.

Bulging fontanelle:

It points towards raised intracranial tension seen in meningitis, intracranial hemorrhage, hydrocephalus.

Jaundice:

Look for jaundice. Physiological jaundice is exaggerated in neonates with septicemia, galactosemia and those with gastrointestinal obstruction, as enteral feeding is withheld in these neonates.

Cataract:

Eyes should be examined for cataract, which appear in galactosemia after 2 to 6 weeks of age.

Temperature:

Presence of fever would suggest septicemia. But, hypothermia is more common in neonates with infection.

Umbilical cord:

Inspect the umbilical cord for the presence of sepsis, which is indicated by pus discharge and redness around the base of the cord. Also count the number of umbilical arteries. Single umbilical artery is associated with congenital anomalies.

Examination of abdomen:

A careful examination of the abdomen is essential. Look for abdominal distension. When it is confined to the epigastrium it suggests upper GI obstruction especially duodenal stenosis/atresia. Generalized abdominal distension would be present in lower intestinal obstruction such as ileal and jejunal atresia, meconium ileus, some cases of anorectal malformation and Hirschsprung disease. Presence of marked distension with engorged veins, soon after birth is characteristic of giant cystic meconium peritonitis and some cases of meconium ileus.

Visible peristalsis in the epigastrium from left to right is in favor of pyloric stenosis. Generalized visible peristalsis all over the abdomen are seen normally in preterms due to thin abdominal wall. It is also seen in neonates with lower gut obstruction.

Guarding of the abdominal wall is absent in newborns with peritonitis, but erythema of the abdominal wall indicates intraperitoneal infection.

Abdomen should be carefully palpated for a lump in newborns especially with persistent vomiting. In case of pyloric stenosis, a firm lump is felt of the size of an olive in the epigastrium or right hypochondrium just above and to the right of the umbilicus beneath the liver edge. In cases of meconium ileus intestinal coils loaded with meconium may be felt.

One must also palpate for hepatosplenomegaly seen in cases of galactosemia.

Examination of genitalia:

In neonates with persistent vomiting, dehydration and failure to thrive one must examine the genitalia for ambiguity. Virilization in a female infant would suggest congenital adrenal hyperplasia.

Per-rectal examination:

Rectal examination yields valuable diagnostic information. Apart from revealing presence or absence of meconium in rectum. The examination may also give important clue about tight and incapacious rectum suggestive of microcolon, which is present in intestinal atresia and meconium ileus.

C. Investigations

After arriving at a tentative diagnosis relevant investigations should be carried out to arrive at a final diagnosis.

Complete blood count:

Polymorphonucleocytosis is present in neonatal septicemia. The total count is usually above 15000/cumm in cases of neonatal infection. Counts below 5000/cumm or absolute neutropenia below 1000/cumm indicates a serious prognosis. Band cell count above 20% and C-reactive protein level above 8 mEq/ml are considered abnormal.

Cultures:

In order to isolate organisms responsible for infection cultures should be taken from blood, urine, CSF, swabs from septic umbilical cord and any other focus of infection.

Plain X-ray chest and abdomen:

The most helpful single investigation, where vomiting appears to be due to a surgical cause is plain X-ray of chest and abdomen in an upright position. This helps in diagnosing not only the presence of intestinal obstruction, but also the level of obstruction and in most cases the cause of obstruction.

- In a case of suspected esophageal atresia pass a red rubber catheter through the oral cavity. If it gets stuck in the esophagus, there is esophageal atresia. Take a skiagram of the chest and abdomen to see the position of the tip of the catheter.

- Look for gas in the abdomen. A gasless abdomen indicates esophageal atresia without tracheoesophageal fistula.

- If only 2 gas shadows are seen in the upper abdomen and rest of the abdomen is gasless, it is characteristic of duodenal atresia conventionally known as 'Double-bubble appearance'.

- Presence of fluid levels indicate intestinal obstruction and the number of levels gives some idea of the location of obstruction. In high obstruction it sometimes happens that an X-ray taken just after a vomit or nasogastric aspiration of the gastric contents does not indicate the fluid levels clearly. In such cases, injection of 20 mL of air into the stomach through a nasogastric tube and taking an X-ray after half an hour is very helpful.

- Presence of calcifications in the skiagram of abdomen indicates meconium peritonitis with antenatal perforation of bowel.

- Soap-bubble appearance in the terminal ileum suggests meconium ileus.

- In neonates with necrotizing enterocolitis X-ray of the abdomen will show distended loops of gut in the initial stage, later on gas would be seen in the wall of the intestines known as pneumatosis intestinalis.

X-ray Chest:

Chest X-ray is very useful in two conditions: Firstly in cases of diaphragmatic hernia. Presence of bowel loops in the chest with dextrocardia is diagnostic. Secondly, presence of cardiomegaly would indicate myocarditis.

Abdominal USG:

It should be done in neonates, where the cause of vomiting seems to be due to pyloric stenosis. The tumour mass can be identified on USG. It is also helpful in cases of congenital adrenal hyperplasia. A Doppler ultrasound is useful in neonates suspected to have malrotation of gut.

Urine examination:

In suspected galactosemia urine examination for reducing substance should be done followed by urinary chromatography for galactose.

Serum electrolytes, pH and arterial blood gases:

Serum electrolytes, pH and arterial blood gases should be done in patients with persistent vomiting, neonates seriously ill and in shock and in neonates suspected to be suffering from congenital adrenal hyperplasia.

Radioactive milk scan:

In most cases gastroesphageal reflux is physiological and resolves by itself. But if it is severe associated with failure to thrive a milk scan should be done to assess the degree of reflux and decide the line of management.

VOMITING IN INFANTS AND CHILDREN

As age advances, possibilities of vomiting as a symptom of congenital obstructive anomalies diminishes. The etiologic spectrum now widens and shifts to acquired conditions, which may be grouped as obstructive lesions of the gastrointestinal tract, reflex vomiting, central causes and metabolic disorders.

ETIOLOGY

Table: Causes of vomiting

- Obstructive lesions in gastrointestinal tract (congenital and acquired). Pyloric stenosis, malrotation of gut, volvulus, intussusception, gastroesophageal reflux, Hirschsprung disease, ascariasis, paralytic ileus

- Reflex vomiting-Gastritis, enteritis, peritonitis, pancreatitis, appendicitis, hepatitis, cholecystitis-Nephritis, pyelitis, cystitis

- Central causes: Raised intracranial pressure - meningitis encephalitis, space occupying lesions, pseudotumorcerebri, hydrocephalus, extradural/subdural hemorrhage, cerebrovascular accidents, epilepsy, migraine, cyclic vomiting.

- Metabolic causes: Uraemia, diabetic ketoacidosis, inborn-error of metabolism

- Miscellaneous: Over feeding, drugs, poisons, motion sickness, protein milk allergy

EVALUATION

It is important to keep in mind that, whenever a child presents with vomiting immediate attention is needed in the following situations:

Red flag signs:

1. A child having persistent vomiting, as it can lead to disturbances of fluid and electrolytes.

2. Vomiting associated with altered sensorium.

3. When a child is unable to suck or swallow.

4. Abdominal distension.

5. Bulging fontanelle-headache or convulsions.

A. History

> **Points in history**
> - Age of the child
> - Onset of vomiting
> - Color of vomitus
> - Anorexia
> - Abdominal pain
> - Headache
> - Stool pattern
> - Color of urine
> - Failure to thrive
> - Periodicity of vomiting
> - Drug history
> - Motion sickness

While taking history stress should be given on the following points, which will give us a clue to the probable cause of vomiting.

Age of the child:

The cause of vomiting in a child varies with age. Certain disorders predominate at a particular age. The common causes of vomiting in early infancy include faulty feeding technique, gastroesophageal reflux and infections. During late infancy and childhood disorders such as gastritis, gastroenteritis, gastroesophageal reflux, extracranial and intracranial infections and intestinal obstructions are more commonly encountered.

Onset of vomiting and duration:

Is vomiting of acute onset or is it long-standing? Acute onset vomiting are usually associated with fever. If there is diarrhea it is likely to be gastroenteritis. If associated with headache, it can be either extracranial or intracranial infection. If vomiting is associated with abdominal pain it is likely to be gastroenteritis hepatitis, pyelonephritis, cholecystitis or intestinal obstruction. If there is only vomiting and no fever one must consider intestinal obstruction. Presence of high grade fever suggests acute bacterial infection or viral infection.

If vomiting is of long duration and recurrent with a completely normal interval period causes could be migraine, cyclical vomiting, motion sickness or psychogenic. On the other hand if vomiting is persistent occurring daily one must think of inborn error of metabolism, intracranial tumor or chronic infection. Vomiting in case of pyloric stenosis is projectile.

What is the color of vomitus?

Bile stained vomitus indicates intestinal obstruction distal to ampulla of vater. However, absence of bile stained vomitus does not rule out intestinal obstruction.

Anorexia:

Is there loss of appetite? Does the child vomit with the sight or smell of food? Anorexia accompanies most of the diseases that present with vomiting. But severe anorexia with pain in abdomen is a feature of viral hepatitis.

Children with gastroesophageal reflux and pyloric stenosis feed well inspite of recurrent vomiting.

Abdominal pain:

Is the child having abdominal pain? What is the nature of pain? Dull aching or colicky? Vomiting associated with abdominal pain indicates infective or inflammatory focus in the abdomen. Abdominal pain also accompanies vomiting in conditions such as gastroenteritis and diabetic ketoacidosis. Pain is colicky in nature in intestinal infection and spasm of the ureter.

Headache:

If persistent vomiting is associated with severe headache one must consider the possibility of an intracranial pathology (infection or space occupying lesion.

Stool pattern:

Has there been any alteration in the stool pattern?

Constipation suggests the possibility of intestinal obstruction, while diarrhea suggests intestinal infection.

Color of urine:

What is the color of urine? Is the child passing adequate urine?

High colored urine would suggest hepatitis or concentrated urine. If there is oliguria it indicates dehydration and would call for immediate fluid resuscitation.

Failure to thrive:

Is the child loosingweight. In cases of pyloric stenosis, inborn errors of metabolism, chronic renal failure and Addison disease there is failure to thrive.

Periodicity of vomiting:

Is the child receiving any drugs? It helps in determining the cause, children with intracranial tumors and inborn errors of metabolism are never well and symptoms are continuous. Children with cyclical vomiting and migraine are asymptomatic in between the episodes.

Drug history:

History of drug intake is important. Certain drugs do produce vomiting, because of their unpleasant taste and others by causing gastritis.

Motion sickness:

Vomiting that occurs during or immediately after travel may be due to motion sickness.

B. Examination

Points on physical examination
• Are there signs of dehydration
• Record vital signs
• Assess growth
• Jaundice
• Skin pigmentation
• Systemic examination.
• Does the child look ill, well or lethargic

Appearance:

Does the child look ill or lethargic? Or does the child look well? If the child looks ill it helps the clinician in suspecting a serious illness.

Lethargy disproportionate to the severity of vomiting and accompanying symptoms is indicative of hepatitis, raised intracranial pressure or diabetic ketoacidosis.

A well-looking child with no clinical findings and with a history of repeated episodes of vomiting one must consider migraine, cyclical vomiting and psychogenic vomiting.

Look for signs of dehydration?

If the child has signs of dehydration viz. depressed anterior fontanelle, loss of skin turgor, sunken eyes or dry oral mucosa, it indicates that vomiting is significant and needs hospitalization for correction of fluid and electrolyte imbalance.

Examine the vitals:

Note the pulse rate, respiratory rate and measure the capillary refill time (CRT) and the blood pressure. It will help in detecting impending shock. If the breathing is acidotic suspect diabetic ketoacidosis.

Assess growth:

If vomiting is of long-standing and there is failure to thrive consider inborn errors of metabolism, chronic renal failure or Addison's disease.

Look for jaundice and pigmentation:

Presence of jaundice would indicate hepatitis. Whileskin pigmentation in a child with long-standing vomiting suggests the presence of Addison's disease.

Systemic examination:

Careful examination of the abdomen is very essential in a child with vomiting. Abdominal distension and hyperperistalsis are suggestive of intestinal obstruction. Guarding, rigidity and tenderness would suggest intra-abdominal inflammatory pathology. Feel for any lump in abdomen. A tender hepatomegaly would suggest hepatitis. If a child has vomiting, since early life along with recurrent respiratory infections and abdomen is scaphoid think of congenital diaphragmatic hernia.

Examine for signs of meningeal irritation. If present would suggest meningitis or meningismus.

Fundus examination should be done for presence of papilledema. If present would indicate raised intracranial pressure either due to meningitis or space occupying lesions such as tuberculoma or tumor.

Presence of neurological deficit also points towards an intracranial pathology.

Nystagmus associated with dizziness and vertigo is indicative of vestibular dysfunction. A sick looking child with vomiting, respiratory distress muffled heart sounds and gallop rhythm, one must keep the possibility of myocarditis.

C. Investigations

Every child with vomiting does not need to be investigated. Only patients with persistent or recurrent vomiting should be subjected to investigations.

Complete blood count:

In majority of the cases, vomiting is secondary to acute infectionin the respiratory tract, gastrointestinal tract, urinary tract, etc. Insuch cases CBC should be useful. Leukocytosis would suggestbacterial infection and leukopenia viral infection.

Urine examination:

a. Routine urine examination especially for albumin, pus cells and bacteriuria if one suspects urinary tract infection. In case of diabetes presence of sugar and ketone bodies are important. Presence of bile pigments and bile salts would indicate hepatitis.

b. Urine culture: In cases of suspected urinary tract infection urine culture with colony count is urinary tract infection.

Cerebrospinal fluid examination:

Should be done where the cause appears to be meningitis. Proteins and cells would be raised, while sugar will be reduced especially in purulent meningitis.

Blood biochemistry:

- Blood sugar estimation: It is indicated, where cause of vomiting appears to be diabetic ketoacidosis or an inborn error of metabolism
- Blood urea nitrogen and serum creatinine: These are altered in chronic renal failure
- Liver function tests: Serum bilirubin and SGPT would be raised in cases of viral hepatitis
- Serum calcium, phosphorus, alkaline phosphatase are altered in cases of chronic renal failure.

Abdominal X-ray in erect position:

Abdominal X-ray is an important investigation, where the cause of vomiting appears to be surgical. Presence of multiple air and fluid levels indicate intestinal obstruction. Gas under diaphragm would suggest bowel perforation.

USG of abdomen:

Would be useful in case of lump in abdomen or an organomegaly.

Barium meal and follow through:

It is indicated in children with persistent vomiting, where the cause appears to be partial obstruction in the gastrointestinal tract.

X-ray chest:

Cardiomegaly would be seen in a child with myocarditis.

Presence ofbowel loops in the chest will indicate diaphragmatic hernia.

Electrocardiography and echocardiography:

If vomiting appears to be due to myocarditis an electrocardiography (ECG), an echocardiography is indicated.

Neuroimaging of brain:

It is indicated in cases, where cause of vomiting appears to be due to raised intracranial tension viz. meningitis, intracranial space occupying lesion and cerebrovascular accidents.

Electroencephalogram:

To be done in cases, where vomiting appears to be due to epilepsy.

SUMMARY

Vomiting in the pediatric age group may be a result of a range of causes, including GI etiologies, CNS disease, renal, endocrine and metabolic disorders. Drugs either as side-effects or in overdose. Psychiatric disorders or stress. Can also lead to vomiting in children.

A carefully carried out interrogation of mother, clinical examination of the child and a period of observation will frequently point to the cause of vomiting. Investigations may be necessary in some cases.

Age based approach to a child with vomiting is more convenient and easy to arrive at a diagnosis.

SUGGESTED READING

1. Nausea and vomiting in children. bestpractice.bmj.com.

2. Approach to vomiting. learn.pediatrics.ubc.ca.

3. Vomiting in the pediatric age group. www.medscape.com.

16

ABDOMINAL PAIN

INTRODUCTION

Abdominal pain is one of the most common reasons for a parent to bring his or her child to a physician. The evaluation of a 'tummy ache' can challenge both parents and the physician. Possible causes for a child's abdominal pain range from trivial to life-threatening conditions. It is essential for a physician to be able to diagnose acute surgical conditions, which need immediate referral and intervention, a serious medical disorder requiring hospitalization from a condition that can be managed on an outpatient basis.

ETIOLOGY

Causes can be acute or chronic. Acute would be presenting as a first episode of pain or it can be recurrent with a past history of repeated episodes of acute pain. Chronic abdominal pain is defined as recurrent or persistent bouts of abdominal pain that occurs over a minimum of 3 months. Nearly 10% to 15% of school children experience recurring abdominal pain, which can be due to organic or functional causes.

Table: Causes of abdominal pain

Causes of acute pain

Infections and Inflammations
Commonest causes are acute gastroenteritis, hepatitis, mesenteric lymphadenitis, appendicitis, pyelonephritis.

Less common causes are liver abscess, pancreatitis, cholecystitis, acute peritonitis, acute salpingitis and hematocolpos.

Colics

Three month colic in infants, intestinal colic, renal colic, biliary colic.

Obstruction

Intussusception, intestinal obstruction, volvulus, testicular torsion, torsion of ovaries.

Extra-Abdominal Causes

- Lower lobe pneumonia, pleurisy, pleurodynia
- Pericarditis, subacute bacterial endocarditis
- Acute hemolytic crisis in sickle cell disease and hereditary spherocytosis
- Abdominal epilepsy
- Diabetic ketoacidosis
- Anaphylactoidpurpura
- Porphyria

Causes of Chronic Pain

Constipation, dyspepsia, psychogenic, parasitic infection, tumors, celiac disease, milk allergy.

EVALUATION

A meticulous history and thorough examination will help in arriving at a diagnosis.

A. History

Details of pain can only be elicited from children above the age of 5 years younger children may not be able to localize pain and infants would only present with crying.

> **Points in history**
> - Age of the child
> - Time of onset of pain and progression% Location of pain and radiation
> - Character of pain
> - Exacerbating and relieving factors
> - Any interference with child's daily activity
> - Presence of associated symptoms
> - Feeding history especially in infants
> - Behavioral history
> - Menstrual history in older girls
> - History of blunt abdominal trauma
> - History of medications

Age of the patient

An infant cannot complaint of pain, but would present with episodes of crying. If a healthy infant is brought with a history of crying every evening for 2 to 3 hours since the age of 2 to 3 weeks it is most likely to be '3 month colic'. Functional pain is often seen in school going children. Acute intussusception occurs in children below 2 years especially in infants at the time when weaning has started. Girls may often suffer from severe abdominal pain with each menstrual period especially around menarche.

Onset of pain and progression

One must enquire as to, from when is the child getting pain? Is this the first episode or is there a history of recurrent episodes of pain in abdomen? Sudden onset of pain within minutes and hours suggest a colic. It is usually short-lasting, self-limiting and often recurrent.

In case of recurrent pain one must enquire, how frequently pain recurs? How long does each episode lasts? Duration of pain free intervals? Are recurrences worse than before? Recurrence occurs in worm infestations, urinary tract infections, ulcers, renal calculi, sickle cell disease, fecal impaction, abdominal epilepsy and psychogenic causes. Inflammatory pain may progress over hours or days. If pain lasts longer than 3 hours, it is likely to be due to an organic cause such as appendicitis. Sudden relief in such a case could mean rupture of the appendix. Sudden screaming episodes in an infant often manifesting as episodic crying would suggest acute intussusception. Infant colic is characterized by severe and paroxysmal crying that begins around the age of 2 to 3 weeks and subsides by 3 to 4 months of age. It occurs mainly in the late afternoon. Infant's knees are drawn up and its fists clenched and usually flatus is expelled after which the infant settles down.

Location of pain and radiation

The child should be asked to point out the site of pain. Is pain localized to a quadrant or is it all over the abdomen? Generalized pain is more common and is due to intestinal or peritoneal pathology. Acute generalized pain suggests peritonitis or acute abdomen from surgical cause.

Apley's observation that "the further the pain from umbilicus, the greater the likelihood of organic disease."

Functional abdominal pain is usually periumbilical. Closer the pain occurs to the umbilicus less is the chance of organic disease. Although in some cases of appendicitis to begin with pain is over the periumbilical area and later on is localized over the right iliac fossa. Acute appendicitis and lymphadenitis present with pain in the right iliac fossa. While pain in the right hypochondrium is seen in acute hepatitis, liver abscess, congestive cardiac failure and choledochal cyst. Abdominal pain in kidney disease is usually present in the back, flanks and lower abdomen.

In case of ureteric colic pain typically radiates from loin to groin.

Pericarditis may cause upper abdominal pain. Pain radiating to the right shoulder may suggest acute cholecystitis, while radiation to the left shoulder tip can be from splenic rupture; referred pain in lower chest is from peritonitis. Pain radiating to the back is a feature of acute pancreatitis. Lower abdominal pain in girls could be due to hematocolpos. Pain in the splenic region could be due to subacute bacterial endocarditis. Adolescent children can have duodenal ulcers and they do present with pain in the epigastric or periumbilical region.

Nature of pain

In an older child one could enquire about the type of pain. A dull aching pain indicates a chronic pathology. If it is situated in the periumbilical region in an adolescent it is usually functional. Obstructive lesions of the gut give rise to severe colicky abdominal pain. Colicky pain is due to smooth muscle spasm of a hollow viscus, e.g. intestine, ureters, etc. Stabbing pain is usually felt in pleurisy and peritonitis. In some cases of peritonitis the patient lies still in bed and does not move since movement is extremely painful. As against this, in renal colic the child is restless, rolls and doubles up as he/she cannot find relief in several positions he tries.

Exacerbating and relieving factors

In case of acute gastritis consumption of food may aggravate the pain, while in duodenal ulcer ingestion of food relieves pain. Cough can exaggerate pain in cases of basal pneumonia and pleurisy. In case of peritonitis, movement aggravates pain. Passage of flatus relieves pain from intestinal cause (colic, distension).

Interferences with child's daily activity

Enquiring from parents whether the pain interferes with child's daily activity, is especially useful in children presenting with recurrent abdominal pain. If child is eating and playing well and pain does not occur during sleep, watching television, playing or such pleasurable activity it is less likely to be organic. On the other hand, if the child gets up from sleep with acute pain or stops playing due to pain such a child needs proper investigations for a cause.

Presence of associated symptoms

One must enquire whether pain in abdomen is associated with symptoms such as vomiting, diarrhea, blood and mucus in stools, passing dark colored urine, constipation, fever, dysuria, urinary frequency, polyuria, passage of worms in stools, drowsiness, recent history of sore throat, cough and cold.

Although any severe abdominal pain can lead to non-specific vomiting, it is commonly associated with gastroenteritis. At the onset of hepatitis nausea and vomiting are very common. Vomiting with pain in the right iliac fossa is a feature of appendicitis.

Persistent vomiting especially if bilious is indicative of obstructive lesions of the gut. Recurrent episodes of severe abdominal pain associated with vomiting and drowsiness may suggest abdominal epilepsy. A child with acute abdominal pain, vomiting with history of polyuria could be a case of diabetic ketoacidosis.

Babies on cow's milk can develop allergy to the milk protein and develop colicky abdominal pain, vomiting and diarrhea.

Passage of blood in stools would suggest dysentery. It is also seen in Henoch-Schonleinpurpura (HSP), red current jelly stools is a feature of intussusception.

Passage of dark yellow urine would be seen in hepatitis, port-wine urine in case of porphyria. Hematuria if present indicates anaphylactoidpurpura.

Constipation is a common cause of dull ache in abdomen. If the child is constipated one must enquire about feeding practices and toilet training.

Fever can be associated with several conditions. Viral hepatitis could present with high grade fever. High fever could also be associated with acute gastroenteritis, acute peritonitis, acute mesenteric lymphadenitis, acute pancreatitis, liver abscess and pyelonephritis. Children with tubercular abdomen could present with continuous fever over a long period of time.

Dysuria and increased frequency of micturition would suggest urinary tract infection. History of pain in abdomen with jaundice intermittently could be due to a choledochal cyst.

Recent history of respiratory infection in a child below 2 to 3 years with pain in right iliac fossa or periumbilical region the cause could be mesenteric adenitis.

History of medications

History of recent mediations is important as antibiotics may predispose the patient to intestinal bacterial overgrowth, acne medications may induce oesophagitis and tricyclic antidepressants may cause constipation.

Psychosocial factors

One must bear in mind that the commonest cause of chronic abdominal pain in older children is functional. However, it should only be thought of after organic causes have been ruled out. One must enquire about parent-child relationship, school environment and whether the child is reluctant to go to school, about interpersonal behavior and parental attitudes. Any tensions in any of these situations may be important in determining psychological causes of pain.

A sizeable number of children complain of pain in abdomen as an attention seeking device. He enjoys seeing parents and grandparents pamper him for his pain. Some children often complain of abdominal pain every morning, when it is time to goto school and rest of the day they are fine. Such situations are seen in children who are either scolded by teachers for bad behavior or poor school performance or bullied by peers. Functional abdominal pain is uncommon under 5 years of age.

Menstrual history

In case of an adolescent girl with pain in abdomen, it is important to enquire whether she has dysmenorrhea, which is common around the age of menarche.

History of trauma

Blunt abdominal trauma is the most common cause of acute pancreatitis in childhood. It can also follow an attack of mumps.

History of abdominal distension

Weight loss, deceleration of linear growth, prolonged fever, bile stained or persistent vomiting, chronic diarrhea, dysphagia, nocturnal symptoms, pain persistently located away from the central abdominal area are the "red flag" symptoms and should trigger a search for organic disease.

B. Physical Examination

Before performing a formal examination, it is crucial in pediatric medicine to observe the child patient. Children who have peritoneal irritation would cry if moved, would like to be carried and appear sick. Conversely, a child who walks into the clinic cheerfully interacts brightly is unlikely to have a serious condition. One essential step is to observe the dynamics between children and their parents. Since abdominal pain in children can be a sign of emotional or social difficulty, often within the context of a dysfunctional family unit, this sort of observation is vital and can shed light on a patient whose symptoms are difficult to interpret.

> ### Points on examination
> - General appearance
> - Vitals
> - Pallor/jaundice
> - Rash
> - Ears and throat
> - Hydration
> - Joints
> - Abdominal examination including rectal examination
> - Other systems

Examination should be carried out methodically and calmly. If required preferably an infant and even a preschool child can be examined in the lap of the mother. Distract the child by chatting or with toys.

General appearance

As soon as the child presents it is important to look whether child looks ill and toxic, which may indicate a serious illness such as peritonitis, acute pancreatitis, acute thrombotic crisis of sickle cell anemia.

Vital signs

The child's pulse rate, respiratory rate, blood pressure, presence of acidosis, signs of hydration should be carefully assessed. If patient is in shock an emergency management can be started until the etiology is determined.

Children with diabetic ketoacidosis can present with acute pain in abdomen with shock and acidosis.

Pallor and jaundice

If the child appears pale and sick it points towards an intra-abdominal hemorrhage and would suggest a surgical condition.

Presence of jaundice with abdominal pain would indicate hepatitis, hemolytic crisis in sickle cell disease or spherocytosis.

Presence of rash

If the child has an urticarial rash, which later becomes maculopapular or purpuric distributed mainly over the legs, feet and buttocks with involvement of joints indicate Henoch-Schonleinpurpura.

Examination of abdomen

Etiology of abdominal pain can be determined to a great extent by meticulous examination of the abdomen. Hands should be warm and the examination should be carried out gently.

Generalized abdominal distension is a feature of intestinal disease or the presence of fluid in the peritoneal cavity. Localized distension suggests organomegaly or a tumor. The presence of visible peristalsis favors intestinal obstruction. Horizontal stretching of the umbilicus is seen when there is fluid in the abdomen.

Bluish discoloration around the umbilicus and flanks is a sign (Cullen sign) of acute pancreatitis. Rigidity of the abdomen denotes peritonitis. Generalized abdominal tenderness would indicate peritonitis or intestinal obstruction while localized tenderness denotes local inflammatory condition such as appendicitis, hepatitis, salpingitis. Absence of tenderness would suggest a non-inflammatory pathology.

Tenderness in the renal angles will suggest pyelonephritis. If fecaliths are felt in the abdomen the cause of pain is constipation. Exaggerated bowel sounds would indicate obstruction and absence or sluggish bowel sounds would suggest peritonitis. In case of intussusception a sausage-shaped lump can be felt and the right iliac fossa appears empty.

One must examine the genitalia and hernial orifices in boys and girls.

Per-rectal examination is important. The tip of the intussusception can be felt.

Examination of other systems

Respiratory system should be examined for pleural rub and signs of pneumonia.

Cardiovascular system for signs of pericarditis.

The **red flag signs** of organic disease include localized tenderness in right upper or lower quadrants, localized fullness or palpable mass, hepatomegaly, splenomegaly, costovertebral angle tenderness or perianal abnormalities.

C. Investigations

- Complete blood count
- Urine examination
- Stool examination
- X-ray abdomen
- Ultrasonography
- Blood biochemistry
  - Serum bilirubin
  - SGPT- Serum amylase, lipase
  - Blood urea, serum creatinine
  - Blood sugar
  - Blood gases
- Barium enema

Most children with pain in abdomen do not need an extensive laboratory work up. However, children presenting with acute abdomen and those getting recurrent abdominal pain need to be investigated. Investigations that are required in a particular child should be based on the clinical diagnosis.

Complete blood count

Complete blood count is indicated wherever the cause appears to be an infection, inflammatory or a hematological cause.

The presence of leukocytosis with polymorphonuclear preponderance suggests infection or inflammation, e.g. acute appendicitis, acute pancreatitis, peritonitis. Evidence of hemolysis, sickle cell, spherocytes in the peripheral smear would suggest acute hemolytic crisis.

Urine examination

Presence of pus cells and bacteriuria would indicate urinary tract infection, which can be confirmed by urine culture.

Presence of bile pigments and salts would suggest hepatitis. In cases of porphyria, porphobilinogen can be detected.

Stool examination

Presence of pus cells and blood are seen in acute dysentery. Giardia lamblia infection is a common cause of recurrent abdominal pain.

Plain X-ray abdomen

Roentgenogram of the abdomen is helpful when suspected diagnosis is intestinal obstruction, calculi in the kidney, ureters or bladder, intestinal perforation or paralytic ileus.

Free air in the peritoneal cavity (pneumoperitoneum) is a feature of intestinal perforation. Multiple air fluid levels is a sign of paralytic ileus. Radio-opaque shadow in the urinary tract suggests calculus.

Calcification may often be present in tumors especially neuroblastoma and teratoma. In some cases, where intestinal obstruction is due to roundworms, a bunch of roundworms can be seen. In case of an abdominal mass, displacement of bowel may be seen.

Ultrasonography of the abdomen

Ultrasonography is useful in cases of organomegaly and helps wherever the cause is a tumor or a mass, e.g. intussusception, appendicular mass, choledochal cyst, liver abscess, mesenteric lymphadenopathy, ovarian cyst. Presence of gall stones, should be seen in spherocytosis and sickle cell anemia.

Mesenteric lymph nodes should be considered significant only when they are more than 10 mm in size.

Blood Biochemistry

- Serum bilirubin, SGPT, Both are raised in hepatitis
- Serum amylase and serum lipase raised in acute pancreatitis
- Blood urea serum creatinine if raised points towards a renal pathology
- Blood sugar raised in diabetic ketoacidosis
- Blood gases-acidosis in diabetic ketoacidosis

Barium enema

Is indicated in suspected cases of intussusception. Spring coil or claw hand appearance is characteristic.

X-ray Chest

For evidence of pneumonia, cardiomegaly, tuberculosis.

Ascitic fluid analysis

Analysis of ascitic fluid is done to decide whether it is transudate or exudate.

Hemoglobin electrophoresis and osmotic fragility

Hemoglobin electrophoresis is indicated where the cause appears to be a sickle cell crisis and osmotic fragility in cases of spherocytosis.

Electroencephalogram

In suspected abdominal epilepsy, confirmation can be done by an electroencephalogram (EEG).

SUMMARY

Abdominal pain is one ofthe most challenging diagnostic problems in children, particularly the young who can barely describe their feelings. The abdomen has been aptly called The Pandora's box in view of the large number of its contents and therefore many surprises it springs in the diagnosis. Constipation is a common cause of abdominal pain in children. Some more serious causes of abdominal pain in children include appendicitis, lead poisoning, intussusception or malrotation. Recurrent abdominal pain is a condition that affects children aged 4 to 11 years.

As soon as a child is brought with the complaint of pain in abdomen, the physician must first evaluate whether the child has an acute abdomen and needs immediate hospitalization and treatment or whether he/she can be investigated and treated on an outpatient basis.

Clinical diagnosis is largely made by the accompanying symptomatology associated with the abdominal pain followed by confirmation from laboratory and investigative techniques.

SUGGESTED READING

1. Sankaranarayan S. Abdominal pain in children. IAP Textbook of Pediatrics.5th Edition (2013), pg. 523.
2. Morris Green. Abdominal and pelvic pain. Pediatric Diagnosis, 6th Edition, pg. 242.

17   GASTROINTESTINAL BLEEDING

INTRODUCTION

Infants and children often present with gastrointestinal (GI) bleeding. Fortunately majority of cases do not result in serious health consequences. There are three typical, but often overlapping presentations of GI bleeding. Chronic and occult intestinal bleeding present with features of anemia, including pallor and fatigue. Stools are characteristically normal in color and consistency, but tests for occult blood are positive. Acute upper GI bleeding usually presents with hematemesis, which is vomiting of bright red or coffee ground material or with passage of melena, i.e. dark colored, tarry stools that contain digested blood.

Lower GI hemorrhage presents as hematochezia (rectal passage of bright red or maroon-colored blood mixed in with the stool).

This symptom of gastrointestinal bleeding will be discussed under two separate headings viz upper and lower GI bleeding.

UPPER GASTROINTESTINAL BLEEDING

Upper GI bleeding (arising proximal to the ligament of Treitz in the distal duodenum) commonly presents either as hematemesis or melena depending upon site and severity of bleeding.

ETIOLOGY

Table: Causes of upper GI bleeding

- Hemorrhagic disease of newborn
- Esophageal varices - due to extrahepatic or intrahepatic portal hypertension
- Peptic ulcer disease - gastric, duodenal
- Curling ulcer - stress ulcers due to burns, septicemia
- Mallory-Weiss syndrome
- Gastritis due to drugs - salicylates, non-steroidal anti-inflammatory drugs (NSAIDs), corticosteroids
- Nasopharyngeal bleeding - bleeding from nose, mouth or pharynx
- Bleeding dyscrasia; congenital or acquired due to acute or chronic liver disease
- Foreign body ingestion
- Cushing ulcer - secondary to encephalitis, head injury or any condition leading to raised intracranial tension.

EVALUATION

The initial approach to patients with significant GI bleeding should be to ensure patient stability, to establish adequate oxygen delivery, to place intravenous access to initiate fluid and blood resuscitation, and to correct any underlying coagulopathies.

A. History

A detail history has to be taken on the points given below:

Age of the child:

Age of the child is very important as the causes are different at different ages, see table:

Table: Causes of upper gastrointestinal bleeding according to age group

Age group	Upper gastrointestinal bleeding
Neonates	• Hemorrhagic disease of the newborn • Swallowed maternal blood • Stress gastritis (sepsis, trauma) • Coagulopathy
1 month to 1 year	• Oesophagitis • Gastritis • Caustic ingestion • Foreign body ingestion • Duplication cysts • Drugs - NSAIDs
Infants 1 to 2 years	• Peptic ulcer disease • Gastritis • Caustic ingestion
Children above 2 years	• Oesophagealvarices • Gastric varices • Caustic ingestion • Coagulation disorders • Vomiting induced bleeding

In the newborns the predominant causes include coagulation disorders such as Vitamin K deficiency, gastritis from stress, sepsis and trauma from placement of nasogastric tubes. From 1 to 5 years causes include erosive esophagitis due to caustic ingestions, peptic ulcer bleeding, varices and vomiting induced bleeding from a Mallory-Weiss tear.

Colour of vomitus:

What is the colour of vomitus? Is it bright red or coffee ground color? Blood when it comes in contact with the acid in the stomach turns coffee ground.

Amount of blood in the vomitus:

If the child vomits large amount of blood he needs to be evaluated immediately for blood transfusion. In Mallory-Weiss syndrome there is a small quantity of hematemesis preceded by repeated retching.

History of melena:

Does the child pass tarry stools? Melena indicates bleeding from any site above the ileocecal valves. Blood enters the colon slowly and the colonic bacteria converts heme of hemoglobin to hematin and hemochromogens, which are black.

Past history of hematemesis:

In case of portal hypertension there may be history of recurrent hematemesis each time due to rupture of varices. Also in congenital coagulopathies there can be a history of recurrent hemetemesis.

Gastrointestinal symptoms:

Does the child get recurrent abdominal pain, nausea and vomiting? Many children with peptic ulcer disease have vague, poorly localized abdominal pain usually in the periumbilical region and can present with sudden hematemesis. A history of acute appendicitis or primary peritonitis in the past can lead to portal vein thrombosis resulting in portal hypertension and hematemesis.

Nose or gum bleeds:

It is essential to enquire if the child has bleeding from the nose or gums. This can lead to swallowing of blood and subsequently vomiting of altered blood (spurious hematemesis).

History of umbilical sepsis/umbilical vein catheterization:

Did the child have umbilical sepsis in the neonatal period? Was the umbilicus catheterized? Omphalitis or catheterization of umbilical vein during neonatal period can lead to extrahepatic portal hypertension, which can present as hematemesis.

History of chronic liver disease:

Past history of jaundice would point towards cirrhosis of liver. If there is a family history of chronic liver disease one must keep in mind hereditary conditions such as congenital hepatic fibrosis, Wilsons disease, -1-antitrypsin deficiency, galactosemia.

Drug ingestion:

Certain drugs increase the risk of UGI bleeding. These include aspirin, NSAIDs and corticosteroids. NSAIDs increase the risk of UGI bleeding by damaging gastric mucosa and promoting tissue friability. The greatest risk of developing gastric complications typically occurs within 30 days of initiating NSAID therapy. Corticosteroid use in neonates has been associated with increased mortality from GI hemorrhage. Mortality rate among children receiving high dose dexamethasone is high due to development of GI complication.

B. Examination

After taking a detailed history, a thorough examination must be conducted.

> **Points on examination**
> - Assess degree of blood loss - pulse rate, blood pressure (BP), capillary refill time (CRT)
> - Anemia
> - Jaundice
> - Nose and throat for bleeding
> - Purpura, ecchymosis
> - Vascular malformations—hemangioma, telangiectasia
> - Eyes for Kayser-Fleischer (KF) ring, cataract
> - Clubbing, palmar erythema, spider nevi
> - Abdomen—dilated vessels, ascites, hepatosplenomegaly
> - Central nervous system—level of consciousness.

Assessment of degree of blood loss:
Whenever a child with GI bleeding is brought the first step would be to assess the degree of blood loss by recording heart rate, blood pressure and CRT. Tachycardia is the most

sensitive indicator for blood loss in children. Disproportionate tachycardia suggests that the child has lost about 20 percent of blood volume. If the CRT is prolonged then the loss could be 25 percent of the blood volume. Such children need immediate treatment for shock. General presentation should also be noted including confusion, irritability and respiratory distress.

Anemia:

It is important to assess degree of anemia by examining the conjunctiva, mucous membrane of the oral cavity, tongue, nails and palms. Severe pallor with shock would indicate acute massive blood loss. But, if the child's vitals are stable and still has severe pallor it would suggest a chronic loss of blood.

Jaundice:

It is essential to examine the sclera for icterus. The presence of jaundice would suggest a liver pathology.

Examination of the oral cavity:

Look for any focus of bleeding in the mouth, nose and throat. As swallowed blood can lead to spurious upper GI bleeding.

Purpura, ecchymosis:

Presence of purpuric spots and ecchymosis over body would suggest a bleeding diathesis.

Eyes:

Eyes should be examined not only for subconjunctival hemorrhage, but also for KF ring and cataract. The former would be present in Wilson disease, while cataract would suggest galactosemia. Both these conditions would lead to cirrhosis of liver. Presence of jaundice would suggest a liver pathology.

Examination of palms and nails:

Presence of clubbing palmar erythema and spider nevi would suggest chronic liver disease.

Systemic Examination:

Abdomen should be assessed for guarding, epigastric or rebound tenderness and signs and sequelae of chronic liver disease. Presence of dilated veins over abdomen, ascites, firm shrunken liver with splenomegaly will be seen in cirrhosis with portal hypertension.

Altered sensorium with jaundice would suggest hepatic coma.

Encephalitis or head injury are also known to produce Cushing's ulcer leading to hematemesis.

C. Investigations

Investigations to be done

- Complete blood count
- Prothrombin time
- Activated partial thromboplastin time
- BUN level
- Liver enzymes SGPT
- Endoscopy
- Doppler ultrasound of the abdomen

Hemogram:

A complete blood count should be done. Hemoglobin will indicate the degree of anemia due to blood loss. A low platelet count will suggest bleeding due to thrombocytopenia. Leucocytosis with increased band cells may point towards sepsis. A normal hematocrit may provide false reassurance regarding some children with hypovolemia and hemoconcentration.

Prothrombin time and activated partial thromboplastin time:

Elevated PT indicates coagulopathy (i.e. DIC) or profound impairment of liver synthetic function. Prolonged APTT indicates a hemophiliac patient or coagulopathy.

Blood urea nitrogen:

High BUN level, would suggest an upper GI source that has had time to allow the body to reabsorb blood leading to a higher BUN level compared with a lower GI source.

Liver function tests:

In suspected liver dysfunction, one must get the serum bilirubin and SGPT done. It would be raised in hepatitis.

Doppler ultrasound of the abdomen:

This would help in identifying patency of portal vein, direction of flow within the portal system, esophageal varices and cavernous transformation of portal vein.

Endoscopy:

Endoscopy will help in identifying the source of GI hemorrhage, i.e. esophageal or gastric varices, gastric or duodenal ulcerations and vascular malformations.

In case of episodic or obscure bleeding, nuclear medicine radionucleotide studies, arteriography, and wireless video capsule endoscopy are used to assist in identifying the site of blood loss.

SUMMARY

The first thing that should be done when faced with a child presenting as hematemesis is to exclude spurious hematemesis due to swallowed blood from nose or gums.

The next step should be to assess whether hematemesis is a part of generalized bleeding diathesis or a local GI cause. A proper history examination would help in arriving at a tentative diagnosis, which can be confirmed by appropriate investigations.

The differential diagnosis of UGI bleeding in children is determined by age and severity of bleed. In infants and toddlers mucosal bleed (gastritis and stress ulcers) is a common cause.

LOWER GASTROINTESTINAL BLEEDING

Lower gastrointestinal bleeding (LGIB) in infants and children is commonly encountered in clinical practice. Acute lower GI bleeding usually presents with hematochezia, which is the passage of bright red or maroon colored blood in the stool. Occasionally, severe acute upper GI bleeding may present with hematochezia due to very rapid transit through the digestive tract.

ETIOLOGY

Lower gastrointestinal bleeding (LGIB) refers to bleeding distal to the ligament of Treitz and thus includes bleeding sources in the small bowel and colon.

Table: Causes of LGIB

- Anal fissure
- Infection: Dysentery due to Escherichia coli, Salmonella, Shigella
- Polyps: Rectal, intestinal polyps in juvenile familial polyposis, Peutz-Jegher syndrome, Gardener's syndrome
- Intussusception
- Meckel's diverticulum
- Intestinal duplication
- Midgut volvulus
- Henoch-Schonlein pupura
- Bleeding diathesis
- Vascular malformation
- Milk protein intolerance

EVALUATION

An initial question to consider in children presenting with LGIB is whether blood is truly present in the stool. Several foods and medicines may give stool a bloody appearance and create unnecessary anxiety in parents.

Following history must be taken in a child presenting with lower GI bleed.

Points in history
• Age at presentation
• Color of stool
• Associated symptoms
• History of joint pains
• History of ingestion of drugs containing iron, NSAIDs

Patient's age:

The causes vary depending upon the age of the child. In neonates the commonest cause is swallowed maternal blood syndrome followed by hemorrhagic disease of the newborn. In infants the most common cause is anal fissure, while in toddlers and older children the commonest cause is polyps.

Table: Causes of lower gastrointestinal bleeding according to age group

Age group	Lower gastrointestinal bleeding
Neonates	• Anal fissure
	• Necrotizing enterocolitis
	• Malrotation with volvulus
1 month to 1 year	• Anal fissure
	• Intussuception
	• Gangrenous bowel
	• Milk protein allergy
Infants 1 to 2 years	• Polyps
	• Meckel's diverticulum
Children above 2 years	• Polyps
	• Inflammatory bowel disease
	• Infectious diarrhea
	• Vascular disease

Color of stool:

It is important to enquire about the color of stool and the amount of blood passed.

In case of anal fissure, the amount of blood passed is small in quantity and is seen as bright red streaking on the periphery of the stool. In case of milk protein intolerance also there is a history of blood streaked stools. In case of intussusception the child passes typical 'red currant jelly' stool. In dysentery blood is mixed with stool and mucous. In rectal polyp blood is passed after the act of defecation.

Associated symptoms:

Enquire about associated symptoms. Does the child have diarrhea or constipation?

Is there abdominal pain or pain during defecation? Any associated vomiting? What is the color of urine? Is the child running fever? Anal fissure is associated with severe constipation and painful defecation. In case of dysentery the stools are loose mixed with blood and mucus associated with crampy abdominal pain and tenesmus the child can be febrile. Intussusception presents with severe colicky pain, screaming, vomiting and passage of stool, which is red currant jelly like. In rectal polyps bleeding is large in amount, but painless. Hematuria can be present in cases of hemolytic uremic syndrome. Some cases of Henoch-Schonlein purpura can also develop hematuria.Joint pains would suggest Henoch-Schonlein vasculitis.

History of drug ingestion:

If the child is on iron therapy the stools are likely to be black, which may be mistaken for GI bleeding. Ingestion of beet would also give rise to red colored stools. Recent use of NSAIDs or any other medication should also be noted.

B.   Examination

After taking a detailed history one must examine the child thoroughly. A good general examination followed by a local examination of the perianal region would help in arriving at a tentative cause of bleeding.

> **Points on physical examination**
> - Presence of anemia
> - Purpura, telengiectasia
> - Circumoral pigmentation
> - Jaundice
> - Arthritis
> - Visualization of perianal region
> - Lump in abdomen
> - Renal abnormalities

Anemia:

It is important to assess the severity of anemia. Chronic blood loss over a period of time can give rise to severe anemia. Massive hematochezia as in case of Meckel's diverticulum would not only give rise to anemia, but the patient may be in shock.

Presence of purpuric spots or ecchymosis:

Bleeding into the skin, mucous membrane and subcutaneoustissue would point towards a generalized bleeding diathesis. In case of Henoch-Schonlein purpura initially the skin rash is often urticarial, which progresses to a macular-papular appearance, which transforms into symmetric purpuric rash, which is typically distributed on the ankles, buttocks and elbows. Purpuric spots, progress to form larger hemorrhages. It is characterized clinically as palpable purpura. Lesions appear in crops.

Circumoral pigmentations:

Mucosal pigmentation of the lips and gums would suggest Peutz-Jegher syndrome. Special attention should be given to examination of the posterior nose to exclude epistaxis as a source of bleeding.

Jaundice:

Presence of jaundice would point towards hepatic failure.

Arthritis:

In cases of Henoch-Schonlein purpura, arthritis is usually localized to knees and ankles.

Examination of perianal region:

It is important to visualize the perianal region for the presence of anal fissure, any prolapse of rectum or polyp.

Examination of the abdomen:

An abdominal examination should be done for signs of portal hypertension (ascitis, prominent veins), masses or tenderness. Distension of abdomen would be present in case of volvulus of the midgut and in cases of intussusception. The abdomen should be carefully palpated for the presence of lump. A sausage-shaped mass may be felt in the upper mid-abdomen in case of intussusception.

C. Investigations

Apt test:

In the immediate neonatal period swallowed maternal blood is the commonest cause of rectal bleeding. This test which is based on alkali denaturation helps to differentiate adult Hb from foetal Hb and therefore maternal blood from neonatal blood.

Complete blood count:

Hemoglobin level will indicate the degree of anemia. Platelet count would be decreased in cases of thrombocytopenia, but normal in Henoch-Schonleinpurpura. Leucocytosis would suggest infection.

Urine and stool examination:

Urine examination for hematuria. Stool examination for presence of pus cells.

Prothrombin time and APTT:

Done in hemorrhagic disease of newborn and where coagulopathy is suspected to be the cause of bleeding.

Proctoscopy:

Done to exclude rectal polyp.

Skiagram of the abdomen:

In suspected NEC in the newborn bubbles of gas in the bowel wall (Pneumatosis intestinalis) is the hallmark of NEC. It is also done in volvulus and intussusception. A contrast enema is useful in intussusception.

Isotopic scanning:

Isotope scanning using technetium is done to identify gastric mucosa in suspected Meckel's diverticulum.

Angiography:

In selected cases of severe chronic unexplained iron deficiency anemia associated with positive fecal occult blood it may be necessary to perform angiography to localize the source of bleeding.

SUMMARY

In a child presenting with dark tarry stools one must enquire that the child is not receiving iron therapy, before proceeding to investigate. The common causes of rectal bleeding in children are dysentery, anal fissue and rectal polyp. Bleeding that needs urgent attention are children with intussusception and Meckel diverticulum. Majority of the cases can be diagnosed by proper history and examination. A few would need investigative procedures.

SUGGESTED READING

1. Owensky S, Taylor K, Wilkins T. Diagnosis and management of upper gastrointestinal bleeding in children. Journal of the American Board of Family Medic (2015) www.jabfm.org.

2. Wolfram Wayne. Pediatric gastrointestinal bleeding workup (2017).emedicine. medscape.com.

3. Patel N. Lower gastrointestinal bleeding in children: Causes and diagnostic approach. https://www.uptodate.com.

18

CONSTIPATION

INTRODUCTION

Constipation is a frequent problem among infants and children. Most often it is short lived and vast majority of children presenting with constipation have no serious underlying organic pathology. It is generally true that the younger the child the more likely it is that the problem is due to a congenital abnormality of the lower bowel.

DEFINITION

Normal bowel frequency varies widely. The average baby passes three to six stools per day in the neonatal period. One to two stools per day at 1 year of life and approximately one stool per day or every other day in the preschool years.

Any definition of constipation is relative and depends on stool consistency, stool frequency and difficulty in passing the stool. A normal breastfed baby may have a soft stool only every 2nd and 3rd day without difficulty. This is not constipation.

For practical clinical purposes, constipation is generally defined as infrequent defecation, painful defecation or both that has been present for 2 weeks or longer.

The term absolute constipation indicates absence of evacuation of feces and flatus and is due to intestinal obstruction from congenital or acquired conditions. Since this is a surgical emergency, it needs urgent attention. Most common symptom of absolute constipation is vomiting with abdominal distension.

ETIOLOGY

Most children suffering from constipation have no underlying medical condition. They are often labeled as having functional constipation or acquired megacolon.

Table: Causes of constipation

1. **Organic causes:**
   - **Intestinal:** Hirschprung disease, anal stenosis, anal fissure, ectopic anus, fistula-in-ano
   - **Drugs:** Narcotics, vincristine
   - **Endocrine:** Hypothyroidism, panhypopituitarism
   - **Neuromuscular:** Cerebral palsy, mental retardation, spinal cord lesions, myotonic dystrophy.
2. **Functional:**
   - **Dietary:** Poor intake of fluids, low fiber diet, excessive intake of proteins and fat
   - **Poor bowel habits:** Suppression of urge to defecate.

EVALUATION

Thorough history and examination will help to ascertain the cause of constipation.

A. History

Points in history

- Is constipation present since birth or has developed later?
- Type of stool
- Dietary history
- Pain associated with defecation
- History of drug intake
- History of passing blood in stools
- History of faecal incontinence
- History of vomiting
- History of prolonged jaundice, feeding difficulty in neonatal period
- Occupation of parents
- Developmental history

Since when is the child constipated?

The commonest cause of organic constipation with onset usually in the neonatal period is congenital aganglionic megacolon. History is often helpful in discriminating functional constipation from Hirschsprung disease. Asking parents when their child had his/her first bowel movement after birth is important. Nearly half of the infants with Hirschsprung disease do not pass meconium during the first 36 hours of life and are diagnosed with constipation within the first 4-6 months of life. Three important organic causes of constipation since birth are congenital megacolon, anal stenosis and hypothyroidism. Functional constipation typically starts after the neonatal period usually in a child older than 18 months.

Type of stools:

Stools of breastfed baby are golden yellow and loose in consistency, which is due to increased lactose content of human milk. The stool of a baby who is receiving top milk or formula milk are pale and firm in consistency. They tend to be constipated. The stools of an infant with congenital megacolon are pellet or ribbon like.

Dietary history:

A detailed dietary history must be taken. Improper diet is an important cause of constipation in toddlers and older children. Inadequate intake of fluids, cereals, vegetables and fruits, i.e. food with low fiber content can lead to constipation. Also excessive consumption of food stuffs rich in protein and fat can also result in constipation. In young infants functional constipation often develops at the time of a dietary transition (e.g. from breast milk to formula).

Bowel habits:

Enquire about the bowel habits. Does the child avoid going to the toilet? Toddlers are often too involved in their play and hence avoid going to the toilet. In older children it is usually due to lack of time in the morning to go to the toilet due to hurry to go to the school or inadequate facilities in school.

Parents often confuse withholding of stool with pain or excessive straining. Common withholding behaviors in young children are squatting, cross ankles, stiffening of the body, holding on to furniture, flushing sweating and crying.

In toddlers, functional constipation often develops near the time of toilet training. In older children, functional constipation often develops at the time of school entry, because they refuse to defecate while they are at school.

Is pain associated with defecation? Pain in the perianal region would suggest anal fissure or an inflammatory lesion in the perianal region. Any painful condition of the anorectal region can lead to constipation. Because of fear of pain child withholds the stool leading to further absorption of fluid from the gut and hardening of stool. Anal fissure can therefore be both cause and result of constipation.

Certain drugs are known to produce constipation viz. codeine, chlordiazepoxide, imipramine, vincristine.

Presence of a streak of blood on the surface of a hard stool is often seen in anal fissure.

In cases of severe constipation there can be history of encoporesis or faecal soiling. This is overflow soiling caused by passage of fluid stool.

In a child with cretinism there would be a history of feedingdifficulty and prolongation of jaundice in the neonatal period.

In cases of pyloric stenosis there is history of projectile vomiting from 2nd or 3rd week of life associated with constipation.

Occupation of parents:

In a child with chronic constipation one must enquire about the occupation of parents especially if it involves exposure to lead.

Developmental history:

Global developmental delay is an important feature of hypothyroidism also seen mostly in children with mental retardation.

B. Physical Examination

Points on examination

- Assessment of growth
- Presence of anemia
- Look for lead line
- Signs of hypothyroidism
- Examination of perineum and back
- Examination of abdomen
- Per-rectal examination

Assessment of growth:

Failure to thrive in a child would indicate an organic cause of constipation, e.g. in cases of congenital megacolon and pyloric stenosis.

Anemia:

One must look for the presence of anemia. Iron deficiency anemia is often observed in a child receiving mainly milk diet. Such a child would often be brought to the physician for constipation. His weight and height for age would be normal. Anemia would also be present in a child with long-standing constipation especially due to congenital megacolon. Children with chronic lead intoxication would also have anemia.

Signs of hypothyroidism:

Look carefully for signs of hypothyroidism viz. open fontanelle, dry skin, coarse features and short stature.

Examination of perineum and back:

One must look for an ectopic anus, anal fissure, proctitis and the back for meningomyelocele. Confirm the presence of an anal wink.

Examination of abdomen:

Distended abdomen would be seen in congenital megacolon and in cases of hypothyroidism.

Wrinkled abdominal wall in cases of Prune-Belly syndrome. Palpation of the abdomen may reveal fecoliths or a fecal mass in the lower abdomen.

Per-rectal examination:

In all children with constipation a per rectal examination is rewarding. In Hirschprung disease the rectum is empty as against functional constipation, where the rectum is loaded with fecal matter. An anal stenosis can also be diagnosed by per rectal examination.

Examination of CNS:

Examination of central nervous system would be important incases of mental retardation, cerebral palsy and neuromusculardisorders.

C. Investigations

Investigations are seldom required in children with constipation. A good history and clinical examination helps in arriving at a diagnosis in majority of the cases. However, in some situations investigations are needed.

Which investigations to be done?

- Estimation of T3, T4 and TSH
- Barium enema
- Rectal manometry
- Rectal biopsy
- Magnetic resonance imaging of spine

Estimation of T3, T4, TSH:

Whenever hypothyroidism is suspected estimation of T3, T4 and TSH should be done.

Barium enema:

There is no need to do barium enema in all cases of constipation to rule out Hirschsprung's disease. If the clinical suspicion is strong (based on history of delayed passage of meconium and empty rectum on digital examination), then only one should consider getting barium enema done). When barium enema is given in a case of congenital megacolon a transition zone is seen between normal dilated proximal colon and a smaller caliber obstructed distal colon caused by the aganglionic bowel.

Rectal manometry:

Investigations become important when one has to differentiate functional constipation from Hirschprung disease. Rectal manometry is a reliable diagnostic tool in cases of Hirschsprung disease. The accuracy is above 90 percent, but is technically difficult in infants.

Rectal biopsy:

A rectal biopsy would reveal absence of ganglion cells in the submucosa in case of congenital megacolon.

Magnetic resonance imaging of spine:

It is indicated where an intraspinal pathology is suspected.

SUMMARY

Constipation is a common symptom in toddlers and children. However, one must appreciate normal variation in frequency and consistency before starting treatment.The commonest cause for constipation is dietetic. Insufficient intake of water, food and fluids and diet rich in proteins cause constipation. Also babies whose diet is exclusively milk and whose weaning on semisolid feeds are delayed have constipation. Other common causes are neglect of bowel training and painful conditions, in the anorectal region. After excluding non-organic causes one should proceed to identify an organic cause such as congenital aganglionic megacolon.

SUGGESTED READING

1. Tabbers MM, DiLorenzo C, Berger MY et al. Evaluation and treatment of functional constipation in infants and children evidence based recommendations from ESPGHAN and NASPGHAN. J Pediatr Gastroenterol Nutr. 2014;58:258-74.

2. Khanna V, Poddar U, Yaccha SK. Constipation in Indian children: need for knowledge not the knife. Indian Pediatr. 2010;47:1025-30.

3. Poddar U. Approach to constipation. Indian Pediatr (2016);53:319-327.

STRIDOR

INTRODUCTION

Stridor is a harsh vibrating sound of variable pitch caused by partial obstruction of the airway resulting at the level of the supraglottis, glottis, subglottis or trachea resulting in turbulent airflow. It may be inspiratory or expiratory. Inspiratory stridor suggests airway obstruction above the glottis laryngeal level, while expiratory stridor is indicative of tracheobronchial obstruction. Biphasic suggests glottic or subglottic lesion.

Stridor should be differentiated from stertor, which is a low pitched, snoring type sound generated at the level of nasopharynx, oropharynx and occasionally supraglottis.

ETIOLOGY

Stridor is a symptom not a diagnosis or a disease and the underlying cause must be determined. Stridor may be acute, chronic or recurrent. Acute stridor usually results due to an inflammatory cause, trauma or foreign body; while chronic stridor is usually because of congenital anomaly of the larynx and trachea. In children, laryngomalacia is the most common cause of chronic stridor, while croup is the most common cause of acute stridor.

Table: Causes of stridor

1. **Acute stridor**
   - Inflammatory-acute epiglottitis, laryngotracheitis, retropharyngeal abscess.
   - Laryngeal diphtheria.
   - Foreign body in larynx.
   - Laryngeal spasm—tetany.
   - Laryngeal edema—angioneurotic, following instrumentation, anaphylaxis, epiglotitis
   - Bacterial tracheitis
   - Retropharyngeal abscess
   - Peritonsillar abscess

2. **Chronic or persistent stridor**
   a. Laryngeal
      - Laryngomalacia
      - Laryngeal webs, polyps, cysts
      - Vocal cord paralysis—unilateral/bilateral
      - Subglottic stenosis, hemangioma.
   b. Tracheal
      - Vascular ring
      - Tracheal stenosis, hemangioma
      - Tracheomalacia
      - Cystic hygroma.
   c. Recurrent stridor
      - Recurrent croup
      - Recurrent laryngotracheobronchitis.

EVALUATION

The most common presenting symptom is loud, raspy, noisy breathing. Depending on the underlying etiology, the presentation may be acute or chronic and may be accompanied by other symptoms.

A. History

A thorough history may provide helpful clues to the underlying etiology of stridor. When a child with stridor is brought it is essential to first assess whether the stridor is of an acute onset. Such a child if breathless needs immediate assessment and intervention. In case of chronic stridor a detailed history and examination can be done.

Points in history

- Age of onset, duration, severity and progression of the stridor
- Chronicity of stridor
- Birth history
- Developmental history
- History of atopy
- Precipitating factors (e.g. crying or feeding)
- Associated symptoms
- History of psychological stress

Age of onset:

Enquire whether the stridor is present since birth or did it appear later? Stridor present since birth is usually due to vocal cord paralysis, congenital anomalies such as laryngeal web, vascular ring or choanal atresia. Laryngomalacia, which accounts for 90 percent of cases of stridor usually manifests after the first or second week of birth.

The usual age of croup, epiglotitis and foreign body aspiration is 1 to 4 years.

Chronicity:

Has the stridor appeared suddenly or is it present over a period of time? Is the stridor recurrent? Acute onset of stridor is usually seen in case of foreign body aspiration, acute infections such as viral croup, acute epiglotitis and laryngeal diphtheria. Persistent stridor is a feature of congenital anomalies such as laryngomalacia, laryngeal web, vascular ring and laryngotracheal stenosis. Recurrent stridor in a child could be due to angioneurotic edema or recurrent laryngotracheobronchitis.

Birth history:

It is important to enquire about birth history especially if a newborn has stridor. Did the child have a difficult delivery? Was he asphyxiated at birth? Was he resuscitated? Was instrumentation done? Any history of aspiration of meconium or amniotic fluid at the time of birth? Intubation in a neonate can lead to trauma of the larynx, which can present as stidor. Also obstruction due to mucus, meconium or blood can produce stridor. However, such a stridor disappears in 24 hours. A surgical history should be obtained. Previous surgical treatment, particularly if it includes neck or cardiothoracic procedures, puts the recurrent laryngeal nerve at risk of injury.

Developmental history:

A detailed developmental history should be obtained. In addition, a history of color change, cyanosis, respiratory effort and apnea should be elicited to determine the severity of stridor. A feeding and growth history should be evaluated because significant airway obstruction can lead to lack of weight gain and growth. Regurgitation could be a sign of GER, which can cause laryngeal and tracheal mucosal irritation which in turn can lead to oedema and stridor.

Precipitating factors:

Enquire whether any factor relieves or accentuates the stridor. Does the stridor becomes worse on crying? Does any particular position worsen the stridor? Is there any preceding history of upper respiratory infection? Is there any history of sudden choking before the onset of stridor. In case of laryngomalacia and tracheomalacia stridor becomes worse on straining, crying or whenever the child is placed in the supine position and during feeds. It disappears during sleep and rest. In a child with macroglossia or micrognathia, stridor is exaggerated in the supine position and is relieved in the prone position. In viral and spasmodic croup the stridor is worst at night. Worsening of the stridor with feeding is also seen in vascular compression and neurologic disease. Viral croup and bacterial tracheitis is often preceded by upper respiratory infection. History of sudden choking followed by stridor is seen in foreign body aspiration. The common objects aspirated by children are coins and food viz corn, peanuts, etc.

Associated symptoms:

An attempt should be made to enquire whether the child has symptoms other than stridor. Is he coughing? Is there any alteration in the voice or cry of the child? Does the child snore during sleep? Is there any difficulty in swallowing? Barking cough is seen in croup. Brassy cough is a feature of tracheal lesion, weak cry is characteristic of supraglottic obstruction, laryngeal anomaly and neuromuscular disorders. Muffled cry is seen in supraglottic lesion. Hoarseness of voice is typical of croup and vocal cord paralysis. In case of tracheal lesion, the cry and voice are normal. Children with adenoids and hypertrophied tonsils often snore during sleep. Drooling of saliva is seen in epiglottitis, foreign body, esophagus and retropharyngeal or peritonsillar abscess. In case of supraglottic lesion and vascular ring the child can complaint of dysphagia.

History of atopy:

Does the child have a history of atopy? Children with history of allergy can develop acute stridor due to angioneurotic edema. Although the exact cause of recurrent croup is not known allergy is considered to be a probable cause. Other causes are gastroesophageal reflux.

B. Clinical Examination

Points on examination
- General appearance
- Quality of stridor
- Type of cough and cry
- Vitals
- Examination of neck and throat
- General examination
- Examination of the chest

On initial presentation, especially if the symptoms are of acute onset, the child should be immediately assessed for severity of stridor and respiratory compromise. Special attention should be paid to the following:
- Heart and respiratory rates
- Cyanosis
- Use of accessory muscles of respiration
- Nasal flaring
- Level of consciousness
- Responsiveness

Physical examination of a patient with suspected acute epiglotitis is contraindicated. The following if present should be noted:
- Infection in oral cavity, diphtheric membrane
- Masses in soft tissues of the face, neck or chest
- Deviation of the trachea

Observe the character of the cough, cry and voice.

Presence of fever and toxicity implies serious bacterial infection.

Careful auscultation of the nose, oropharynx, neck and chest helps to locate the site of stridor. Assess growth. It is helpful in evaluation of chronic stridor.

General appearance:

Firstly, one must assess whether the child appears sick, toxic and restless. Such an appearance would suggest acute epiglotitis, acute laryngeal diphtheria, acute laryngotracheobronchitis or sudden aspiration of a foreign body. Also observe the position of the child. If he keeps the neck hyperextended it suggests extrinsic obstruction at or above the larynx. Leaning over and drooling is seen in epiglotitis. If the intensity of stridor decreases in prone position it favors laryngomalacia.

Quality of stridor:

Listen carefully whether the stridor is purely inspiratory, expiratory or both? Stridor that is entirely inspiratory is due to lesion above the glottis. The one that is entirely expiratory is due to a tracheobronchial lesion. Biphasic stridor suggests glottic or subglottic lesion. Low-pitched stridor suggests supraglottic lesion, while high-pitched, inspiratory or expiratory stridor denotes severe subglottic obstruction.

Type of cough and cry:

Stridor with barking cough is seen in tracheal lesions. Stridor with hoarse voice or cry is seen in lesions involving glottis. In subglottic or tracheal lesion the cry is normal.

Vitals:

In any child who presents with stridor it is essential to record the vital signs. Presence of tachycardia points towards cardiac failure.

Presence of fever would suggest an underlying infection. Count the respiratory rate and look for signs of dyspnea, especially suprasternal, intercostal and subcostal retraction. Respiratory distress is commonly observed in acute epiglottis, acute laryngitis laryngeal diphtheria and foreign body in the larynx.Presence of cyanosis is usually seen in cyanotic heart disease and also when the obstruction is in the air passage is severe as in case of acute epiglottis, foreign body in the larynx and laryngeal diphtheria.

Examination of neck and throat:

The neck should be examined for presence of a mass, which may cause pressure giving rise to stridor such as cystic hygroma or thyroglossal cyst. A bull neck with cervical lymphadenitis is a feature of diphtheria. Observe for the presence of micrognathia. It leads to obstruction of hypopharynx due to posterior displacement oftongue. In such a situation stridor worsens in supine position. Micrognathia is a feature of Pierre-Robin and Treacher-Collin syndrome. Next look for macroglossia. A large tongue obstructs the hypopharyx. It is commonly seen in several syndromes viz. Beckwith-Wiedemann syndrome, Down syndrome, glycogen storage disease and hypothyroidism. The oral cavity should be examined for hypertrophic tonsils/adenoids as they lead to obstruction of supraglottic airway. The intensity of stridor in this condition is more during sleep.In case of peritonsillar abscess, the child will have difficulty in opening the mouth. In retropharyngeal abscess the child will keep the neck hyperextended. In both the conditions there will be drooling of saliva and dysphagia.

General examination:

Look for cutaneous hemangioma. Its presence may point towards subglottic hemangioma, which may be responsible for the stridor. Presence of urticaria would suggest angioneurotic edema of the larynx tongue, etc. responsible for the stridor. If the child has a peripheral neuropathy vocal cord paralysis could be the cause of stridor.

Examination of the chest:

The chest should be thoroughly examined. A prolonged inspiratory phase suggests laryngeal obstruction, while prolonged expiratory phase, indicates tracheal obstruction. If there is unilateral decreased air entry in the chest, foreign body in the ipsilateral bronchus should be considered.

C. Investigations

Depending upon the probable cause relevant investigations should be done.

Table: Which investigations to be done?

Investigation	Probable Cause
1. X-ray neck	Adenoidal hypertrophy
• Retropharyngeal bulge	Retropharyngeal abscess
• Thumb like thickening	Epiglottis
2. X-ray chest and neck	
• Radio-opaque shadow	Foreign body aspiration
• Steeple sign	Croup
3. Barium swallow	
• Useful in	Compression by vascular anomaly
• Reflux present	GE reflux
4. Endoscopy useful in	Foreign body, laryngeal web, polyp
5. CT scan and MRI done to visualize	Airway and surrounding soft tissue structure
6. CBC	
• Leucocytosis	Abscesses

Radiological assessment:

Anterior and lateral views of neck are useful in the assessment of adenoidal and tonsillar size, epiglottic size and shape, retropharyngeal profile, subglottic and tracheal anatomy. Soft tissue bulge in the posterior pharyngeal wall will suggest retropharyngeal abscess. Thumb-like thickening will be seen in epiglotitis. X-ray chest anteroposterior (AP) and lateral views is diagnostic in case of radio-opaque foreign body. It also helps in concomitant pulmonary disease. Foreign body can lead to air trapping producing hyperlucent lung field on ipsilateral side and shift of mediastinum to the opposite side. In case of croup X-ray neck reveals characteristic narrowing of the subglottic region known as the 'steeple sign' also called as wine bottle sign.

Barium swallow:

Barium swallow of the esophagus is done to rule out extrinsic compression by vascular anomaly. It is also useful in case of gastroesophageal reflux.

Endoscopy:

Flexible and rigid endoscopy is indicated in case of foreign body aspiration and vocal cord paralysis. It is also indicated in laryngeal webs, polyps, etc.

Computed tomography and magnetic resonance imaging:

Computed tomography scan and magnetic resonance imaging - are done to visualize airway and surrounding soft tissue structure including any evidence of vascular compression.

Complete blood count:

Complete blood count - indicated where cause of stridor is infective.

Throat swab examination:

If a membrane is present in the throat smear examination and culture should be done for C. diphtheriae.

SUMMARY

Stridor or noisy breathing is generally due to upper airway obstruction. Although it may be the result of a relatively benign process, it may also be the first sign of a serious and even life- threatening disorder. Stridor can be inspiratory, expiratory or biphasic. Laryngomalacia is the most common cause of stridor in children followed by viral croup. If a child presents with acute stridor the possibility of foreign body in the larynx should be kept in mind.

SUGGESTED READING

1.   Benson BE, Ravindhra G, Ellure et al. Stridor. Emedicine. Medscape.

COUGH

INTRODUCTION

Cough is the most common presenting symptom in primary care settings. It is a protective mechanism which, serves to expel foreign matter inhaled by accident and to remove secretions from the air passage to keep it clear.

Cough can impact a child's activity level and ability to sleep, play or attend school and is often a source of parental anxiety.

Cough in children differs in several ways from that in adults. Expectoration does not ordinarily accompany cough in children. They often vomit the phlegm or swallow it. Cough as a symptom is rare in a newborn. In an older infant however, it is almost always a symptom of lower respiratory tract infection and therefore shouldnot be dismissed lightly.

ETIOLOGY

Table: Causes of cough

1. Infections of respiratory tract:
   a. Upper respiratory tract: Common cold, sinusitis, pharyngitis, laryngitis
   b. Lower respiratory tract: Bronchitis, bronchiolitis, pneumonias, pertussis, measles, bronchiectasis, lung abscess.
2. Hyperactive airways: Allergic rhinitis with postnasal drip, asthma.
3. Aspiration syndrome: Gastroesophageal (GE) reflux, cleft palate, mental retardation, epilepsy, esophageal stricture,tracheoesophageal (TO) fistula, palatopharyngeal incompetence, neuromuscular in-coordination.
4. Foreign body inhalation: Aspiration of peanut, corn, seeds, etc.
5. Congenital anomalies: Congenital lobar emphysema, cystic adenomatoid malformation.
6. Mediastinal compression: Lymph nodes, tumors, cysts, aberrant vessel.
7. Pulmonary edema: Large left to right shut, left sided failure.
8. Defects of mucus clearance: Cystic fibrosis, ciliarydyskinesias.
9. Drug: Angiotensin-converting enzyme (ACE) inhibitors.
10. Functional.

EVALUATION

There are several causes of cough in children, but the commonest cause in office practice is viral infection of upper respiratory tract. Hyperactive airway disease is the next common cause.

Certain conditions need immediate attention such as an infant who presents with cough (as cough reflex is absent in very young infants), a child having respiratory distress and where there is a history of foreign body aspiration.

Approach to a child with cough is best done by enquiring about the duration of cough and age of the child. Acute cough is one that lasts for less than 4 weeks. Chronic cough lasts for more than 4 weeks. Most cases of acute cough in children are associated with viral upper respiratory infection. Preschool children continue to cough for nearly 3 weeks after a respiratory tract infection. While school age children continue to cough for 10 days after the onset of common cold. There are specific causes of chronic cough enumerated in table on the basis of the age of the child.

Table: Common causes of chronic cough based on child's age

	Children (< 5 years)	Older children (> 5 years)
1.	Infections (viral)	Asthma
2.	Gastroesophageal reflux	Infection
3.	Congenital malformation	Post nasal drip
4.	Asthma	Environmental pollution
5.	Environmental pollution	Bronchiectasis
6.	Foreign body inhalation	Psychogenic cough

Non specificcough is dry cough in the absence of an identifiable respiratory disease of known aetiology. Majority of the cases are due to non seriousaetiology, e.g. post viral cough and/or increased cough receptor sensitivity and may spontaneously resolve. Specific cough is associated with other symptoms and signs suggestive of an underlying problem.

Indicators of the presence of specific cough

- Coughing initiates suddenly with a choking episodes
- Coughing is progressive
- Shortness of breath chronic or exertional
- Failure to thrive
- Hypoxemia
- Constitutional symptoms
- Clubbing
- Hemoptysis
- Chest wall deformity
- Noisy breathing and / or abnormal lung auscultation
- History of recurrent pneumonia
- Cough in neonatal period
- Swallowing difficulty
- Craniofacial abnormality
- Neuromuscular disorder
- Wet cough lasting more than 3 to 4 weeks

A. HISTORY

Points in history

- Age of the child
- Onset and duration of cough
- Type of cough
- Is it wet or dry?
- Any history of fever
- Is there running nose, earache, sore throat, etc.
- Aggravating and relieving factors
- Any history of allergy, asthma, tuberculosis, heart disease
- History of choking and snoring
- Is cough associated with wheezing?
- History of taking drugs
- History of contact with tuberculosis.

Age of the child:

Causes of cough vary according to age, younger the infant more significant is the cough. In a child with chronic cough, with onset since birth one must think of congenital anomalies such as H-type tracheoesophageal fistula, laryngeal webs, vascular rings, etc. Cough starting in 1st month could be due to congenital infections leading to interstitial pneumonia. If the onset of cough is since early infancy one must consider the possibility of gastro-esophageal reflux. With onset in late infancy one must consider hyperactive airway disease, cystic fibrosis and whooping cough. In a toddler, common causes are viral infections of the respiratory tract, hyperactive airway disease, foreign body aspiration, chronic suppurative lung disease. Causes that can give rise to cough at all ages are asthma, tuberculosis, viral bronchitis, whooping cough and foreign body aspiration.

Onset and duration:

If cough persists beyond 2 to 3 weeks, it is considered chronic or persistent. Acute onset is usually seen in viral respiratory infections, asthma or pneumonias. Abrupt onset of cough without any other symptoms suggest foreign body aspiration.

Is cough recurrent or persistent?

It is very important to find out whether the cough is recurrent or persistent, i.e. whether the child becomes absolutely normal in between episodes of cough. If such is the case the cause most likely is bronchial asthma. Other causes could be aspiration syndromes or recurrent respiratory infections in immunodeficient patients. If cough is persistent over several weeks one must consider pressure over tracheobronchial tree due to lymph node or tumors.

Other reasons could be chronic sinusitis, foreign body aspiration, pertusis syndrome, GE reflux, endobronchial tuberculosis, cystic fibrosis and bronchiectasis.

Type of cough:

Ask about the nature of cough. Paroxysmal cough is seen in bronchial asthma, adenoviral infection, foreign body inhalation and pertusis.

A barking brassy cough suggests laryngitis, while anirritative cough could be a feature of pharyngitis. Cough is feeble in neuromuscular disease. Cough of psychogenic nature has a honking character. Throat clearing cough is seen in cases of postnasal drip.

Is the cough productive or non-productive?

Usually infants and young children do not expectorate, although the cough may be associated with secretions in the throat. A bout of cough is often followed by vomiting in infants and children.

In older children presence of copious purulent sputum, suggests suppurative lung disease such as bronchiectasis or lung abscess.

Hemoptysis is uncommon in children and if present indicates bronchiectasis.

History of fever:

If a child develops cough with high fever it often indicates acute viral infection. Fever will also be a symptom in pneumonias.

Whenever a child with chronic cough gets fever tuberculosis should be thought of. Even in suppurative lung disease, the child will have persistent or recurrent fever with cough. Is cough associated with running nose, earache or sore throat? Presence of these symptoms would indicate that the cough is due to upper respiratory tract involvement, either viral or bacterial.

Aggravating and relieving factors:

Timing of the cough also gives clue to the cause of cough. Dry cough, which is mainly nocturnal or in the early hours of the day suggest bronchial asthma. Cough, which is more at night can also be due to postnasal drip seen in sinusitis.

In infants if the cough worsens during feeds and the child gets choked the cause could be aspiration seen in GE reflux. Cough, which appears on lying down is also a feature of GE reflux.

If exercise or dust induces cough, it points towards hyperactive airway disease. In case of functional cough usually seen in little older children cough subsides during sleep and is much less when distracted. If cough is relieved by bronchodilators, it suggests hyperactive airway disease.

History of choking:

If there is a history that the child gets choked with a bout of cough it could be whooping cough or aspiration in a patient with GE reflux or following esophageal stricture. It is also a feature of H- type tracheoesophageal fistula.

Snoring and mouth breathing:

Snoring and mouth breathing could be because of adenoidal hypertrophy.

Associated wheezing:

Cough associated with wheezing, the cause is hyperactive airway disease.

History of drugs:

Child receiving ACE inhibitors can have cough.

History of contact:

In a child with cough persisting over several weeks, one must enquire for history of contact with an open case of pulmonary tuberculosis. If there is a suspicion of whooping cough, a history in other siblings or children in the neighborhood with a similar cough should be enquired.

History of malabsorption:

Does the child pass large bulky stools. This may indicate mucoviscidosis.

History of allergy:

Is cough seasonal? Is it associated with sneezing? Does the child get urticarial rash? Allergy is the cause of cough if it is seasonal and often associated with sneezing and running nose. A history of atopy may also be obtained in such cases.

B.   EXAMINATION

Points on examination

- Assessment of growth
- General appearance
- Facies
- Anemia, cyanosis, clubbing
- Lymphadenopathy
- Eyes
- Ear, nose and throat
- Noisy breathing
- Systemic examination
- Evidence of infection other than the respiratory tract

Cough can be classified as acute or chronic, specific and non-specific. Dry cough can be converted to wet cough when airway secretions increase. Young children rarely expectorate sputum, so wet cough rather than productive cough is the preferred term. Wet cough indicates an underlying cause of mucous hypersecretion or impaired mucociliary clearance whereas dry cough indicates an underlying cause of airway irritation or inflammation. Wet cough warrants detailed investigation whenever it becomes chronic or associated with other manifestations e.g. failure to thrive or clubbing.

Growth assessment:

Assessment of growth is very important in a child with chronic cough. Failure to thrive would be observed in a child with tuberculosis, suppurative lung disease, mucoviscidosis and heart disease with cardiac failure.

General appearance:

Sick emaciated appearance would suggest a chronic illness. In an acute attack of bronchial asthma, the child is dyspneic and has difficulty in speaking.

In case of hypertrophied adenoids, one must look for adenoid facies, which is characterized by long narrow face, short upper lip mouth breathing and in some nasal speech.

Anemia / cyanosis / clubbing:

Anaemia would indicate a chronic illness. Clubbing points towards suppurative lung disease and cyanotic heart disease. Presence of central cyanosis would suggest a cyanotic heart disease.

Lymphadenopathy:

The child should be carefully examined for lymphadenopathy. Enlarged tender lymph nodes in the neck could be a feature of upper respiratory tract infection such as tonsillitis. Matted lymph nodes with sinuses would point towards tuberculosis. If the lymph nodes are significantly enlarged and firm think of lymphoma, in such a situation cough could be due to enlarged lymph nodes in the mediastinum causing compression.

Examination of eyes, ears, nose and throat:

The presence of subconjunctival hemorrhage in a child with paroxysmal cough suggests whooping cough. The ears, nose and throat should be carefully examined for rhinitis, otitis, pharyngitis, tonsillitis and postnasal drip. Tenderness over frontal and maxillary sinuses would indicate sinusitis.

Noisy breathing:

Presence of stridor or hoarseness of voice would suggest laryngeal involvement. Grunting is observed in alveolar pathology, while wheezing is present in hyperactive airway disease and cystic fibrosis.

Systemic examination:

The respiratory system should be carefully examined for signs of consolidation, collapse, emphysema, pneumothorax.

Presence of bilateral crepitations would suggest bronchopneumonia, while scattered rhonchi all over is a feature of hyperactive airway disease. Silent chest in a child who comes with cough and respiratory distress is a feature of an acute attack of bronchial asthma.

Look for murmur, cardiomegaly, evidence of congestive cardiac failure, which may be responsible for the cough.

Examine the child carefully for any neuromuscular disease, especially if the cough is weak.

C. INVESTIGATIONS

S. No.	Investigations	Probable Diagnosis
1.	Complete blood count	
	• Leucocytosis	Bacterial infection
	• Leucocytosis with absolute lymphocytosis	Whooping cough
	• Eosinophilia	Hyperactive airway disease
2.	Skiagram chest	
	• Persistent patch at same spot	Tuberculosis, congenital anomaly, foreign body
3.	Skiagramparanasal sinuses	
	• Haziness present	Sinusitis
4.	Skiagramnasopharynx	Adenoids
5.	Bronchoscopy	Foreign body aspirationEndobronchial tuberculosis
6.	Milk scan	
	• Reflux present	Gastroesophageal reflux
7.	Mantoux test	
	• Positive	Tuberculosis
8.	2-D Echocardiography	Heart disease
9.	CT scan of chest	Congenital anomalies, tumour, lymph nodes

Complete blood count:

Leukocytosis will be present in cases of bacterial infection.

Whooping cough is characterized by elevated leukocyte count with absolute lymphocytosis. Eosinophilia could be seen in cases of hyperactive airway disease.

X-ray chest:

Skiagram of the chest is done in almost all cases of chronic or persistent cough. If X-ray shows a persistent patch at the same spot it could be due to tuberculosis, congenital anomaly or foreign body. If the picture is that of multifocal lesions one must consider aspirations, bronchial asthma or mucociliary defects. Focal lesions could be due to tumor, cyst, lymph nodes in majority of the cases.

X-ray paranasal sinuses:

Indicated in suspected cases of chronic sinusitis.

X-ray nasopharynx:

A lateral view of nasopharynx should be done to look for adenoidal hypertrophy.

Bronchoscopy:

In suspected foreign body aspiration and endobronchial tuberculosis bronchoscopy should be considered.

Milk scan / barium swallow:

If the cause of cough appears to be due to a GE reflux milk scan is indicated.

MantouxTest:

A tuberculin test is indicated in all cases of chronic cough, to rule out tuberculosis.

2-D Echocardiography

Indicated in children with heart disease.

Computerized Tomography of the Chest:

It is informative in structural abnormalities such as congenitalanomalies, tumors, lymph nodes.

SUMMARY

Cough is the commonest presentation of respiratory disease in children. The nature of cough and its accompanying symptoms and signs should be closely observed as they often provide a clue to diagnosis. The commonest cause of cough in children is common cold (coryza), followed by hyperactive airway disease. Cough in a young infant especially under 6 months of age is unusual and should be evaluated. If a child presents with sudden onset of cough with respiratory distress one should rule out foreign body aspiration, while a child with persistent cough needs thorough clinical evaluation and investigation.

SUGGESTED READING

Haya Alsubaie, Abdullah Al. Shamrani. Approach to cough in children. International Journal of Pediatrics and Adolescent Medicine 2015;2:38-43.

CRYING

INTRODUCTION

Crying is the normal physiological response to many stimuli in non-verbal children. Healthy children cry for about 3 hours per day on an average at 6 weeks of age. There is little consensus about the definition of abnormal cry in the literature. Various terminologies used for abnormal cry, incessant cry, persistent cry, excessive cry and problem crying. The incidence is high beyond 6 months of age. Incessant crying is one of the common reasons for many emergency visits during infancy which often leads to considerable parental stress.

Incessant crying can lead to parental frustration disturbed parent child relationship and problems like shaken baby syndrome resulting in brain damage.

ETIOLOGY

Children of all ages cry, but frequency is more in a younger child. Mostly the causes are trivial or non-organic.

Causes of crying

- **Non-organic / trivial:**

  Hunger, sleep and feeding disturbances, thirst, loneliness, wet diaper, tired, loud noise, excess heat or cold, overclothing, light clothing, soiled napkin, sudden noise, strong light on face, sudden change in position, stranger anxiety, separation from mother or care giver, stopping of pleasurable activity, fall, punishment, dispute with playmates, attention seeking device

- **Organic causes:**
  - GIT: Infantile colic, constipation, anal fissure, GE reflux, intestinal obstruction, intussusception
  - Genito-urinary system: UTI, torsion testis, urinary retention, obstructed hernia (inguinal and femoral)
  - Infections: AOM, meningitis, herpes, cellulitis, pneumonia
  - Musculoskeletal: Trauma, child abuse, septic arthritis, osteomyelitis
  - Other causes: Foreign body, burns, diaper rash, cow's milk allergy, sickle cell crises, DPT immunization, insect bite, pseudotumor cerebri

---

EVALUATION

The causes of incessant crying range from trivial illness to life threatening diseases hence examination and arriving at a diagnosis is always a concern. The following are pointers for underlying organic cause:

- High pitched / abnormal sounding cry
- Lack of diurnal rhythm
- Presence of frequent regurgitations, vomiting, diarrhea, blood in stools, weight loss, failure to thrive
- Family history of migraine, asthma, atopy, eczema
- Positive physical examination
- Persistence of crying past 4 months of age

A. History

Although some infants cry more than others, the triggers for crying remain a puzzle.

> **Points in history**
> - Duration, frequency of crying
> - Periodicity & intensity
> - Aggravating and alleviating factors
> - Co-morbid medical conditions
> - Insect bite
> - Sibling and family history
> - Recent vaccination
> - Feeding and sleep behavior
> - Mother-infant relationship
> - Maternal fatigue and stress

Age of the child:

Causes vary according to age of the child. It is often a challenge to diagnose the cause of crying in a young infant. Crying in an infant does not have the same meaning as it does in an older child. It has many meanings not just pain, sadness or frustration. In the early weeks, some of the reasons for crying are hunger, wet napkin, tight clothes and loneliness. After the first 2 to 3 weeks until 3 to 4 months most babies keep fussing and crying. Some of them cry limited to one period in the evening or afternoon. Such babies are thought to be suffering from colic. Infantile colic is defined as paroxysmal crying more than 3 hours/day occurring more than 3 days/week, lasting for more than 3 weeks in an otherwise healthy child who is more than 3 weeks and less than 4 months of age. Colic is diagnosis of exclusion. The period from birth to about 3 to 4 months is one of adjustment of the baby's immature nervous and digestive system. Other babies cry anytime during the day or night. Crying in older children is more understandable. It is either due to pain, sadness or frustration.

Onset and duration of crying:

One must enquire since when is the child crying? Is this the first time that the infant is crying or does he/she invariably cry daily for a few hours? Does the child cry during any specific time of the day or night? If the parents complaint of inconsolable crying in their infant since the past few hours, it indicates acute pain usually due to a colic or earache. It is often observed in case of otitis media that the child wakes up from sleep with unconsolable crying. There is usually a preceding history of upper respiratory infection. Such unconsolable crying is also seen in some children following DPT vaccination.

Neonates with intracranial hemorrhage, meningitis or encephalitis may cry continuously. As the child grows crying may arise from situations where his pride is hurt or where he faces a frustrating experience.

Aggravating and relieving factors:

It is essential to enquire whether certain factors aggravate crying. Also find out what soothes the baby?

Is the child tired? The more the child is fatigued the more he/ she cries. Any history of illness in the baby? Just before the onset of illness the child may cry excessively. Even after a prolonged illness the child is irritable and cranky and wants to be picked up. Is the crying relieved as soon as the infant passes flatus. Most infants cry when they are hungry. But settle down as soon as they are fed. Others cry violently if there is some delay in giving the food and refuse feeding altogether. The mother should also be asked whether the child cries after feeds? Does he get restless? Does he vomit? In case of GE reflux the child after feeds becomes restless, irritable, cries and vomits. This is because of the intense burning of the esophagus due to reflux of gastric contents. Most infants cry when they are lonely and quieten down the moment they are picked up.

Infants and toddlers often cry when the mother goes out. This occurs on a regular basis till the child gets used to the caregiver. The child is otherwise healthy.

Behaviour of the child:

Enquire about the behaviour of the child. Is he a very demanding child? Does he keep throwing temper tantrums?

Many infants and children cry incessantly for petty things and are very demanding. Some cry and hold their breath if their wish is not fulfilled.

Co-morbid conditions:

Enquire for co-morbid conditions such as earache, vomiting, diarrhea, trauma, swelling and pain in any part of the body.

B. Physical Examination

Physical examination should first ascertain whether the infant is healthy or ill-looking as life threatening conditions are not uncommon with incessant crying.

> **Point on examination**
> - Healthy or sick
> - Vital signs
> - Head to foot examination
> - Systemic examination

Examination should first ascertain whether the infant is healthy or ill-looking. Recording of vitals should be done followed by top to toe examination. Eyes should be examined for redness and eyelids everted for any foreign body. The type of cry also needs to be documented as it often gives a diagnostic clue e.g. high pitched incessant cry may indicate central nervous system infection. Continuous cry associated with grunting may indicate respiratory infection / foreign body. Screaming and pulling at the ears may indicate AOM. Intermittent bouts of cry associated with pallor and drawing of the knees over abdomen may indicate intussusception. Paroxysmal crying episodes in the evening in a healthy infant would indicate infantile colic.

Incessant crying beyond 3 months of age associated with hyperactivity, cognitive deficits, poor fine motor abilities may point towards a mentally challenged child. Cry of a full term baby is lusty, while cry of a premature baby is weak. Croupy cry is seen in laryngotracheobronchitis. In Cri-du-chat syndrome cry is cat like.

One must look for bulging tympanic membrane, anal fissure, obstructed hernia, torsion testis, rib fracture open diaper pin injury, tender swollen gums during teething, bulging fontanelle, signs of meningeal irritation, abdominal distension, lump in the abdomen and diaper rash.

C. Investigations

The role of investigations in identifying the cause of crying in infants is limited. It may help in only 3 to 5% cases where history and examination findings are inconclusive. In nearly all cases clinical assessment should guide decision making about sequential investigations.

Following are some of the investigations which may be needed.

- Urine examination: microscopic and culture
- Stool examination for occult blood
- Milk scan in suspected GERD
- USG abdomen in suspected intussusception and intestinal obstruction

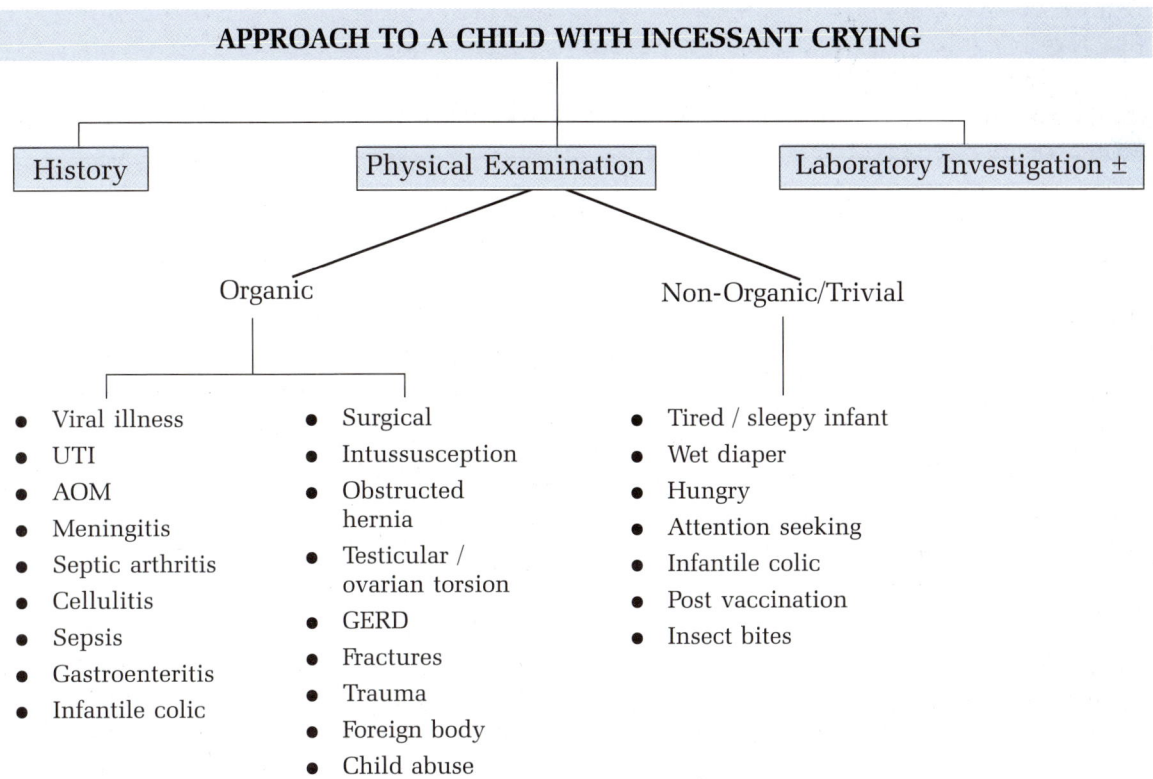

APPROACH TO A CHILD WITH INCESSANT CRYING

History | Physical Examination | Laboratory Investigation ±

Organic | Non-Organic/Trivial

Organic:
- Viral illness
- UTI
- AOM
- Meningitis
- Septic arthritis
- Cellulitis
- Sepsis
- Gastroenteritis
- Infantile colic

- Surgical
- Intussusception
- Obstructed hernia
- Testicular / ovarian torsion
- GERD
- Fractures
- Trauma
- Foreign body
- Child abuse

Non-Organic/Trivial:
- Tired / sleepy infant
- Wet diaper
- Hungry
- Attention seeking
- Infantile colic
- Post vaccination
- Insect bites

SUGGESTED READING

1. Arumugam J, Sivandam S, Vijaylakshmi AM: Evaluation and management of incessantly crying infant. Sri Lanka Journal of Child Health 2012;41(4):192-198.

22

JOINT PAINS

INTRODUCTION

Joint pain is a common symptom for which a child often comes to a pediatrician.

The term arthritis denotes inflammation of the joint manifested by pain, heat, redness, swelling and limited motion, while arthralgia means simply pain in joints with full range of motion.

ETIOLOGY

Table: Causes of arthritis

- Infections: Arthritis (viral, septic, tubercular), osteomyelitis
- Trauma
- Acute rheumatic fever
- Rheumatological disorders-Juvenile idiopathic arthritis, systemic lupus erythematosus (SLE), Kawasaki disease, dermatomyositis, Henoch Schonlein-purpura
- Scurvy
- Blood diseases-sickle cell disease, hemophilia, leukemia
- Reactive arthritis
- Malignancies
- Psychogenic

EVALUATION

A. History

Points in history

- Mode of onset and duration of joint involvement
- Whether there is involvement of single or multiple joints?
- History of trauma, illness or drug intake
- History of fever or other systemic manifestations
- Relationship of pain to activity and sleep
- History of bleeding diathesis
- Is the child suffering from any blood diseases?
- Dietary history
- Family history

Mode of onset and duration of joint involvement:

One must enquire about duration of illness at the time of presentation. If the duration is less than 2 weeks, it is acute, subacute if the duration is 2 to 6 weeks and chronic if the duration is more than 6 weeks. Conditions presenting as acute arthritis are acute rheumatic fever, septic arthritis, Henoch-Schonleinpurpura, trauma and transient synovitis. Subacute onset is seen in reactive arthritis, arthritis associated with SLE, dermatomyositis, polyarteritisnodosa, leukemias, sickle cell disease and hemarthrosis. Chronic arthritis is a feature of juvenile idiopathic arthritis, tubercular arthritis and psoriasis.

Joint involvement:

How many joints are affected single or multiple? Which joints are affected?

Single joint affection is usually seen in cases of tuberculosis, septic arthritis and trauma. Multiple joint involvement is seen in systemic disease.

Large joints are affected in most of the conditions, but small joint affection is seen in juvenile idiopathic arthritis, sickle cell disease (hand-foot syndrome) and also in tubercular dactylitis.

History of preceding illness or trauma:

Did the child sustain injury? Did he/she suffer from upper respiratory infection in the recent past? Did he/she suffer from any viral infections? Did he/she receive any drugs?

Trauma can give rise to pain in several ways. It can lead to hemarthrosis, effusion, strained ligaments, sprained muscles, dislocation or fracture. A preceding history of upper respiratory catarrh would suggest transient synovitis. It is a self-limiting condition characterized by sudden onset of pain in hips, thighs and knees following an upper respiratory infection. Viral infections such as mumps, chickenpox, infectious mononucleosis, hepatitis B are known to give rise to monoarticularsynovitis. Drugs such as penicillins, immunoglobulins and antitoxins are known to give rise to arthritis/arthralgia.

History of fever:

Does the child have fever with joint pains? Since how long? Is fever high grade or low grade?

A history of acute onset of high grade fever with chills and joint swelling would suggest septic arthritis. In tubercular arthritis also there would be fever of long-standing, usually low grade and continuous. Prolonged high grade irregular fever with remissions would suggest idiopathic arthritis or SLE. Prolonged fever with joint involvement would also be seen in leukemias.

Relationship of pain to activity and sleep:

Pain that is worse on activity is indicative of destructive joint disease, whereas pain and stiffness early in the morning and which decreases by evening isindicative of juvenile idiopathic arthritis.

History of bleeding:

Is there bleeding from any site?

Bleeding from gums would suggest scurvy. Bleeding with hemarthrosis on trivial injury would suggest hemophilia.

Bleeding per rectum with pain in abdomen is characteristic of Henoch-Schonleinpurpura.

Progression and character of pain:

Progression of joint involvement and character of pain must be enquired. Migratory symptoms present in one joint for a few days and then remit only to reappear in some other joint is classically seen in rheumatic fever. If new joints are progressively involved while initial joints being affected at the same time i.e. additive symptoms is seen in SLE, JIA and psoriatic arthritis. Intermittent joint involvement in which the symptoms appear and disappear with completely asymptomatic periods in between are seen in reactive arthritis.

History of blood diseases:

Is the child suffering from any blood disease such as sickle cell disease, leukemia or hemophilia.Hemarthrosis is seen in bleeding disorder and hand foot syndrome in sickle cell anemia.

Dietary history:

A detailed dietetic history should be elicited especially when there is a suspicion of scurvy.

B. Clinical Examination

After having elicited a thorough history, it is essential to carry out examination of the joints involved. Apart from local examination of the joints, a thorough systemic examination is essential to exclude a systemic disease responsible for joint involvement.

Physical signs
- Local examination of joint/joints involved
- Examination of the spine
- Examination of the muscles
- Presence of rash/subcutaneous nodules
- Lymphadenopathy/sinuses
- Eyes
- Oral cavity
- Desquamation of fingers
- Any focus of infection
- Organomegaly
- Cardiovascular system

Examination of joints:

Joints should be thoroughly examined for swelling, pain, tenderness and range of movements.

It is essential to differentiate arthralgia from arthritis. If there is only pain in the joints it is arthralgia and if pain is associated with joint swelling it is arthritis. Next one must see which are the joints affected. Involvement of a single joint is more likely to be due to infection or trauma, while multiple joint involvement suggests generalized disease. Involvement of large joints of the lower extremities, i.e. knee and ankle are seen in oligoarticular type of idiopathic arthritis. While large and small joints of both upper and lower extremities is characteristic of polyarticular type of idiopathic arthritis. Spindle-shaped fingers are seen in rheumatoid arthritis. Diffuse swelling of the entire dorsum of the hand and foot would suggest sickle cell disease.

Position of the limb at rest should also be observed:

In case of septic arthritis because of pain there may be pseudoparalysis (inability to move joint because of pain).

In tuberculosis of the hip joint the limb is flexed, abducted and medially rotated.

Scorbutic beading of the costochondral junction is seen in scurvy.

Examination of the spine:

The spine should be examined for the presence of kyphosis or scoliosis, which can be seen in tuberculosis (TB) of the spine.

Examination of the muscles:

Wasting of muscles above and below the affected joints is seen in idiopathic arthritis, or any joint that has been affected for a long time (disuse atrophy). Tenderness of muscles is a feature of dermatomyositis.

Skin rash:

Skin rash is seen in several conditions associated with joint involvement.

Erythema marginatum is a feature of acute rheumatic fever. In juvenile idiopathic arthritis one may observe evanescent macular rash. Typical butterfly rash over the malar eminences is seen in systemic lupus erythematosus. Palpable purpuric rash over the extensor portion of the extremities is characteristic of Henoch- Schonleinpurpura. Characteristic heliotrope discoloration over he upper eyelids is seen in juvenile dermatomyositis.

Purpuric and ecchymotic patches would suggest leukemia. Presence of subcutaneous nodules over the skin, extensor aspect of upper extremities and in the suboccipital region would suggest rheumatic fever.

Lymphadenopathy:

Presence of lymphadenopathy would suggest tuberculosis, leukemia and collagen disease. If the lymph nodes are matted and there are sinuses the likely etiology is tuberculosis.

Eyes:

The presence of pallor and jaundice along with symmetrical painful swelling of hands and feet (Hand-foot syndrome) would suggest sickle cell disease. The presence of iridocyclitis would indicate idiopathic arthritis. High fever with conjunctival injection suggests Kawasaki disease.

Oral cavity:

Spongy gums are present in scurvy, while swollen tongue and lips are seen in Kawasaki disease. Desquamation of fingers is seen in Kawasaki disease.

Organomegaly:

Hepatosplenomegaly is seen in collagen disease, leukemias, disseminated tuberculosis. Splenomegaly is seen in sickle cell disease.

Cardiovascular system:

Blood pressure should be recorded. There can be hypertension in SLE. The heart should be carefully auscultated for a pericardial rub. Pericarditis is seen in rheumatoid arthritis and SLE. While myocarditis occurs in rheumatic fever and Kawasaki disease.

Any focus of infection:

One must carefully look for a focus of infection viz. boils, abscesses, etc. This could lead to septic arthritis especially in infants.

C. Investigations

Table: Which investigations to be done?

Sr. No.	Investigations	Probable Cause
1.	Complete blood count	
	• Leucocytosis with polymorphonuclear predominance	Septic arthritis
	• Leukopenia with lymphopenia	Systemic lupus erythematosus
	• Leucocytosis with immature cells	Leukemia
	• Thrombocytosis	Idiopathic arthritis
2.	Erythrocyte sedimentation rate	
	• Raised	Collagen disease
	• Decreased	Sickle cell anemia
3.	Coagulation factors deranged	Coagulopathy
4.	Mantoux test – positive	Tubercular arthritis
5.	Skiagram of affected joint useful in	Scurvy, tuberculosis, idiopathic arthritis

6.	Serology	
	• RA factor – positive	Polyarticular rheumatoid arthritis
	• ANA – positive	SLE
	• Anti-DNA antibody – positive	SLE
	• ASO titer rising titer	Acute rheumatic arthritis
7.	Synovial fluid culture – positive	Septic arthritis

Complete blood count:

In sickle cell disease and leukemia hemoglobin would be low.

In septic arthritis there will be leukocytosis with polymorphonuclear predominance. In SLE there will be leukopenia with lymphopenia.

Reticulocyte count would be increased in sickle cell disease.

Thrombocytopenia is seen in leukemia, while thrombocytosis is a feature of idiopathic arthritis.

In Henoch-Schonleinpurpura the platelet count is normal.

Anemia of chronic inflammation will be seen in collagen vascular disease.

Erythrocyte sedimentation rate:

Erythrocyte sedimentation rate (ESR) is raised in collagen diseases and acute rheumatic fever, while it is decreased in sickle cell anemia.

Estimation of coagulation factors:

Whenever there is hemarthrosis with prolonged clotting time estimation of coagulation factors must be done.

Mantoux test:

Tuberculin test must be done in suspected cases of tuberculosis.

Skiagram of the affected joint:

X-ray of the lower end of the femur in cases of scurvy is diagnostic. Bone has a ground glass appearance, with pencil thin cortex, signet ring appearance of epiphysis and metaphysis shows a whiteline of calcified cartilage known as Frenkel line. X-ray of the affected joint would also show changes in tuberculosis, idiopathic arthritis and tubercular dactylitis.

Estimation of RA Factor, ANA/Anti-DNA antibody:

Rheumatoid factor is increased in polyarticular type of rheumatoid arthritis.

The hallmark of the SLE is the presence of antinuclear antibodies. Presence of antidouble strained DNA antibodies is highly specific of SLE.

ASO titer:

It should be done in cases of rheumatic arthritis. Rising ASO titer indicates recent streptococcal infection.

C-reactive protein:

C-reactive protein is raised in acute rheumatic arthritis.

Throat swab examination:

Throat swab culture for isolation of Beta-hemolytic streptococci is done in suspected cases of rheumatic arthritis.

Urine examination:

A routine urine examination especially for albumin and hematuria is indicated in cases of collagen disease.

Synovial fluid aspiration:

Synovial fluid aspiration for microscopy and culture is indicated, if septic arthritis is suspected.

Imaging techniques:

Ultrasonography and magnetic resonance imaging of the joint is indicated in certain situations such as septic or tubercular arthritis and in cases of hemarthrosis.

SUMMARY

Arthritis in childhood is common with monarthritis being more common than polyarthritis. The pattern, presentation, duration of arthritis help differentiate between various possible diagnosis. Eighty percent of rheumatological diagnosis comes from clinical history, 15% from examination and only 5% from investigations. Laboratory investigations by themselves have very little role in arriving at a diagnosis. They must always be directed by clinical presentation.

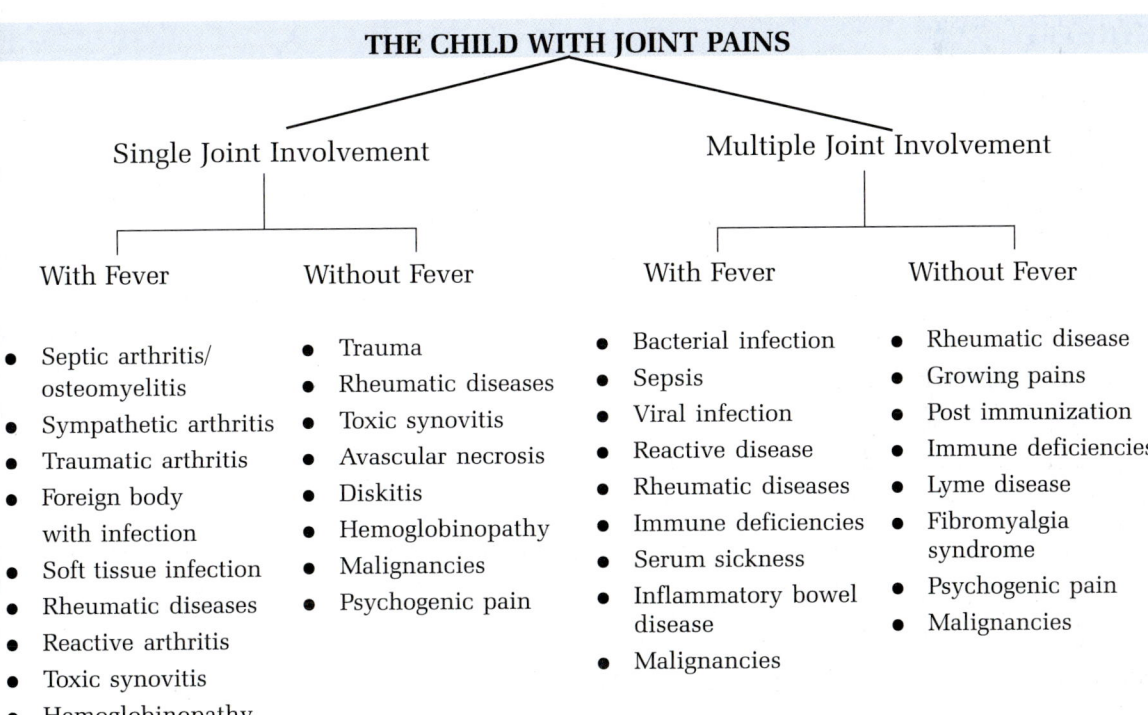

THE CHILD WITH JOINT PAINS

Single Joint Involvement

With Fever
- Septic arthritis/ osteomyelitis
- Sympathetic arthritis
- Traumatic arthritis
- Foreign body with infection
- Soft tissue infection
- Rheumatic diseases
- Reactive arthritis
- Toxic synovitis
- Hemoglobinopathy
- Malignancies

Without Fever
- Trauma
- Rheumatic diseases
- Toxic synovitis
- Avascular necrosis
- Diskitis
- Hemoglobinopathy
- Malignancies
- Psychogenic pain

Multiple Joint Involvement

With Fever
- Bacterial infection
- Sepsis
- Viral infection
- Reactive disease
- Rheumatic diseases
- Immune deficiencies
- Serum sickness
- Inflammatory bowel disease
- Malignancies

Without Fever
- Rheumatic disease
- Growing pains
- Post immunization
- Immune deficiencies
- Lyme disease
- Fibromyalgia syndrome
- Psychogenic pain
- Malignancies

SUGGESTED READING

1. Balan S, Prabhu AS. Approach to a child with monoarthritis. Indian J. Pediatr. (2010) 77: 997-1004.

2. Singh S, Mehra S. Approach to polyarthritis. Indian J. Pediatr. (2010) 77:1005-1010.

23

FAILURE TO MOVE A LIMB

INTRODUCTION

Pathology in a limb can either present as failure to move a limb or as a limp. It is usually due to pain or paresis. The causes range from as trivial as a thorn in the heel to as serious as malignancy.

ETIOLOGY

Causes of failure to move a limb can be classified on the basis ofsite of anatomical involvement.

Table: Causes of failure to move a limb

- **Skin and soft tissue**: Foreign body (thorn, nails), cellulitis
- **Muscles and ligaments**: Sprains, viral myositis, dermatomyositis
- **Bones**: Fractures, osteomyelitis, scurvy, syphilis, bone tumors, leukemia
- **Joints:** Transient synovitis, reactive arthritis, septic arthritis, sickle arthropathy, congenital dislocation of hip, Perthe's disease
- **Vascular**: Deep vein thrombosis
- **Neurological:** Herpes zoster (pre-exanthematous), Guillain - Barre syndrome, poliomyelitis, postdiphtheritic palsy, spinal cord lesions, lesions of nerve root, post-traumatic nerve injury.

EVALUATION

Whenever a patient is brought with the complaint of inability tomove a limb or a limp one should first decide, whether it is a true paralysis or pseudoparalysis. In order to arrive at a definitive cause a thorough history and examination is mandatory.

A. History

While recording the history emphasis should be laid on the following points:

Points in history

- Age of the patient
- Mode of onset and duration of illness
- Is there pain?
- Diurnal variation in pain
- History of trauma
- History of fever
- History of receiving injection
- Any problem with the shoe?
- Dietary history
- History of vaccination

Age of the child:

In newborns and infants the commonest cause is septic arthritis. Congenital syphilis can also present with failure to move the limb. This is because of syphilitic osteitis and periosteitis. If a neonate is unable to move his upper extremity and there is a history of difficult labor the possibility of Erb's palsy must be borne in mind. Traumatic deliveries can also give rise to fractures leading to inability to move the affected limb. This would be associated with crying and irritability due to pain.

In a toddler one must keep in mind developmental dysplasia of the hip giving rise to a limp during walking. Other causes at this age could be scurvy, poliomyelitis, injuries. In a school child transient synovitis, tuberculosis of the hip, psoas abscess and acute appendicitis can give rise to pain and limping. In an adolescent common causes are injury, tuberculosis hip and Perthe's disease.

Guillain-Barre, septic arthritis and osteomyelitis are common at all ages.

Onset of illness:

What was the mode of onset of illness? Was it acute, subacute or chronic. Since how long is the child unable to move the limb?

An acute onset, i.e. within hours and days is seen in acute poliomyelitis, Guillain-Barre syndrome, sprain, transient synovitis, septic arthritis, deep vein thrombosis and sickle cell arthropathy. A subacute onset is over days and weeks would suggest viral myositis, reactive arthritis, scurvy and osteomyelitis. If the onset of disease is over several weeks or months the usual causes are juvenile idiopathic arthritis, congenital dislocation of hip and Perthe disease.

Is there pain?

Is there pain in the affected limb?

In an infant one could elicit history of pain by asking, whether the infant is fretful and cries on being handled. The limb is painful in cases of sprains, synovitis, septic arthritis,

reactive arthritis, deep vein thrombosis, scurvy, osteomyelitis, viral myositis, juvenile idiopathic arthritis. In case of root pains the cause is usually a tumor, which can be malignant or pre-exanthematous stage of herpes zoster.

If there is no pain, the cause is neurological such as poliomyelitis, Guillain-Barre syndrome, peripheral neuritis or congenital dysplasia of hip.

Any diurnal variation in pain:

Is there any diurnal variation in pain?

If there is pain and stiffness in the morning, which tends to become less as the day passes by it is likely to be juvenile idiopathic arthritis. Pain increases at the end of the day in cases of mechanical problems. Bone pains at night suggests malignancy.

History of trauma:

Did the child sustain any injury? In case of newborn is there any history of birth injury? Was the baby delivered by breech? Was there shoulder dystocia at birth?

Such traumas during the process of birth can be responsible for Erb,s palsy, Klumpke paralysis, fracture of the clavicle, humerus or femur. In an infant and older child it is important to ask for history of fall, pull or blow.

History of fever:

Did the child have fever before the onset of illness? Is he/she presently having fever?

The pattern and severity of fever must also be asked.

Presence of fever will always indicate infective or inflammatory etiology. In transient synovitis there is preceding history of sore throat and fever.

History of injection:

Has the child received any intramuscular injection before the onset of illness? It can be responsible for traumatic nerve injury. Sciatic nerve injury is often observed if an infant is given intramuscular injection in the gluteal region. Sometimes following intramuscular injection especially after DPT injection child can have local pain and swelling causing him to limp.

Shoe problem:

One should not forget to ask in a child with a limp if he/she has any problem with his shoes. This can happen in ill-fitting new shoes.

History of vaccination:

If an infant or a child has been brought with inability to move his limb or limbs one must enquire, whether he has been immunized against poliomyelitis and diphtheria. Poliomyelitis can give rise to paresis and following diphtheria the child can develop post-diphtheritic paralysis. If he/she has not been immunized against these diseases one must keep the possibility of these conditions in mind.

B. Examination

The examination should be focused on whether the limp or inability to move the limb in the child is due to true paralysis or pseudoparalysis.

Pseudoparalysis means inability to move a limb, in absence of any neurological lesions. Muscle power is essentially normal and whenever movements cause pain, child will resist active and passive movements of that limb.

> **Points on examination**
> - Appearance of the child
> - Is the child febrile?
> - Posture and gait
> - Examination of the affected limb
> - Skin
> - Asymmetry of gluteal creases
> - Examination of spine
> - Inguinal lymphadenitis
> - Scorbutic changes
> - Examination of foot
> - Neurological examination
> - Examination of the abdomen

Appearance of the child:

One must observe whether the child looks sick and toxic or well. A sick look indicates an infective etiology or malignancy. While if the child appears well the cause could be neurological, congenital condition or transient synovitis. In an infant if there is pain he/she is fretful and crying and does not like to be handled.

Is the child febrile?

Fever with chills would be a feature of septic conditions such as arthritis, osteomyelitis, abscess. Low grade irregular fever may indicate tuberculosis of the joint or juvenile idiopathic arthritis.

Posture and gait:

It is important to observe the posture of the affected limb. In case of scurvy the child may be lying in a frog position.

In case of deep vein thrombosis the child is unable to move the limb, the extremity is cold and pulses are weak or absent.

If the child is limping observe the limbs that are affected. Is there involvement of one limb only? Is the gait hemiplegic? Toe walking is seen in children with mild cerebral palsy.

In tuberculosis of hip joint intermittent slight limp with pain is an early sign. Pain is usually referred to the knee or medial side of thigh. In Perthe's disease, there is limitation of only abduction and internal rotation.

An attempt should be made to determine whether the cause is in the spine, hip, knee, ankle, foot or soft tissues.

One must also look for asymmetry in size of the legs.

Examination of the affected limb:

The affected limb should be thoroughly examined to determine, whether there is pain or paralysis. In case of pain one must find out whether the pain is due to lesion in the soft tissue such as cellulitis or abscess or in the bone or joint (arthritis). Is there swelling? Is the local temperature raised. Is there restriction of joint movements? Is there muscle wasting above and below the joint. One must differentiate periarticular swelling from arthritis.

Skin:

Presence of pallor and petechiae would indicate leukemia.

Asymmetry of gluteal crease:

In suspected cases of congenital dislocation of hip one must look for asymmetry of thighs, gluteal and knee creases and also check for inability to abduct the hip. Further confirmation can be done by Ortolani's sign and Barlow's maneuver, which would be positive.

Examination of the spine:

The spine must be thoroughly examined. Presence of scoliosis can give rise to limp.

Examination of the foot:

The foot should be examined for presence of corn, blisters, paronychia or an ingrowing toe nail, which may be responsible for the limp.

Clinical features of scurvy:

If there is a clinical suspicion of scurvy, one must look for signs of scurvy such as scorbutic beading, bleeding and spongy gums.

Neurological examination:

Once pseudoparalysis is excluded and the cause appears neurological one must ascertain, whether it is a lower motor neuron type or upper motor neuron type of paralysis. Examination of power, tone and reflexes would help in deciding the same. Muscle wasting, loss of tendon reflexes and hypotonia would be features of lower motor neuron type of paralysis, while in upper motor neuron lesion there would be spasticity, hyperreflexia and extensor plantar response. Common lower motor neuron lesions are poliomyelitis, polyneuritis, postdiphtheritic neuritis, traumatic neuritis. In the neonate Erb's palsy is common following difficult delivery.

One must also look carefully for involvement of respiratory muscles, palatal and pharyngeal muscles, which indicate ascending paralysis. Isolated palatal palsy would suggest post diphtheritic polyneuritis.

Examination of the abdomen:

The abdomen must be carefully examined. Abdominal pain may cause the child to limp, especially when there is peritoneal irritation as in appendicitis, salpingitis and psoas abscess.

C. Investigations

Depending upon the clinical cause the following investigations can be done. Which investigations to be done?

Investigations	Probable diagnosis
1. Complete blood count	
• Polymorpholeucocytosis	Suppurative lesions
• Raised leucocyte count with immature WBCs	Leukemia
2. Hemoglobin electrophoresis	Sickle cell arthropathy
3. X-ray of affected bone and joint	Tuberculosis, Perthe's disease, scurvy, congenital syphilis
4. Ultrasound of joint	Useful in arthritis
5. Cerebrospinal fluid examination	
• Albuminocytological dissociation	Guillain Barre Syndrome
6. Nerve conduction studies	Polyneuritis
7. MRI of the affected joint	Distinguishes traumatic from infective aetiology

Complete blood count:

In cases of suppurative lesions the count is raised. There is usually polymorpho-nuclearleuocytosis. In case of leukemia not only is the count raised, but the peripheral smear would reveal immature white blood cells (WBCs).

Hemoglobin electrophoresis:

Blood for sickling phenomenon and hemoglobin electrophoresis should be done in suspected cases of sickle arthropathy.

X-ray of the affected limb/joint:

X-ray is useful in cases of tuberculosis, Perthe's disease, septic arthritis and scurvy.

In scurvy the radiological findings are very characteristic. There is ground glass appearance due to rarefaction of the bone, signet ring appearance of epiphysis, white line of Frankel and penciling of the cortex.

X-ray of the knee is also diagnostic in cases of congenital syphilis. There is osteitis, periosteitis with moth-eaten appearance known as the Vimberger's sign.

Ultrasound of joint:

Ultrasound of the affected joint is indicated whenever there is suspicion of arthritis.

Cerebrospinal fluid examination:

Cerebrospinal fluid examination would reveal albuminocytological dissociation in cases of Guillain-Barre syndrome.

Nerve conduction studies:

In suspected polyneuritis nerve conduction studies would be helpful.

Neuroimaging:

Magnetic resonance imaging is indicated whenever there is involvement of the joint.

It helps to distinguish traumatic from infective etiology.

SUMMARY

If a child is unable to move a limb, we need to ascertain if it is 'true paralysis' or 'pseudoparalysis'. A painful condition prevents a child from moving his limb, such as in bone or soft tissue injury or trauma and is termed as pseudoparalysis. True paralysis is associated with a neurological condition of the brain, spinal cord, peripheral nerves or muscle.

Initially, when the child is brought one must determine whether it is a 'pseudo' or 'true' paralysis. Subsequently, one must proceed to determine the cause on the basis of history, clinical examination coupled with appropriate investigations.

SUGGESTED READING

1. P. Parekh: Failure to move a limb. Manual of Pediatric Differential Diagnosis (2013) 220-228.

2. Moris Green: Limb and Musculoskeletal pain. Pediatric Diagnosis (2001) 419-422.

ACUTE FLACCID PARALYSIS

INTRODUCTION

Acute flaccid paralysis (AFP) is a medical emergency requiring rapid assessment, systematic evaluation and immediate stabilization. Prompt etiological diagnosis of AFP is important for both management and prognosis. If untreated AFP can rapidly progress and lead to death due to paralysis of respiratory muscles.

DEFINITION

Acute flaccid paralysis (AFP) is a clinical syndrome characterized by rapidly evolving weakness, which may include weakness of the respiratory and bulbar muscles, advancing to maximum severity within several days to weeks usually 15 days. AFP is thus a syndromic diagnosis and not an etiological diagnosis.

WHO has defined AFP as "any child under 15 years of age with AFP or any person of any age with paralytic illness if polio is suspected".

ETIOLOGY

Causes of AFP can be classified on the site of involvement of neuroaxis.

Guillain-Barre syndrome remains the most common cause of AFP in children after polio eradication.

Other common causes are diphtheritic polyneuropathy and transverse myelitis.

Table: Causes of AFP

Site of lesion	Disease
Spinal cord	• Cord compression
	- Trauma
	- Extradural hematoma
	- Epidural abscess
	- Pott's spine
	• Inflammatory myelitis
	- Acute transverse myelitis
Anterior horn cell	• Viral
	- Polio virus infection
	- Non-polio enterovirus
	- Neurotropic viruses, enteroviruses

	• Vascular
	- Anterior spinal artery infarct
Peripheral nerves/roots	• Immune mediated
	- Guillain-Barre syndrome
	- Acute inflammatory demyelinating polyradiculoneuropathy
	- Acute motor axonal neuropathy
	• Toxin
	- Porphyria
	- Post-diphtheritic polyneuropathy
	• Trauma
	- Sciatic nerve injury following injection
Neuromuscular junction	• Immune mediated
	- Myasthenia gravis
	• Toxins
	- Snake venom
	- Organophosphates
	- Botulism
Muscle	• Infection
	- Viral myositis
	• Dyselectrolytemia
	- Hypokalemia

EVALUATION

The first step is to determine if an unwell child actually has muscle weakness. Many children with weakness present with non-specific symptoms. Information is derived from the history and focused neurological examination.

A. History

Points in history

- Fever at onset
- Progress of paralysis
- Trauma
- Exposure to toxins

- Preceding infections
- Vaccination
- Precipitating factors
- Bowel bladder involvement
- Alteration in speech
- Receiving intramuscular injection

Fever:

Fever at presentation suggests an inflammatory pathology. It can be seen in polio, other enteroviral infections, transverse myelitis, viral myositis, epidural and extradural abscess and Pott's spine. Fever is low grade with an insidious onset in case of TB spine.

Progress of weakness:

It is important to enquire about the progress of weakness. Is it symmetrically involving both the lower limbs? Is the weakness progressing from above downwards. Descending weakness suggests diphtheritic polyneuropathy, myasthenia gravis and botulism. Symmetrical and ascending weakness suggests diagnosis of Guillain Barres yndrome, rabies or inflammatory myelitis. Fluctuating weakness, diurnal variation is seen in myasthenia gravis.

Trauma:

If there is history of trauma or symptoms and signs suggestive of spinal cord compression such as asymmetric weakness, spinal deformity, sensory or bladder dysfunction it suggests compressive myelopathy. Unilateral lower limb paresis with past history of intramuscular injection at gluteal region suggests traumatic sciatic neuropathy.

Infections:

Preceding history of upper respiratory infection, acute gastroenteritis can be present in acute transverse myelitis, GBS, polio and polio like illness.History of throat pain and neck swelling in an unimmunized child suggests diphtheritic polyneuropathy.

Drugs and toxins:

Exposure to drugs, organophosphorus compounds, animal bites, consumption of honey by infants and ingestion of canned food can lead to flaccid paralysis.

B. Examination

After immediate stabilization of the child a focused history and examination is necessary for localization, etiological investigation and definitive management.

Points in clinical examination

- Assessment of respiratory muscle weakness
- Assessment of bulbar weakness
- Fever
- Examination of neck
- Assessment of sensorium
- Cranial nerve involvement
- Lower limb paralysis
- Sensory involvement
- Bladder and bowel involvement
- Deformity or tenderness of spine

Younger children with weakness present often with non-specific signs and symptoms such as lethargy, irritability, frequent falls and refusal to stand or walk. An attempt should be made for assessment, quantification and distribution of weakness.

As soon as a child comes to the emergency ward the first thing to assess is respiratory muscle weakness. This is done by counting the respiratory rate and observing chest expansion. Tachypnoea and use of accessory muscles of respiration may be absent due to extreme weakness of respiratory and diaphragmatic muscles hence serial blood gas monitoring is essential.

Assess for bulbar weakness:

Alteration in voice, weak cry, pooling of secretions in the throat, nasal regurgitation and inability to swallow would indicate bulbar weakness.

Encephalopathy:

Assess the level of consciousness. Profound encephalopathy, flaccid paralysis, respiratory weakness, pin point pupils and fasciculation suggests organophosphorus poisoning

---

Flaccid paralysis, respiratory weakness, ptosis and external ophthalmoloplegia suggests snake envenomation.

Throat should be examined for the presence of a membrane which would suggest diphtheritic polyneuropathy.

Assessment should be done for cranial nerve involvement especiallyfacial, ocular, neck and trunk muscles, deep tendon reflexes and plantars. Bladder and bowel involvement and level of sensory involvement if any should be assessed.

Spine should be examined for tenderness and deformity.

Table: **Clues from history and examination**

Points in history and examination	Remarks
1. Fever at onset	Polio or enteroviral myelitis Transverse myelitis, epidural abscess
2. Trauma: Head/neck	May lead to spinal compression in patients with cervical vertebral instability
3. Exposure	Toxins: Lead, arsenic Snakes envenomation
4. Preceding infections	GBS, transverse myelitis, sore throat, swelling in neck – prodrome / vaccination diphtheritic polyneuropathy History of Honey exposure – botulism
5. Precipitating factors	Diarrhoea: Hypokalemia, enteroviral myelitis Intramuscular injections: traumatic sciatic neuritis
6. Sensory loss/level	Compressive myelopathy, transverse myelitis
7. Early bowel/bladder involvement	Compressive myelopathy, transverse myelopathy
8. Prominent autonomic signs and symptoms	GBS, acute myelopathy
9. Ascending weakness	GBS, ascending myelitis
10. Descending weakness	Diphtheria, botulism
11. Prominent and early ptosis	Myasthenia gravis, botulism
12. Facial weakness	GBS, myasthenia gravis, botulism
13. Fluctuating symptoms, fatiguability	Myasthenia gravis
14. Muscle tenderness	Myositis, GBS

15.	Tendon reflexes	Absent: GBS, polio, diphtheritic neuropathy, spinal shock, at level of spinal cord damage.
		Preserved: Myasthenia gravis, periodic paralysis, botulism. Exaggerated: Lesion below spinal level
16.	Spinal tenderness, painful spine movement	Spinal trauma, epidural abscess, extradural compression
17.	Neck stiffness	Polio, enteroviral myelitis, GBS, transverse myelitis

C. Investigations

Which investigations to be done?

Based on the clinical diagnosis investigations are planned.

Investigations in acute flaccid paralysis

- Lumbar puncture
- Serum electrolytes
- CSF examination
- MRI spine
- Nerve conduction
- Electromyography
- Enzyme studies
- Throat swab-culture

Table: Clues from investigations

Investigation	Clinical condition
1. CSF examination	Bacterial infection - Protein elevated, low glucose, polymorpholeucocytosis
	Guillain-Barre syndrome - Albumino-cytological dissociation
	Acute polio - Lymphocytic pleocytosis PCR on CSF and stool
2. Electrolyte abnormalities	Childhood periodic paralysis – hypokalemia
3. MRI spine	Contrast enhanced MRI spine for spinal cord compression and trauma MRI shows specific changes for inflammatory myelopathy, demyelinating disorders, abscess, spinal artery infarct, neoplasm

4.	Nerve conduction studies	Helps in diagnosis of Guillain-Barre Syndrome and diphtheritic polyeneuropathy which shows predominantly demyelinating polyneuropathy
5.	Electromyography	Helps in diagnosis of anterior horn cell myelitis, myasthenia gravis and botulism
6.	Serial blood gases	These are required for monitoring especially when there are signs of respiratory muscle and bulbar weakness
7.	Enzyme studies	Creatine kinase enzymes are elevated in infectious, inflammatory or viral myositis. In organo phosphorus intoxication plasma or red blood cell acetylcholinesterase activity may be indicated

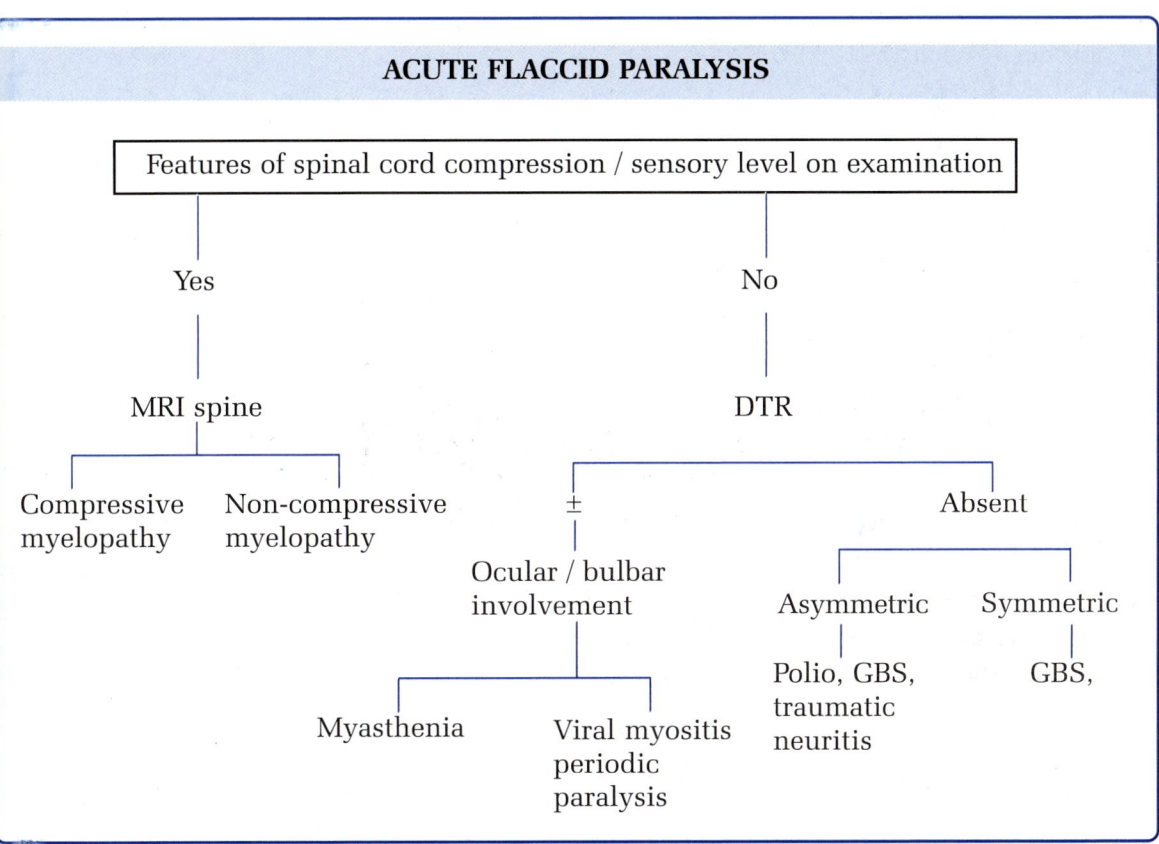

ACUTE FLACCID PARALYSIS

Features of spinal cord compression / sensory level on examination

Yes — No

MRI spine — DTR

Compressive myelopathy — Non-compressive myelopathy

± — Absent

Ocular / bulbar involvement

Asymmetric — Symmetric

Polio, GBS, traumatic neuritis — GBS,

Myasthenia — Viral myositis periodic paralysis

SUMMARY

Acute flaccid paralysis is a medical emergency. It is a syndrome with a number of differential diagnosis. As soon as the child arrives a quick evaluation should be done to assess the extent of paralysis and its tentative cause. As the evolution of the illness can be rapid it is essential to observe the involvement of vital centres in the brain. Hence, a child with AFP should be kept in the PICU for the first few days. After the eradication of poliomyelitis, GBS, transverse myelitis and non-polio myelitis are common causes of acute flaccid paralysis.

SUGGESTED READING

1. N. Sankhyan, R. Suthar. Approach to a child with acute flaccid paralysis. Indian JPF 2016;18(2):101.

2. Singh SC, Sankhyan N, Shah R, et al. Approach to a child with acute flaccid paralysis Indian J Pediatr 2012;79:1351-7.

Chapter
25

HEADACHE

INTRODUCTION

Headache is a common symptom in childhood and adolescence. Most often it is benign, but at times the cause can be a serious intracranial disease. Headache in infancy is rare, but may present as irritability and head banging.

It is one of the most common cause of referral to the neurology clinic. Migraine, tension type headache and cluster headache are common. Headache may be secondary to increased intracranial pressure. Cranial neuropathies and primary facial pain syndromes account for the third category of headache.

ETIOLOGY

The brain meninges and bony skull are insensitive to pain. Pain appreciated as headache arises from intra and extracranial blood vessels, cranial and spinal nerves, cranial and cervical muscles and adjacent structures (teeth, sinuses and ears). The neurogenic hypothesis is currently favoured over the vascular hypothesis (vasoconstriction producing an aura followed by painful vasodilatation) in the pathogenesis of migraine.

Based on the temporal patterns, headache can be categorized into acute and recurrent, chronic non-progressive and progressive.

Table: Causes of headache

1. Acute: Fever, systemic illness, head and neck infections, meningitis, rupture of vascular malformations, dyselectrolytemia, hypertension, trauma.
2. Acute and recurrent: Migraine, cluster headache, migraine variants.
3. Chronic and non-progressive: Chronic migraine, tension headache, depression.
4. Chronic and progressive: Intracranial space occupying lesions, hydrocephalus

CLINICAL EVALUATION

A. History

Clinical assessment is the most effective screening procedure in children with headaches. Children older than eight years of age can usually give a detailed account of their symptoms. Younger children require the assistance of their parents.

Points in history

- Duration and onset
- Nature of pain
- Site of pain
- Diurnal variation
- Associated features
- Family history
- Precipitating and relieving factors
- History of occult head trauma

Onset and duration:

Since, when is the child having headache? Is it the first attack or is he getting recurrent episodes? Long standing recurrent episodes would point towards migraine, while long standing near continuous headache would suggest refractive error, sinusitis hypertension or stress. Recurrent headache is also seen in cases of psychological stress. Acute onset with fever is seen in both extra and intracranial infection. Acute headache is also a feature of hypertension and intracranial hemorrhage.

The commonest cause of chronic headache is tension and depression. Other conditions that should be considered are raised intracranial tension due to tumor, subdural hemorrhage or pseudotumorcerebri. It is also seen in sinusitis.

Chronic progressive headache is a feature of space occupying lesion.

Nature of pain:

Most children are incapable of describing the nature of pain. Terms such as 'throbbing' and 'splitting' more often describe the intensity than the character of pain. The parents can be asked, whether the headache is disabling and the child is unable to attendschool. Does the child look sick during the episode of headache, which may suggest migraine. The pain in migraine is usually throbbing, pulsating or pounding. In tension headache pain is dull and diffuse and aching and constant, but not progressive. It is usually not severe enough to interrupt the child's daily activities. Eye strain also results in dull aching pain behind the eyes.

Site of pain:

The site of pain should be enquired. In case of migraine pain is unilateral (frontal/temporal) in two-thirds of the cases in the rest,

it is bilateral. It is most intense in the region of the eyes, forehead and temple. In chronic hypertension there is occipital headache, it is also a symptom of posterior fossa tumor. In case of tension headache pain is localized mainly to the back of the head and neck.

Diurnal variation:

Is there any diurnal variation in pain?

Expanding intracranial lesions and benign intracranial hypertension (pseudotumorcerebri) produce headaches that are present on waking and are aggravated by coughing, sneezing and straining at stool. The headaches associated with these conditions are progressive with frequency and severity increasing over time. Morning headache is also seen in hypertension and sinusitis. Tension headache grows as the day advances and subsides with sleep.

Associated symptoms:

Various symptoms can be associated with headache. Enquiring about them would help in evaluating the cause of headache.

Does the child get an aura, before the onset of headache? Is fever associated with headache? Does the child get recurrent respiratory infections especially rhinitis with running nose? Have the parents noticed any personality change such as irritability in the child since onset of headache?

Is headache associated with vomiting or seizures?

Presence of aura is a feature of migraine. The presence of preceding aura can be established by asking the child whether he or she gets any warning before the headache starts. Auras include flashing lights (photopsia), visual field defects (scotomata) and distortions of size (micropsia or macropsia). Children with migraine often look unwell and pale during an attack.

Presence of fever would suggest infection. If fever isassociated with drowsiness, it is likely to be an intracranial infection.

High fever with headache and severe myalgia is a feature of dengue fever.

History of recurrent respiratory infections would suggest sinusitis, while in cases of brain abscess and mastoiditis one must ask for history of otorrhea.

Subtle neurological manifestations, such as irritability, mood and personality changes, drowsiness, gradual deterioration in school performance, indicates an intracranial pathology. Headache that disrupts sleep should be thoroughly investigated.

If headache is associated with persistent vomiting, one must consider raised intracranial tension. Headache is a common observation after lumbar puncture. It occurs on assuming an upright position and disappears on lying down. Any history of seizure should also be enquired.

B. Examination

Family history:

Is there a history of headache in parents. Migraine is a hereditary disorder. It has been observed that atleast one parent gives a history of migraine in 90 percent of cases.

History of head trauma:

Parents should be specifically asked for a history of subtle head trauma in the recent past, which they may not volunteer. Headaches may occur acutely following trauma or as part of a post-concussion syndrome.

Aggravating and relieving factors:

Are there any situations, which aggravate the headache? What relieves the headache?

Migraine is often precipitated by emotional stress, flickering lights, food substances such as caffeine, chocolates, cheese, inadequate sleep, bending forward from sitting position. Is it relieved after sleep?

Vomiting often relieves headache associated with raised intracranial tension due to space occupying lesions.

Stress, academic difficulties and social adjustment issues are associated with tension headache.

Psychological problems:

Some children may complaint of headache as an attention-seeking device or as a pretext for not going to school or taking permission from the teacher to return home.

C. Clinical Examination

> **Points on clinical examination**
> - Appearance of the child-sick/well
> - Record vital signs-pulse, temperature and blood pressure
> - General examination with special emphasis on ear, nose and throat
> - Central nervous system (CNS) examination-level of consciousness, signs of meningeal irritation, tone and reflexes, any neurological deficit, cranial nerve palsies, fundoscopy.

Appearance:

If the child has a first attack of headache and appears acutely ill, the possibility of extracranial or intracranial infection must be kept in mind.

In case of migraine, the child appears sick during the attack, but is perfectly normal in between the attack. Children having a space occupying lesion with chronic raised intracranial tension may not appear acutely ill, but have subtle personality changes such as irritability, mood swings and sleep disturbances. Overall growth and development must be assessed.

Vitals signs:

Pulse, temperature and blood pressure must be recorded. Bradycardia would suggest raised intracranial pressure, while high blood pressure is a feature of hypertension and raised intracranial pressure.

General examination:

During a routine general examination one should especially look for purulent nasal discharge or postnasal drip, which would suggest sinusitis. Any tenderness over frontal or maxillary sinuses. The ears should be examined for evidence of chronic otitis media.

One must look for evidence of pallor, petechiae, which may suggest meningococcemia. Presence of neurocutaneous markers would suggest neurocutaneous syndrome.

The oral cavity should be examined for any infection in the teeth.

Examination of eyes:

In a child with chronic headache, eyes should be examined for refractive error and problems of accommodation. Refractive error must be considered if headache is precipitated by reading or relieved by rest.

Examination of central nervous system:

In children most intracranial tumors arise in the posterior fossa or suprasellar region so assessment of gait and coordination as well as eye movement, visual acuity and visual fields must always be assessed.

The nervous system should be examined with special referenceto the following:

- Level of consciousness - if a child with headache develops altered sensorium, it points towards an intracranial lesion such as meningitis, encephalitis, encephalopathy, intracranial hemorrhage.

- An attempt should be made to elicit signs of meningeal irritation. Presence of these signs would suggest meningitis, subarachnoid hemorrhage. If the neck is stiff with a head tilt, one must consider posterior fossa tumor.

- A positive Macewan sign in an older child points towards raised intracranial pressure.

- Cranial nerves should be examined for any palsies. Sixth nerve palsy usually indicates raised intracranial pressure.

- Examine for tone, reflexes and any evidence of neurologic deficit such as hemiparesis.

- Fundus should be carefully examined for evidence of raised intracranial tension, which would manifest as papilledema. Presence of hypertensive changes and retinal hemorrhage should be looked for.

D.   INVESTIGATIONS

Since the cause of headache in most children is benign detailed investigations are not required in majority of the cases.

Table: Features of headache that indicate the need for investigations:

- Young age (< 5 years) of onset
- Increasing severity and/or frequency
- Early morning headache with or without vomiting
- Focal neurological signs or symptoms during or after the headache
- Localised pain
- Headaches not relieved by analgesics
- Headaches that wake the child from sleep
- Abnormal neurological examination e.g. abnormal gait
- Constant daily headache
- Change in behavior or loss of skills

Table: Which investigations to be done

Sr. No.	Investigation	Probable Cause
1.	Complete blood countPS for malarial parasiteLeucocystosis	Malaria Acute infection
2.	Cerebrospinal fluid examination Increased protein, increased cells	Meningitis
3.	Neuroimaging	Space occupying lesions
4.	X-ray paranasal sinuses	Sinusitis

Clues from Investigations

Complete blood counts:

Complete blood count is indicated in children with acute onset of fever with headache. The peripheral smear should be properly screened for the presence of malarial parasite, leucocytosis.

Cerebrospinal fluid examination:

Lumbar puncture should be done in all cases of suspected meningitis. In case of meningitis proteins and cells will be raised. However, it should only be done after fundus examination. If CSF is positive, it should also be sent for culture.

Neuroimaging:

Computed tomography (CT)/magnetic resonance imaging (MRI) of the brain is indicated in patients with clinical evidence of raised intracranial tension or those with worsening symptoms.

X-rays of paranasal sinuses:

In children, where the cause of headache seems to be due to sinusitis. X-rays/CT of paranasal sinuses is indicated.

SUMMARY

Headache is a common symptom in children. It is less common in younger children below 5 years, but when present should be carefully evaluated as a possible cause of underlying organic disease. Younger the child with headache, more sinister is the cause. Headache, which is severe, recurrent or persistent should be evaluated to rule out any serious cause especially raised intracranial tension due to meningitis or tumor.

Common causes of headache are sinusitis, refraction errors, migraine and psychogenic stress.

SUGGESTED READING

1. G.M. Fenichel. Clinical Pediatric Neurology. A signs and symptoms approach: Headache 5th Ed. p. 77-89.

2. SangeethaYoganathan. Childhood Migraine.Ind. J. Prac.Pediat. 2016;18:186-92.

3. Gupta Piyush et al. Headache.Textbook of Pediatrics, 1st Ed. P. 487-8.

INTRODUCTION

Seizures is a common neurologic disorder in the pediatric age group. Five percent of children are estimated to experience one or more seizures in childhood, but less than one percent have epilepsy.

Seizures are the clinical manifestations of aberrant, abnormal electrical activity in the cortical neurons. Thus, they can be regarded as a symptom of cerebral pathology and are not in themselves a disease.

The term epilepsy is not synonymous with seizures. Seizures occurring during the course of an acute illness are termed as provoked seizures. Febrile seizures are the most important cause of provoked seizures.

At times a child may present with a condition that can mimic or be misinterpreted as a seizure. These conditions include syncope, decerebrate posturing, dystonia and migraine. A seizure has to be differentiated from these conditions as misdiagnosis may lead to unnecessary therapy.

Since the etiology and clinical presentation of seizures in the neonatal period are different, it will be discussed separately.

I. SEIZURES IN INFANCY AND CHILDHOOD

ETIOLOGY

Causes of seizures fall into 4 groups. Firstly febrile seizures, secondly due to intracranial pathology, thirdly metabolic and lastly epilepsy.

Epilepsy is defined as two or more unprovoked seizures in a time frame of >24 hours.

Seizures are considered acute symptomatic if they occur within 7 days of cerebrovascular disease, trauma, CNS infections or anemia.

For acute symptomatic seizures due to metabolic illnesses, the blood sample on which classification is based is defined as within 24 hours of the seizure.

Table: Causes of seizures

1. Febrile convulsions - simple benign, atypical febrileseizures.

2. Intracranial causes:
   - Trauma: Cerebral concussion, contusion, laceration, focal or generalized edema, extradural or subdural hematoma, subarachnoid hemorrhage.
   - Infections:Congenital - TORCH (where, T=Toxoplasmosis, O=Other infections, R=Rubella, C=Cytomegalovirus, H=Herpes simplex virus-2)
   - Acquired - encephalitis, meningitis, subdural effusion, abscess, neurocysticercosis.
   - Cerebrovascular accidents: Rupture of congenital aneurysm, hemorrhagic disease, thrombosis or embolism of

cerebral vessels as in cyanotic heart disease, sickle cell anemia, severe dehydration, arteriovenous malformations.

- Neurocutaneous syndromes: Sturge-Weber, tuberous sclerosis.
- Malformations: Agenesis of corpus callosum, lissencephaly, holoprosencephaly.
- Encephalopathy: Postvaccinial, hypertensive, toxins. Degenerative disorders.
- Brain tumors.

3. Metabolic—Hypoglycemia, inborn errors of metabolism, electrolyte disturbances, uremia, anoxia.

4. Epilepsy.

EVALUATION

The following points have to be kept in mind while evaluating a child with seizure activity.

- Whether the event is a seizure?
- Is it the first time or recurrent.
- Febrile or afebrile.
- Focal or generalized.
- Symptomatic or idiopathic.
- Syndromic.
- Co-morbidities.

Approach to a child with convulsions will depend on whether the child is brought with seizures or has come in the interseizure period and is stable. In the former situation it is essential to first control his seizures and take care of the vitals. Look for acute intracranial infections such as meningitis and encephalitis. Look for head injury and subsequently take a detailed history. When the child is brought in the interseizure period one could proceed systematically by first recording the history and later a detailed examination.

Whenever a child with convulsions is brought it is essential to elicit a good description of the seizures followed by a neurological examination.

A. History

Points in history

- Age of the child
- Duration of seizures
- History of fever
- Detail description of the seizures/precipitating factors
- Postconvulsive phenomenon
- Any specific time when the child gets seizures
- Perinatal history
- Developmental history
- Family history
- Is the child on any drugs?

One has to decide whether the spell in question is a seizure? What type of seizure? And cause of seizure. Was there any warning before the spell? If so what was the warning. Did the child complain of abdominal discomfort, fear or any other unpleasant sensations before the spell? What was the child doing before the spell? Was the child asleep or awake prior to the event? Was the child well before the spell or was there fever or illness? Did the child remember what occurred during the episode? Were there any repetitive behavior during the spell such as lip smacking, constant rubbing of objects, etc. Were there any body movements? How long did the spell last?

Age of the child:

Age of the child is very important. Causes of seizures in the newborn are completely different and hence will be discussed separately.

Febrile seizures usually occur between the ages of 6 months to 5 years.

Benign childhood epilepsy is common between 2 and 13 years. Infantile spasms usually occur between 3 to 8 months of life. Peak prevalence of absence seizures is between 6 to 8 years.

Duration of seizures:

Since when is the child getting seizures? Is this the first attack? If the child is getting seizures since long. Has the frequency of seizures increased or decreased.

History of fever:

Does the child get fever before the onset of seizures?

Febrile convulsions are common in children. They are not related to the degree of temperature rise, but are frequent if temperature rises abruptly. In simple benign febrile convulsions, fits occur within 24 hours of the onset of fever.

Fever would also be an important feature in fits associated with central nervous system infections such as meningitis and encephalitis.

Detail description of the seizures:

Was the seizure generalized or partial (focal). If seizures are generalized whether they are tonic, clonic, absence attacks (petitmal), atonic, akinetic or myoclonic? Generalized tonic-clonic seizures are the most frequent form of epilepsy. In absence seizures the child has a brief abrupt lapse of consciousness. He may show sudden cessation of the activity being performed with staring spell, eye fluttering or rhythmic movements. There is no loss of posture and the child resumes the activity he was doing. Infantile spasms is characterized by sudden dropping of the head and flexion of arms.

In case of partial seizures, it is important to ask whether the seizures are associated with loss of consciousness? In simple partial seizures there is no loss of consciousness, in complex partial there is impairment of consciousness accompanied with motor manifestation or automatism. Partial seizures with secondary generalization also occur.

One must also enquire whether the seizure is preceded by an aura and followed by any postconvulsive phenomenon such as sleep, headache, abnormal behavior or transient weakness of limb (Todd paralysis).

How long does the seizure last?

Did the child at any time develop status epilepticus?

Timing of seizure:

Is there a specific time of the day when the child gets a seizure? During sleep or just after getting up from sleep.

Perinatal history:

Perinatal insult such as prolonged and difficult labor, premature delivery, birth asphyxia, hyperbilirubinemia and perinatal infections can give rise to seizures in the neonatal period or later.

Developmental history:

Developmental history in all the four domains viz. gross motor, fine motor, language and personal social must be enquired in detail. Were the milestones normal before the onset of seizures? Acute loss of milestones occurs with conditions such as encephalitis, raised intracranial tension due to any cause and rarely encephalopathy related to metabolic derangements. Subacute loss of milestones is related to chronic raised intracranial pressure. A gradual loss of milestones is indicative of degenerative disease of the brain. If the milestones are delayed since the beginning it points towards brain damage from early life due to cerebral malformations or intrauterine infections.

Family history:

History of seizures in other family members must be enquired. Intrafamilial recurrence of convulsions especially simple febrile convulsions and some epilepsies is common.

History of drugs:

Is the child receiving any antiepileptic drugs? In case he is receiving, which drugs? Since when? Dosage and drug compliance?

Other symptoms:

Is there any history of headache or vomiting, which would suggest raised intracranial tension?

History of head injury:

After head injury the child can develop convulsions in the acute phase and even subsequently may develop epileptic seizures after several months or years.

B.   Physical Examination

A general examination followed by detailed neurological examination is important.

Points in history
• Observe the seizure
• Vitals
• Specific odor/pallor/cyanosis/purpuric spots/clubbing
• Head circumference
• Any facial dysmorphism
• Neurocutaneous markers
• Any congenital anomalies
• Neurological examination
• Look for organomegaly
• Examination of cardiovascular system

Observation of seizure:

If the child is brought with convulsions one must observe whether seizure is generalized or partial. Pattern of seizure tonic - clonic, tonic or clonic. If seizure is partial whether there is loss of consciousness. Any automatism, which would point towards temporal lobe epilepsy. Following seizure whether the child becomes normal or goes into sleep.

Salaam spells are very typical. The head drops forward and the arms flex. Duration of each seizure is a few seconds the child often gets such hundreds in a day.

Head circumference:

The head circumference must be measured. Is there microcephaly? Microcephaly could be primary or due to intrauterine infections, which could be the cause of seizures. If there is macrocephaly one must look for sutures and fontanelle. If the fontanelle is wide for the age of the child with separation of sutures the possibility of hydrocephalus must be considered. In such a situation one must look for sunset appearance of eyes. A tense bulging fontanelle indicates raised intracranial pressure seen in meningitis, encephalitis, hydrocephalus, subdural effusion, cerebral edema and intracranial hemorrhage. In older children separation of sutures can be suspected by percussion of the skull, which would elicit a cracked pot sound.

Neurocutaneous markers:

Any child who presents with seizures, one must look for neurocutaneous markers such as cafe-au-lait spots. More than six in number, each over 5 millimeter in diameter are significant. Adenoma sebaceum on the face would indicate tuberous sclerosis. A facial hemangioma points towards Sturge-Weber syndrome. Other markers that should be looked for are shagreen patches and subungual fibromas.

Neurocutaneous disorders causing seizures in infancy

- Incontinentia pigmenti
- Linear nevus sebaceous syndrome
- Neurofibromatosis
- Sturge-Weber syndrome
- Tuberous sclerosis

Vital signs:

Recording of vital signs is especially important if child is brought with seizures. Pulse, temperature, respiration and blood pressure should be monitored. If there is bradycardia one must suspect raised intracranial pressure.

Acidotic breathing points towards a metabolic cause.

If there is hypertension either there is raised intracranial pressure or the convulsions are due to hypertensive encephalopathy.

Congenital anomalies:

In every case of seizure, one must look for any facial dysmor-phism, which may suggest a chromosomal aberration. Other anomalies which may point towards an intrauterine infection are microphthalmia, microcornea, cataract, coloboma, glaucoma, etc.

General examination:

The skin should be examined for pallor as severe anemia could lead to anoxia and seizures. The presence of cyanosis and clubbing suggests cyanotic congenital heart disease. The presence of purpuric spots points towards a bleeding diathesis, which

may also be responsible for intracranial bleed and seizures. Presence of specific odor suggests an inborn error of metabolism.

Central nervous system examination:

A detail central nervous system (CNS) examination must be done with emphasis on the following. If the child is conscious assess whether the child is mentally challenged. Assess the development whether it matches with the chronological age of the child or are the milestones delayed.

If the child has presented with altered consciousness look for signs of meningeal irritation. If signs of meningeal irritation are present it points towards meningitis. Next look for signs of raised intracranial pressure, which is suggested by tense bulging fontanelle, decerebrate posture, sixth nerve palsies, bradycardia and hypertension. Assess for neurological deficits. Focalneurological deficit prior to seizures needs to be evaluated for an abscess, granuloma or tumor.

If the child has spastic hemiplegia, diplegia, etc. before seizures, it would suggest cerebral palsy. Acute hemiplegia with seizure points towards a cerebral stroke.

A lot of information can be obtained by fundus examination.

Look for presence of papilledema indicating raised intracranial pressure. Look for hemorrhages and hypertensive changes. Salt pepper appearance is typical of rubella syndrome.

Presence of cherry red spot indicates Tay-sach disease,

Niemann-pick disease, metachromatic leucodystrophy. It is also seen in mucolipidosis.

Examination of abdomen:

The abdomen should be examined for hepatosplenomegaly.

Presence of it would indicate intrauterine infections. It is also a feature of certain metabolic disorders.

Examination of cardiovascular system:

The cardiovascular system should be examined especially for presence of a cyanotic congenital heart disease which could present with seizures.

C. Investigations

Investigations should be used judiciously.

Cerebrospinal fluid examination:

Lumbar puncture is indicated whenever the cause of seizure appears to be an intracranial infection (meningitis and encephalitis). It is also indicated in the first febrile seizure in infants so as not to miss meningoencephalitis. It is contraindicated in raised intracranial tension.

Biochemical investigations:

- Blood glucose, serum calcium and magnesium estimation should be done in infants as hypoglycemia and hypocalcemia are common causes of seizures in this age group

- Determination of pH and arterial blood gases, blood ammonia, blood and CSF lactate/pyruvate levels are indicated if inborn errors of metabolism are suspected and in familial seizures

- Electrolyte estimation should be done whenever the cause of seizure appears to be due to dyselectrolytemia.

Electroencephalography:

Electroencephalography (EEG) is a valuable investigational tool for seizure disorder if used appropriately. It could provide vital information such as type of seizure in selected patients with epilepsy or subjects with unprovoked seizures and in some seizure types.

It would differentiate seizures from non-seizures. In intractable epilepsy it helps to localize epileptogenic focus. It is especially helpful for making the diagnosis of absence attacks, herpes encephalitis and myoclonic epilepsies.

It is not required in febrile convulsions. It should only be done if fever triggered epilepsy is suspected.

EEG patterns change with age, sleep state, physiologic and pathologic states. Accurate interpretation and good recording are fundamental. It should never be done in the immediate postictal period.

Video EEG: It is reserved for complicated cases with protracted or unresponsive seizures and when the seizure type cannot be ascertained.

It is important in all cases of non-febrile seizures as neurocysticercosis is an important cause of epilepsy in our country.

Neuroimaging:

Transfontanellar ultrasonography can be done in infants where the cause appears to be hydrocephalus, subdural effusion / hematoma.

Computerized tomography (CT scan): CT scan is useful for anatomic lesion identification. It helps to distinguish symptomatic epilepsies of partial/generalized nature from idiopathic epilepsy.

Some of the symptomatic causes that CT helps to identify are granulomas, tumors, porencephalic cyst, atrophies and gross migrational disorders. It is therefore, indicated in temporal lobe epilepsy and cortical epilepsy. Intracranial calcification is seen in tuberous sclerosis, Sturge-Weber syndrome and congenital toxoplasmosis. Neuroimaging is also indicated in children with focal seizures, uncontrolled seizures despite optimum therapy, focal neurological deficits, loss of acquired milestones and features of raised intracranial tension.

Magnetic Resonance Imaging (MRI): It helps in better identification of epileptogenic lesion, diagnosis of live cysticercus cysts, heterotropias, migration defects and small tumours. It is essential in the workup of intractable epilepsy (hippocampal evaluation).

Positron Emission Tomography (PET Scan): PET scan is useful for localization of an anatomic focus in presurgical work up of intractable epilepsy.

Complete blood count:

Complete blood count (CBC) is indicated if cause of seizures appears to be due to cerebral malaria, sickle cell anemia or blood dyscrasias.

II. SEIZURES IN NEWBORN

The most prominent feature of neurological dysfunction in the neonatal period is the occurrence of seizures. Determining the underlying etiology for neonatal seizures is critical. Etiology determines prognosis and outcome and guides therapeutic strategies.
In this section, only differences from seizures in older children will be discussed. Seizures are more common in the newborn period than at any other time in life. This increased susceptibility to seizures is due to transient overdevelopment of excitatory systems compared to inhibitory systems.

Newborns do not manifest febrile seizures. Jitteriness is common in newborn babies and needs to be differentiated from seizures. It is characterized by symmetrical tremors of extremities, which are provoked by stimulus and aborted by restraining the limbs. There are no associated eye movements, behavioral phenomena or electroencephalography (EEG) abnormalities.

ETIOLOGY

Table: Causes of neonatal seizures

1. Perinatal injuries: Birth asphyxia, intracranial hemorrhage.

2. Central nervous system infections: Intrauterine infections (TORCH), neonatal meningitis.

3. Metabolic disturbances: Transient— Hypoglycemia, hypocalcemia, hypo/hypernatremia, hypomagnesemia, pyridoxine dependency. Inborn errors of metabolism.

4. Developmental defects: microcephaly, hydrocephalus, disorders of neuronal migration (heterotopias, lissencephalus), disorders of neuronal organization (polymicrogyria).

5. Benign seizures: Benign neonatal sleep myoclonus, benign familial neonatal convulsions.

TYPES OF SEIZURES

Clinical manifestations of neonatal seizures differ in several ways from those in older children. The seizures in the newborn are more subtle and pleomorphic and motor manifestations are often disorganized. Generalized tonic clonic convulsions are not seen in neonates. This is due to incomplete development of axons, dendritic processes, arborization and poor myelination. Severity of convulsive movements is related to the size of the baby. Larger the baby more powerful are the twitchings. Manifest seizures are uncommon in premature babies. The clinical type of seizures generally offers little clue to the etiology.

Clinical subtypes:

Clinical seizure types may be categorized broadly into 4 groups. In many cases more than one type of seizure occurs over time in a newborn.

Subtle seizures:

Over half of the seizures in the newborn are subtle. They present as behavioral phenomena such as deviation of eyes, fluttering of eyelids, roving movements of eyes, staring look, chewing, sucking, lip smacking. Initially, there is tachycardia followed by bradycardia and apnea at times. This orofacial and lingual phenomenon is due to advanced maturation of the limbic system.

Focal clonic seizures:

Focal seizures in a newborn are a manifestation of bilateral cerebral disturbances. Common causes of focal clonic seizures are metabolic disturbances, birth trauma and cerebral infarction.

Multifocal clonic seizures:

Clonic movements migrate from one limb to another haphazardly. The commonest cause of such seizures is hypoxic-ischemic-encephalopathy (HIE).

Tonic seizures:

They are characterized by decerebrate or decorticate posturing of the body and often associated with stortorous breathing and eye signs. They are often associated with intraventricular hemorrhage and kernicterus. The prognosis in general of tonic seizures is poor.

Myoclonic seizures:

These seizures are characterized by sudden jerky movements. They are associated with diffuse usually serious brain dysfunction resulting from inborn errors of metabolism, perinatal asphyxia and developmental defects of the brain.

Apneic seizures:

Seizures in the newborn can manifest as apneic attack. The difference from apnea of prematurity is that during convulsive apnea the heart rate remains normal or there may be tachycardia. It is often associated with eye movements.

EVALUATION

While evaluating a newborn with seizures emphasis should be laid on the following.

A. History

> **Points in history**
> - Family history
> - Maternal history
> - Perinatal history
> - Day of onset of seizures

Family history:

Did any of the siblings or family members suffer from seizures?

Seizures in siblings would point towards a hereditary metabolic disorder or benign familial neonatal seizures.

Maternal history:

Is the mother diabetic? Did she suffer from infection during pregnancy? Is the mother suffering from hyperparathyroidism? Is she an epileptic? If yes, is she receiving anticonvulsant drugs?

Infants of diabetic mothers do develop hypoglycemia and hypocalcemia giving rise to seizures. Congenital intrauterine infections (TORCH) can present with seizures. Maternal hyperparathyroidism induces transient neonatal hypoparathyroidism, which would lead to hypocalcemia and seizures. If the mother is receiving anticonvulsant drugs during pregnancy it leads to increased catabolism of vitamin D which in turn leads to vitamin D deficiency, hypocalcemia and seizures.

Perinatal history:

Was the baby asphyxiated at birth? Did he need resuscitation? Was the labor prolonged? Was there premature rupture of membranes? Did the mother suffer from fever during labor?

Neonate who has sustained birth asphyxia is likely to develop seizures any time. The neonate is predisposed to sepsis and meningitis,if the mother has infection during labor, or the labor is prolonged or the membranes rupture prematurely.

Feeding history:

Has the baby been fed since birth? Is he breastfed or top fed?

Delayed feeding especially in low birth weight infants can lead to hypoglycemia and seizures. Babies receiving animal milk can develop seizures due to hypocalcemia.

Day of onset of seizures:

In case of birth asphyxia seizures can develop within the first few hours to as late as several weeks after birth.

In preterm babies seizures are common during first three days due to hypoglycemia and hypocalcemia. Infants of diabetic mothers can develop seizures during the first 24 to 48 hours due to hypoglycemia. Late onset hypocalcemia usually present with seizures at the end of the first week.

B. Physical Examination

Points on examination
- General appearance
- Assessment of growth
- Examination of head
- General examination
- Systemic examination

General appearance:

Is the neonate dull, lethargic with hypotonia or is he active and normal in between seizures? Dull lethargic neonate would suggest an encephalopathy following asphyxia or sepsis and meningitis.

Assess growth of the newborn:

A neonate with intrauterine growth retardation is likely to develop hypoglycemia and hypocalcemia. An infant of a diabetic mother is large for date, plethoric and is also susceptible to develop hypoglycemia and hypocalcemia.

Examination of head:

Measure circumference of skull for evidence of micro and macrocephaly.

Tense bulging fontanelle indicates raised intracranial pressure, which could be due to hydrocephalus, meningitis or intracranial hemorrhage. Microcephaly would point towards intrauterine infection or a genetic cause.

General examination:

Look for icterus, purpuric spots and congenital anomalies which suggest intrauterine infections.

Systemic examination:

In suspected TORCH infection look for hepatosplenomegaly and fundus examination.

C. Investigations

Biochemistry:

Hematocrit, blood glucose, calcium, phosphorus, magnesium, sodium must be estimated in all cases of neonatal seizures as hypoglycemia, hypocalcemia, hypomagnesemia, dyselectrolytemia are common causes of seizures in the newborn.

Complete blood count and CSF examination:

along with blood culture must be done in all cases to exclude sepsis and meningitis.

Electrocardiogram: EKG can be done to rapidly diagnose hypocalcemia. It gives rise to prolonged QTc interval (> 0.2s).

Cranial ultrasound: It is indicated especially in cases of intracranial bleed and in suspected hydrocephalus.

MRI and CT scan is indicated in structural and developmental defects like cerebral dysgenesis, lissencephaly and neuronal migration disorders.

Serology for TORCH infections: It should be done where the cause of seizures appears to be intrauterine infections.

Screening for inborn errors of metabolism:

If the cause of seizures appears to be an inborn error of metabolism, then an ABG, blood ammonia, lactate/pyruvate level, plasma and urinary amino acid levels are indicated.

Electroencephalography: EEG recording with videomonitoring is very useful in some cases. In Herpes encephalitis, EEG shows a multifocal periodic pattern. Neonates with pyridoxine dependency have generalized 1 to 4 Hz sharp and slow wave activity. Comb rhythm on EEG is suggestive of Maple syrup urine disease.

SUMMARY

Seizures are a symptom of an underlying disorder of the CNS requiring investigations to determine the cause and plan a course of treatment. Epilepsy is recurrent seizures that is not related to any acute cerebral disease or fever. There are certain conditions that can mimic seizures such as syncope, dystonia, decerebrate posturing. These conditions need to be recognized or else the patient may receive unnecessary drugs.

The commonest age group for seizures is the neonatal period. Pattern of seizures is also different in this age group. Subtle seizures are common in the neonatal period. It is essential to learn to identify them. Also tremulousness is physiological in this age group and needs to be differentiated from seizures.

Between the ages of 1 to 5 years, febrile convulsions are common. All cases of seizures do need to be investigated to arrive at a definite diagnosis and to subsequently plan therapy.

SUGGESTED READING

1. Seizures in children: Types, symptoms, causes and treatment. www.emedicinehealth.com.

2. Seizures in children: Diagnosis, causes, signs, treatment www.webmd.com.

3. Neonatal seizures: (2016) emedicine.medscape.com.

27

COMATOSE CHILD

INTRODUCTION

Altered sensorium is one of the commonest emergency, for which a child is brought to the pediatric ward. Although there are several causes of coma, when faced with an unconscious child a quick assessment and immediate action is important.

The word coma is derived from a Greek word 'koma' meaning deep sleep. Clinical definition of coma means an altered state of consciousness combined with a reduced capacity for arousal and decreased responsiveness to visual, auditory and tactile stimulation.

Comatose patients have no eye opening as opposed to states of transient unconsciousness. Coma must last for at least 1 hour.

ETIOLOGY

Traumatic brain injury leading to coma is much more common than non-traumatic coma.

Table: Causes of coma

1. Traumatic Coma
2. Non-traumatic coma
   - Central nervous system infections: Meningitis (purulent/ tubercular), encephalitis, septicemia, intracranial abscess
   - Cerebrovascular accidents:
     a. Hemorrhage, rupture of arteriovenous (AV) malformations
     b. Thrombosis: Cyanotic congenital heart disease, sickle cell anemia; venous sinus thrombosis—sepsis, dehydration
     c. Embolism: Bacterial endocarditis
   - Brain tumor: Hemorrhage in the tumor
   - Hypertensive encephalopathy
   - Postictal coma
   - Metabolic: Diabetic ketoacidosis, Reye's syndrome, hepatic coma, uremia, hypoxemia, inborn errors of metabolism, hypernatremia, hyponatremia
   - Drugs and poisons: Barbiturates, phenothiazine, narcotics, lead poisoning, salicylate
   - Heat stroke.

EVALUATION

As soon as an unconscious child is brought to the ward, the first thing that should be done is to evaluate his airways, breathing and circulatory status and attend to it. An intravenous access should be obtained. If respiratory depression or circulatory collapse is present, one should immediately prepare for intubaton, assisted ventilation and vasopressor support. Only after having done this should a detail history and examination be performed.

A. History

Points in history
• Age of the child
• Onset—acute or gradual
• Any history of trauma
• History of fever
• History of contact with tuberculosis
• History of headache and vomiting
• History of illness
• History of failure to thrive
• History of drug intake

Age of the child:

In a newborn the commonest cause of altered sensorium is hypoxic ischemic encephalopathy followed by meningitis and encephalitis. In an older child, the commonest cause would be intracranial infections.

Onset:

Was the onset of coma acute or gradual? Sudden onset usually follows head injury, cerebrovascular accidents, especially hemorrhage and postictal phase. Gradual onset usually seen in cases of intracranial infections and metabolic causes.

History of trauma:

Did the child sustain any head injury?

History of fever:

Large number of infections affect the nervous system. Does the child get fever? If yes, since when? Is it high grade? Is fever associated with chills and rigors? High grade fever with chills and rigors usually suggests cerebral malaria. In purulent meningitis and encephalitis onset of illness is associated with fever. In tubercular meningitis there is usually history of low grade fever for several weeks before the child goes into coma.

History of headache and vomiting:

Did the child complain of headache? Was there associated vomiting? Presence of headache and vomiting would suggest raised intracranial tension.

History of illnesses:

It is essential to enquire whether the child is an epileptic because the child may be in the postictal phase.

A history of diabetes, renal disease, hepatic disease, sickle cell anemia and heart disease must also be enquired.

Failure to thrive:

History of failure to thrive would suggest an inborn error of metabolism.

History of drug intake:

Is the child receiving any drugs such as sodium valproate or phenobarbitone? Has he consumed any drug accidentally?

B. Examination

Aim of physical examination is to determine both the anatomical site of disturbed cerebral function and its cause.

Points on physical examination
• Assess level of unconsciousness
• Vital signs - temperature, respiration, pulse and blood pressure
• General examination
• Neurological examination
• Examination of other systems

Assess the depth of unconsciousness:

It is essential to assess the degree of altered sensorium. It is classified in four stages:

• Stage I or stupor: In this stage, patient

can be aroused briefly and shows verbal or motor responses to stimuli.

- Stage II or light coma: Patient can only be aroused with painful stimuli.
- Stage III or deep coma: There is no response to painful stimuli.
- Stage IV or brain death: All cerebral functions are lost. Pupillary reflexes are absent. Local spinal reflexes may be preserved.

This staging helps in following the course of illness in the child. Whether his consciousness is improving or deteriorating.

Vital signs:

Recording the temperature, respiration, pulse and BP is very important.

Respiration: Count the respiratory rate and assess the type of respiration. Cheyne-Stokes respiration, in which periods of hyperpnea alternate with periods of apnea, is usually caused by bilateral hemispheric or diencephalic injuries, but can result from bilateral damage anywhere along the descending pathway between the forebrain and upper pons. The brainstem is intact. Hyperventilation occurs in metabolic coma with acidosis and in brainstem lesions. Irregular or ataxic breathing indicates involvement of respiratory centre in the medulla.

Pulse: Count the pulse. Presence of bradycardia would suggest raised intracranial pressure. Tachycardia could be due to fever, hypovolemic or septic shock, heart failure or arrhythmias. Presence of fever suggests an infective process e.g. sepsis, pneumonia, meningitis, encephalitis or a brain abscess, but may also indicate heat stroke. Tachypnea with respiratory distress indicates lung pathology e.g. pneumonia, pneumothorax, empyema or asthma. Tachypnea without distress may be present in diabetic ketoacidosis, uremia or poisoning. Hypertension could be due to hypertensive encephalopathy or raised intracranial pressure. Hypotension could be due to sepsis or cardiac dysfunction.

General examination:

In the general examination of an unconscious child, one must look for jaundice, as it would indicate hepatic coma. Presence of pallor with high fever and altered sensorium would suggest cerebral malaria. Petechiae with shock and altered sensorium is a feature of meningococcemia.

Rash could be seen with measles encephalitis. Peculiar smell would suggest inborn error of metabolism, diabetic ketoacidosis, hepatic coma.

One must look for signs of dehydration especially in a child with diarrhea. Dyselectrolytemia could result in altered sensorium.

Neurological examination:

Level of consciousness must be recorded

Pupillary light reflex: Reaction of pupils to light must be examined. Small equal reactive pupils would suggest toxic or metabolic cause of coma. Moderately dilated pupils with no reaction to light would suggest midbrain damage. Pinpoint pupils indicate pontine lesion or morphine poisoning. Bilateral fixed dilated pupils suggests terminal stage or severe ischemic brain damage or datura poisoning. Unilateral dilated unreactive pupil indicates third nerve damage, which is often associated with transtentorial herniation of the temporal lobe.

Brainstem function:

- **Look at the position of eyeballs.** Tonic lateral deviation of both eyes indicates irritative lesion in the cortex on the opposite side of the gaze, whereas destructive lesion produces conjugate deviation of the eyes to the ipsilateral side.

- **Doll's eye response:** This should be elicited in every child with altered sensorium. When the head is suddenly turned to one side, there is conjugate deviation of the eyes in the opposite direction. This response occurs if the brainstem is intact. Doll's eye movement is not seen in normal conscious infants and is absent, when brainstem centers for eye movements are damaged.

- **Oculovestibular response:** After eliciting the Doll's eye response one should elicit the oculovestibular response. This reflex is elicited by irrigating the external auditory canal with cold water. The eyes normally deviate towards the stimulated side. The presence of this reflex indicates that much of the brainstem is intact.

Motor responses:

Observe the trunk and limb position at rest, spontaneous movements and response to noxious stimuli.

Spontaneous movements of all limbs generally indicates a mild depression of hemispheric function without structural disturbance.

Monoplegia or hemiplegia with or without hemifacial weakness suggests structural disturbance of the contralateral hemisphere involving cortical or subcortical motor centres. In a comatose child, these motor abnormalities may manifest as alteration in muscle tone, deep tendon reflexes or

decreased spontaneous activity, when compared with the contralateral side. If the child is lying in a decorticate posture, i.e. with flexion of both upper extremities with extension of lower limbs, it indicates a cortical or subcortical disturbance with the brainstem preserved.

If the child is lying with extension of all the extremities, i.e. decerebrate posture, it indicates brainstem compression and should be considered an ominous signs. Decerebrate rigidity can result from increased intracranial pressure, metabolic disease, Reye syndrome and cerebral hypoxia. Both decorticate and decerebrate posturing are stimulus, sensitive and may require the induction of pain for their appearance. Flaccidity occurs, when both the cortical and brainstem function have ceased.

Signs of meningeal irritation:

Signs of meningeal irritation must be elicited in all unconscious children. Presence of meningeal signs would suggest meningitis. Kernig's and Brudzinski's signs are more reliable signs of meningeal irritation.

Systemic examination:

The cardiovascular system must be examined for heart disease and the abdomen for evidence of liver disease. Enlarged spleen with anemia would suggest cerebral malaria.

C. Investigations

Laboratory evaluation should be individualized not every test is essential for each clinical situation.

Table: Clues from investigation

	Investigations	Probable Diagnosis
1.	Blood chemistry	
	• Blood glucose	
	Low levels	Hypoglycemic coma
	Raised	Diabetic coma
	Serum electrolytes deranged	Dyselectrolytemia
	• BUN and serum creatinine	
	Raised	Uremia
	• Liver function test deranged	Hepatic dysfunction
	• Serum ammonia and lactate raised	Diabetic coma, in-born errors of metabolism
2.	Urine examination	
	• Sugar and ketone bodies present	Diabetic ketoacidosis
	• Proteinuria present	Renal cause
3.	Complete blood count	
	• Leucocytosis	Sepsis
4.	Cerebrospinal fluid examination	
	• Proteins raised	Meningitis / encephalitis
	• Cells raised mainly polyps	Purulent meningitis
	• Increased lymphocytes	Tubercular meningitis / viral meningitis
5.	CT scan head informative in	Head trauma and intracranial space occupying lesion
6.	Electroencephalogram	
	• Periodic lateralizing epileptiformdis charges in temporal lobe	Herpes encephalitis

Biochemical tests, urine examination and a complete blood count must be done in all unconscious patients.

Biochemical tests:

Estimation of blood glucose should be done for hypo and hyperglycemia.

Serum electrolytes for dyselectrolytemia. Blood urea nitrogen and serum creatinine for uremia.

Liver function tests for hepatic dysfunction. Serum ammonia, lactate, arterial blood gases in suspected diabetic coma and inborn error of metabolism.

Estimation of serum calcium and phosphorus are also indicated.

Urine examination:

It should be done for reducing substance ketone bodies, which would be present in diabetic ketoacidosis. Presence of proteinuria suggests a renal cause.

Blood examination:

Complete blood count (CBC) should be done for evidence of sepsis. Peripheral smear should be carefully examined for malarial parasite, if the cause is febrile coma. Blood culture is also indicated.

Cerebrospinal fluid examination:

Cerebrospinal fluid examination must be done if the cause is an intracranial infection, i.e. meningitis/encephalitis. Apart from routine examination of CSF, culture should also be done.

Computed tomography of head:

It is indicated where the cause of coma is head trauma, there is evidence of raised intracranial pressure, focal neurological deficits, unexplained altered sensorium and features of herniation.

Electroencephalogram:

Electroencephalogram is useful in herpes encephalitis, in which case EEG shows periodic lateralizing epileptiform discharges in one temporal lobe. It may be useful in absence or complex partial status also.

SUMMARY

Coma is a medical emergency which presents diagnostic as well as therapeutic challenges. The causes are numerous and can result from intracranial or extracranial causes. The critical window for diagnosis and effective intervention is short. Diagnosis can often be made from a good history, careful examination and simple investigations.

SUGGESTED READING

1. Sharma S, Kochar GS, et al. Indian J Pediatr. 2010;77:1279-1287.
2. Fenichel M. Gerald: Altered states of consciousness. Clinical Pediatric Neurology, 5th Edition, 2007; 47-75.

28 FLOPPY INFANT

INTRODUCTION

Floppy infant syndrome is a term used to describe infant, presenting with marked hypotonia. It has a diverse etiology. A floppy infant is recognized by abnormal posture, decreased resistance to passive movement and abnormal range of joint movement due to hypotonia. The motor milestones are also delayed.

ETIOLOGY

Acquisition of normal tone is dependent upon an intact central and peripheral nervous system. Floppy infant often termed floppy infant syndrome is not a disease but a clinical condition associated with a large number of diseases and disorders. These infants usually present with floppiness, decreased motor activity and/or certain complications like feeding difficulty and pneumonia.

Table: Causes of floppy infant

1. Central causes:
   - Atonic cerebral palsy due to perinatal asphyxia
   - Kernicterus
   - Chromosomal anomalies such as Down syndrome, metabolic defects-gangliosidosis
   - Cerebral dysgenesis
   - Cerebral or spinal cord trauma
2. Peripheral Causes:
   - Anterior horn cell disease-spinal muscular atrophy, poliomyelitis
   - Peripheral nerves-peripheral neuropathies, Guillain-Barre syndrome, diphtheritic paralysis
   - Myoneural junction-myasthenia gravis, infantile botulism
   - Muscles-congenital myopathies (central core disease and nemaline myopathy) glycogen storage disease (Pompe's) congenital myotonic dystrophy, benign congenital hypotonia
3. Miscellaneous:
   - Protein energy malnutrition,Rickets, Prader-Willi syndrome
   - Ehlers-Danlos syndrome, Cutislaxa, Cretinism

EVALUATION

The first step in diagnosis is to determine whether the disease is situated in the brain, spine or motor unit. More than one site may be involved.

A. History

Points in history
- Age of onset of floppiness
- Mode of onset
- Any feeding problem
- Any alteration in voice
- Mother's perception of fetal movements
- Perinatal history
- Developmental history
- Family history of similar illness
- Presenting symptoms

Age of onset:

Is floppiness since birth or has it appeared later? At birth hypotonia could be due to several causes. If the neonate appears sick the cause could be birth asphyxia, sepsis, drugs given to the mother during delivery such as $MgSO_4$/diazepam. If the neonate is well, but hypotonic must consider Werdnig-Hoffman disease, congenital myopathies, Down syndrome and hypothyroidism. Hypotonia in infancy and childhood could be due to spinal muscular atrophy, congenital myopathies, neuropathies, metabolic causes or hypotonic cerebral palsy.

Mode of onset and course of the disease:

Was the onset of weakness acute or slow? Is it progressive orstatic?

Developmental disorders are slow in onset and progressive.

Cerebral or spinal cord injury due to trauma is usually acute in onset. The disease is progressive in spinal muscular atrophy type 1 (SMA 1) and static in SMA II, SMA III, congenital myopathy, cerebral palsy and neuropathies.

If the child was perfectly well and suddenly develops fever followed by weakness of limbs, the cause could be Guillain-Barresyndrome or poliomyelitis but not a neuromuscular disorder.

Feeding history:

Does the child have any difficulty in sucking, chewing or swallowing? Is the voice hoarse? Feeding problems with recurrent pneumonias would indicate neuromuscular disorders.

Antenatal history:

At what period of gestation did the mother perceive fetal movements?

Whether the fetal movements were normal or decreased?

Any history of polyhydramnios? Absence or reduction in fetal movements along with polyhydramnios is a feature of spinal muscular atrophy and is due to intrauterine swallowing difficulty.

Perinatal history:

Did the child sustain birth asphyxia? Did he have hyperbilirubinemia leading to kernicterus? Was there sepsis? In all these conditions, the neonate can be hypotonic. Birth asphyxia and kernicterus can later on lead to hypotonic type of cerebral palsy.

Developmental history:

Developmental history must be enquired. Beyond the neonatal period floppy infants usually present with delay in motor milestones. If there is associated mental retardation one must think of central causes of hypotonia. Delay of motor milestones with normal intellectual development suggests a possible defect in the motor unit.

Family history:

Is any other member in the family having a similar illness?

History of similar illness in other family members would point towards a genetic disease. It would also help to determine the pattern of inheritance.

Presenting symptoms:

The usual symptoms with which these babies present are weakness, poor sucking, feeble cry, lethargy, reduced spontaneous activity and delayed motor development.

B. Physical Examination

Points on examination

- Confirm hypotonia
- Look for facial dysmorphism
- Is the baby obese?
- Is there weakness?
- What about tendon reflexes?
- Is there sensory involvement?

- Any developmental retardation
- Respiratory movements?
- Any fasciculations or fibrillations
- Is the child grossly malnourished?
- Any evidence of rickets.

Confirm hypotonia:

In a floppy baby there is hypotonia of the skeletal muscles, which can be recognized by the posture of the infant. The infant assumes a frog like posture, in which there is abduction of the hips and flexion of the knees. The baby slips under the fingers, when held upright from the axilla, there is diminished resistance to passive movements and excessive range of joint mobility.

Facial dysmorphism:

Dysmorphic face could be seen in congenital muscular dystrophy. Typical facies in Down syndrome and Prader-Willi syndrome, coarse facies would be a feature of cretinism.

Presence of ptosis would suggest myasthenia gravis.

Is the baby obese?

Obesity would point towards Prader-Willi syndrome.

Is the baby alert?

If the baby is alert in comparison to the weakness he has, one must suspect SMA.

Look for fasciculation:

Presence of fasciculation on tongue would suggest nerve disease.

Look for degree of weakness:

While assessing muscle power one must assess the degree and extent of weakness and also whether involvement is more in the proximal or distal group of muscles. Whether the weakness is symmetrical or asymmetrical.

Degree of weakness of muscles can be assessed by observation of the movements of limbs. If the muscle power is proportionate to the degree of hypotonia, one must suspect muscle/nerve disease. Disproportionate weakness indicates the cause in the central nervous system, systemic illness, metabolic or connective tissue disease.

It is important to compare extent of weakness of arms, legs and face. Extreme weakness of arms and legs would suggest anterior horn cell disease, peripheral nerve involvement or neuromuscular junction disease. Involvement of the face is also seen in neuromuscular junction disorder. In myopathies involvement of the face is variable. Presence of ptosis and limited eye movements would suggest myasthenia gravis. Compare the proximal versus distal muscle involvement. In peripheral nerve involvement, weakness is more in the distal group of muscles.In neuromuscular disease weakness is equal in both the groups while in myopathies proximal muscle involvement is more than in the distal muscle.

Deep tendon reflexes:

Deep tendon reflexes can be normal or exaggerated in central nervous system disorder, absent in anterior horn cell disease.They are decreased in peripheral nerve involvement and muscle disease.

The reflexes are normal in neuromuscular junction disorder such as myasthenia. In hypotonic cerebral palsy, there ishypotonia with brisk reflexes. In chromosomal aberrations there is hypotonia, dysmorphic features, but no exaggeration of deep reflexes.

Sensory abnormalities:

Sensory involvement would indicate presence of neuropathy.

Respiratory movements:

Respiratory movements should be carefully evaluated for weakness of intercostal and diaphragmatic muscles. These muscles are more affected in spinal muscular atrophy.

Floppy Infant   203

Assessment of growth:

It is important to assess the growth of the child. Severe malnutrition can lead to hypotonia. Even children with rickets can have generalized hypotonia.

Table: Investigations to be done

	Investigations	Probable Cause
1.	Nerve conduction velocity	Neuropathies
2.	ElectromyographyCharacteristic EMG patterns	Distinguish denervation from myopathic involvement
3.	Muscle biopsy	Distinguish neurogenic from myopathic process, also identifies specific myopathy
4.	Tensilon test positive	Myasthenia gravis
5.	Molecular genetic markers	Hereditary myopathies and neuropathies
6.	Neuroimaging – MRI	Useful where cause is central
7.	Metabolic screen	In-born errors of metabolism
8.	Karyotyping	Chromosomal anomaly
9.	Creatine kinase	Myopathies

In all case of hypotonia nerve conduction studies and electromyography (EMG) are useful to establish a neuromuscular cause, either denervation process or a myopathy. This should be followed by biopsy, serum enzymes as well as EMG may be completely normal in some of these infants.

Muscle biopsy:

Muscle biopsy is the most important and specific diagnostic study of most neuromuscular disorders.

Not only neurogenic and myopathic processes distinguished but also the type of myopathy and specific enzymatic deficiencies may be determined.

Histochemical studies of frozen sections of the muscle are useful in some cases.

If the cause is myasthenia gravis, the tensilontest would be positive.

C. Investigations

After having made a clinical diagnosis patien should be subjected to appropriate investigatior to reach a final diagnosis.

Many DNA markers of hereditary myopathies and neuropathies are now available. In a suspected case of metabolic error certain tests are indicated viz. serum ammonia levels, venous pH, serum aminoacids, urine aminoacids and organic acid estimation.

Karyotyping:

Karyotyping is indicated, where cause appears to be a chromosomal anomaly. In a newborn if the cause of generalized hypotonia appears to be due to sepsis than a septic screen is indicated. A complete bloodcount, blood culture, cerebrospinal fluid (CSF) examination andculture should be done.

Creatine Kinase:

Creatine kinase is characteristically raised in certain diseases. Nerve Conduction Velocity Neuropathies of various types are detected by decreased conduction.

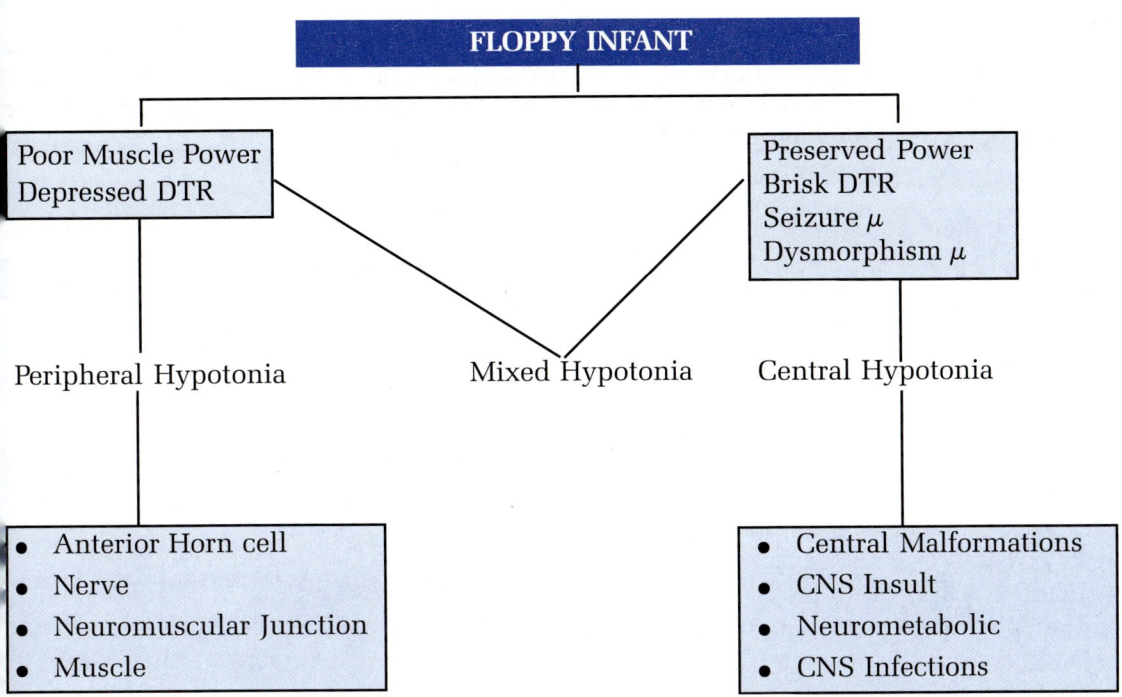

FLOPPY INFANT

- Poor Muscle Power
  Depressed DTR

- Preserved Power
  Brisk DTR
  Seizure μ
  Dysmorphism μ

Peripheral Hypotonia   Mixed Hypotonia   Central Hypotonia

- Anterior Horn cell
- Nerve
- Neuromuscular Junction
- Muscle

- Central Malformations
- CNS Insult
- Neurometabolic
- CNS Infections

SUMMARY

An infant with marked hypotonia is labeled as a floppy infant. The cause can be in the central nervous system, spinal cord, peripheral nerves or in the muscles. A clinical diagnosis of hypotonia is first made based on abnormal postures of the infant, relative immobility and excessive range of joint mobility. Depending upon the clinical diagnosis, relevant investigations are carried out to confirm the diagnosis.

SUGGESTED READING

1. Floppy infant in Textbook of Pediatrics. Ed. Piyush Gupta 2013, 1st Ed. 498-502.

2. Bibek Talukdar. Floppy infant – Clinical approach. IAP Textbook of Pediatrics. 5th Ed. 378-381.

Chapter

29 GLOBAL DEVELOPMENTAL DELAY

INTRODUCTION

A child is often brought to a clinician for delayed achievement of developmental milestones. In such a situation one has to firstly determine, whether the delay is restricted to a specific area or is it global? Secondly, whether the development is delayed or regressing. The latter may at times be difficult to assess in an infant because in static encephalopathy new symptoms may appear such as seizures and involuntary movements giving an impression that the infant has a progressive neurological disorder. Also delayed achievement of milestones without other neurological deficit is sometimes the initial manifestation of progressive disorder.

In this chapter we shall be only discussing about a child with global developmental delay.

DEFINITION

Global developmental delay is defined as significant delay by atleast 2 standard deviation (SD) in four different components of development viz gross motor, fine motor or adaptive, language and personal social.

The term global developmental delay is usually reserved for children less than 5 years of age.

ETIOLOGY

Table: Causes of delayed development

Organic:

- Maternal factors: Exposure to teratogen (alcohol, drugs, radiation, etc. in pregnancy. Intrauterine infections - CMV, Rubella, Toxoplasmosis, HIV Placental dysfunction, toxemia, APH.

- Fetal factors: Chromosomal disorder (fragile X chromosome, Down' syndrome), congenital CNS malformations, extreme prematurity metabolic disorders (hypoglycemia galactosemia, mucopolysaccharidosis phenylketonuria).

- Hypothyroidism

- Natal factors: Hypoxic-ischemic insult birth injuries, intracranial hemorrhage

- Postnatal causes: Meningitis, encephalitis malnutrition, hypoxia, kernicterus, stroke CNS disorders: Cerebral palsy neurocutaneous syndrome, degenerative brain diseases

Environmental:

- Psychosocial deprivation
- Nutritional deprivation
- Child abuse

EVALUATION

An approach to making a diagnosis involves a detailed history and physical examination Specific points in the history and physical examination are given below:

Evaluating a child for development needs patience and time. One could choose a screening test, with which one is comfortable. Severe developmental disorders can be picked up in early infancy on the first occasion. However, periodic assessment is essential.

A prerequisite to assess development in any child is to develop a rapport with the parents and the child.

A. History

- Family history (3 generations)
- Consanguinity
- Previous pregnancy outcomes
- Ethnic background
- Prenatal history
- Perinatal history
- Postnatal history
- Pattern of development

Parents observation should always be taken into account:

Is the development normal or delayed?

Is the delay in development in all the areas or is it restricted to a specific area? Is there any loss of milestones?

Delayed development is quite different from that of psychomotor regression. Slow progress in the attainment of developmental milestones may be caused by either static or progressive encephalopathies.

At times static encephalopathies of the nervous system may appear progressive due to appearance of new symptoms such as seizures and involuntary movements. Whenever there is a clear history that the milestones, which the child had attained are lost it is a definite evidence of progressive disease of the nervous system. Several inborn errors of metabolism in infancy present as delayed development. It is only later in the course of the disease that regression of milestones is identified.

Family history:

Enquire about family history of birth defects, childhood deaths, mental retardation, speech delay, learning disabilities, autism and known genetic conditions.

Family history should be recorded in the form of a pedigree. Seeing the family history in pictorial form makes the pattern of inheritance more apparent. For boys with developmental delay, particular interest is in looking for evidence of X-linkage. Consanguinity is common in certain ethnic groups and may not be mentioned unless specifically queried. If present makes autosomal recessive inheritance more likely.

Prenatal history:

Potential teratogens, including alcohol, medications, vitamins, maternal infection (Rubella, CMV, toxoplasmosis, varicella) maternal diabetes, hyperthermia, maternal phenylketonuria during pregnancy are known to affect the developing brain leading to developmental delay.

Perinatal history:

Premature birth, traumatic delivery infections, birth asphyxia needing resuscitation, hyperbilirubinemia and kernicterus, intrauterine growth retarded baby are likely to sustain brain injury leading to developmental delay. Poor feeding, hypotonia in the neonatal period are pointers of cerebral insult in the neonatal period.

Postnatal history:

History of illness in the neonatal period viz. meningitis, encephalitis, encephalopathy of any origin is important. Any history of seizures, increased or decreased tone. Overall growth movements, coordination should be asked. A detailed developmental history (milestones) including vision and hearing and school performance should be enquired. Evidence of regression of milestones may be a clue to inborn error of metabolism or neurodegenerative process.

Environmental deprivation:

History pertaining to the environment, in which the child is living is also important. Is he an abandoned child? Is he neglected due to parental conflicts? Does he stay in an orphanage or away from parents? How are the caretakers?

Emotional deprivation due to any cause can lead to slow development primarily because of lack of stimulus.

Nutritional history:

In a developing country like ours, malnutrition is common in rural and urban slums. Severely malnourished children in infancy and early childhood can present with global developmental delay. Hence, it is essential to take a dietetic history.

B. Clinical Examination

An attempt should be made to classify the child into syndromic versus non-syndromic developmental delay. Although sometimes clear-cut, this may not be so easy if the patient is generally non-syndromic, but has one or two unusual features e.g. hypotonia or short stature.

Points on examination
- Developmental assessment of the child
- Growth assessment
- General examination
  - Dysmorphic features
  - Stigmata of intrauterine infection.
- Systemic examination

Developmental assessment:

A developmental assessment should be first done using any of the developmental screening tests to determine, whether the child has a global developmental delay.

Initially adequate time should be spent observing the child, when the baby is with the mother. Points to be observed are alertness, concentration, social responsiveness and hyperactivity.

Growth assessment:

Record the weight, height and head circumference of the child. Failure to thrive is a feature of inborn errors of metabolism such as maple syrup urine disease and those with HIV. Growth retardation is also seen in infants with TORCH infections, chromosomal aberrations and hypothyroidism.

Children with homocystinuria are tall thin and may have a Marfan syndrome habitus.

Microcephaly is a feature of chromosomal aberrations and intrauterine infections. It is also seen in babies who had sustained severe birth asphyxia and those with cerebral malformations.

Head circumference is above 50th percentile in children with fragile X-syndrome and those with hydrocephalus.

Growth parameters especially head circumference should be compared with those of other family members. Familial megaloencephaly, for e.g. is particularly common and may not be significant if one of the parents also has a large head. An assessment of body proportions is also important. Is there any asymmetry between left and right? Are the limbs and trunk in proportion. It is important to look at the shape of the head.

General examination:

Try to first determine whether the child looks like either of the parents or siblings. Often this is done by general gestalt, rather than looking at each feature separately. If the child looks significantly different try to analyze each feature separately. Sometimes a comment about the face in general is adequate (i.e. coarse, myopathic) whereas in other situations more specific description of each feature is required e.g. widely placed eyes (hyperteloric), anteverted nares (upturned). Single palmar crease (simian crease) common in many genetic syndromes as well as the general population, whereas cutaneous syndactyl (webbing) between the fingers is far less common and is helpful in pinpointing a diagnosis. Other clues to common causes of developmental delay may be found by carefully examining the skin for hyper or hypopigmentation. Café-au-lait spots may signal neurofibromatosis, while hypopigmented lesions may suggest other neurocutaneous disorders e.g. tuberous sclerosis. Vascular tumors or hemangiomas may suggest certain genetic disorders or syndromes.

Other unusual findings such as anomalies of the genitalia, connective tissue and/or joint abnormalities and internal anomalies especially cardiac and renal should be noted. In addition a detail ophthalmic checkup, audiometry, cardiac and psychometric evaluation are helpful in assessing all children with developmental delay.

Typical mongoloid facies in case of Down syndrome, coarse features in hypothyroidism, chubby round face in glycogen storage disease.

Coarse brittle hair would suggest maple syrup urine disease.

Musty odor of the skin is a feature of phenylketonuria. The eyes should be examined for anomalies like cataract and dislocation of lens. The latter is seen in homocystinuria.

Dysmorphic features—special effort should be made to look for dysmorphic features. Chromosomal aberrations are often associated with multiple minor face and limb abnormalities. Individual abnormalities may not be important, but in combination they assume diagnostic significance. Following are some examples.

Trisomy 721—Mongoloid facies (upward slant of eyes, epicanthal folds, midfacial hypoplasia, small dysplastic pinnae), brushfield spots, simian crease, short broad hands, hypoplasia of middle phalanx of 5th finger.

Trisomy 18—Closed fists with index finger overlapping the middle finger, 5th digit overlapping fourth, prominent occiput, short sternum, rocker bottom feet, micrognathia.

Trisomy 13—Midline cleft lip, poly dactyl, ocularhypotelorism, bulbous nose, microphthalmia, genital anomaly.

Fragile X-syndrome—Males are mainly affected. Some of the typical features are a high forehead, long jaw, large protuberant ears, hyperextensible joints and large testis.

Stigmata of intrauterine infection—Look for stigmata of intrauterine infection. Apart from intrauterine growth retardation and microcephaly, other features of TORCH infection are cataract, coloboma, chorioretinitis, rash, jaundice, etc.

Systemic examination:

A careful systemic examination must be done in all cases of developmental delay.

Abdomen should be examined for hepatosplenomegaly. Presence of organomegaly is seen in intrauterine infections [cytomegalovirus (CMV), HIV, rubella, etc.] and storage disorders.

Cardiovascular system - Presence of congenital heart disease would suggest rubella and chromosomal aberrations such as trisomy 21.

Central nervous system:

Look whether child is hyperactive, does he have signs of autistic spectrum disorders. Check for sensorineural deafness seen in rubella and Down's syndrome.

Any visual impairment.

Muscle tone should be carefully assessed. Generalized hypotonia is seen in abnormalities of autosomal chromosomes.

Spasticity is seen in cerebral palsy and certain inborn errors of metabolism.

Focal neurological deficits would suggest cerebral palsy, maple syrup urine disease and homocystinuria.

C. Investigations

While the list of potential investigations for mental retardation is large, the choice of tests can usually be targeted based on information gathered during the evaluation.

Investigations would depend on whether child is non-syndromic or syndromic.

Non-syndromic child:

The basic work-up for a non-syndromic, delayed child who has normal growth and no birth defects is as follows:

- Chromosomal analysis and DNA testing for Fragile-X syndrome. Cytogenetic abnormalities are present in a large number of mentally retarded non-dysmorphic children especially sex chromosome aneuploidy (XXX, XXY, XYY), subtle deletions, duplications or chromosome re-arrangement.

- Metabolic screening such as plasma amino acids and urine organic acids: It is not recommended in children presenting with undifferentiated mental retardation.

- CT / MRI of the brain: In general it is not considered necessary unless there are other unusual features such as neurological signs, macro or microcephaly.

Syndromic child:

In addition to the investigations listed above, a child who presents with unusual features, whether they may be related to disturbances in growth, specific birth defects, dysmorphic features unusual behavior or so on, may warrant specific targeted investigations.

- Dysmorphic with or without congenital anomalies:
  - FISH analysis for specific chromosomal microdeletion syndromes
  - Specific gene analysis
  - Search for occult anomalies (renal USG, echocardiogram)
  - CNS imaging – MRI
- Overgrowth
  - Bone age
  - Beckwith Wiedmann syndrome – abdominal USG for organomegaly
  - Sotos syndrome – MRI brain
- Disproportionate short stature
  - Skeletal survey radiographs
  - Specific DNA analysis for suspected gene (e.g. FGFR3) for achondroplasia
- Unusual head shape (craniosynostosis) - CT brain
- Coarse facies
  - TSH
  - Skeletal survey
  - Urine for mucopolysaccharidosis

SUMMARY

Approach to a child with global developmental delay will depend whether the child is syndromic or non-syndromic.

1. First step would be to assess whether the child has a global developmental delay; which means a delay in all the four fields of development.

2. From history and clinical examination determine whether the child is syndromic or non-syndromic.

3. Investigations will be tailored depending on the above.

SUGGESTED READING

1. Wendy S. Meschino: The child with developmental delay: An approach to etiology. https://www.ncbi.nim.nih.gov/pmc/articles/PMC2791071.

INTRODUCTION

Children with ataxia are often brought by parents with the complaint that suddenly their child after getting up from sleep is unable to sit or walk. Some may be brought to the physician for staggering gait or clumsiness. Assessing such a child at times may be challenging. One must not forget that ataxia is a symptom of an underlying disease.

DEFINITION

Ataxia is a broad term that refers to disturbances in the smooth performance of voluntary motor acts. It is due to disturbances in the fine control of posture and movements.

This control is normally maintained by the cerebellum and its connections with the frontal lobes and posterior column fibers of the spinal cord. Therefore, ataxia can arise from disorders of:

• Cerebellum

• Sensory pathways (posterior column, dorsal root ganglia, peripheral nerves)

• Frontal lobe lesions (via frontocerebellar associative fibers)

ETIOLOGY

Causes of ataxia can be grouped into three. In the first group are causes which present with acute onset of ataxia. The second group are conditions with insidious onset and the course remains static or may be progressive.

While in the third group are illnesses which give rise to recurrent, intermittent or episodic ataxia.

Table: Causes of ataxia

1. Acute ataxia
    • Drug ingestion (anticonvulsants, antihistaminics)
    • Post infections: acute cerebellar ataxia
    • Brain stem encephalitis
    • Trauma
    • Sudden hemorrhage in a tumor
    • Acute labyrinthitis
    • Cerebral hemorrhage (vascular lesions AVM)
    • Conversion reaction

2. Chronic / progressive
    • Brain tumors: Cerebellar astrocytoma, cerebellar hemangioblastoma, ependymoma, medulloblastoma, neuroblastoma, supratentorialtumors
    • Abscess
    • Hereditary ataxias
        - Autosomal ataxia telangiectasia
        - Friedrich's ataxia
        - Refsum's disease
        - Wilson's disease
        - Abetalipoproteinemia
        - Vitamin E deficiency
        - Autosomal dominant spinocerebellar ataxia

- Congenital malformations
  - Basilar impression
  - Cerebellar aplasia
  - Dandy walker malformations
  - Vermian aplasia
  - Arnold Chiari malformation

3. Recurrent ataxia (episodic)
   - Metabolic / inborn errors of metabolism
     - Hartnup disease
     - Maple syrup urine disease
     - Pyruvate dehydrogenase deficiency
   - Basilar migraine
   - Benign paroxysmal vertigo
   - Dominant recurrent ataxia

CLINICAL EVALUATION

Initial evaluation must focus on excluding serious causes of acute ataxia. Must rule out mass lesions, central nervous system infections and hydrocephalus.

A. History

In addition to a thorough history, the following pertinent questions must be included:

> **History in a case of ataxia**
> - Age at disease onset
> - Onset of illness
> - Progression of the disease
> - Accompanying symptoms
> - History of ingestion of drugs, toxins, etc.
> - History of trauma
> - Recent immunization
> - Symptoms suggesting raised intracranial pressure

> - Any change in mental status
> - History of similar episodes in the past
> - Family history of similar illness
> - Illness in the neonatal period
> - Psychomotor development

Age:

It is essential to enquire at what age of the child did the parents notice onset of symptoms. Congenital malformations of the posterior fossa usually present in infancy. Acute cerebellar ataxia which is the commonest cause of ataxia in childhood affects children between 2 and 7 years of age. Accidental ingestion of drugs is common between the ages 1 to 5 years. The mean age of onset of neuroblastoma is 18 months range being 1 month to 4 years. Eighty five percent of primary brain tumorsin children 2 to 12 years old are located in the posterior fossa. Supratentorialtumors predominate in children younger than 2 years and older than 12 years. In case of ataxia telengiectasiatruncal ataxia develops during the first year of life and telengiectasias appear after the age of 2 years.

Dominant recurrent ataxia manifest between 5 and 7 years. Presentation of ataxia in maple syrup urine disease is usually between 5 months and 2 years, on the other hand pyruvate dehydrogenase deficiency begins after 3 years of age.

Onset of illness and progression:

Was the child perfectly alright before the onset of ataxia? Did the child suddenly develop unsteadiness of gait and inability to sit or was it a gradual onset? Are the symptoms progressing, static or regressing? Is there any history of previous episodes of ataxia? Chief complaint of ataxia is usually refusal to walk, "staggering gait" or clumsiness. Sudden onset of ataxia is commonly seen in post infectious acute cerebellar ataxia and following intake of drugs especially phenytoin and antihistaminics. Hemorrhage in a tumor or rupture of an arteriovenous malformation can give rise to acute ataxia. Brain stem encephalitis and trauma are other causes of acute onset ataxias. Insidious onset with gradual progression are observed in children with brain tumors, cerebellar abscess and hereditary ataxias while in congenital malformations such as cerebellar and vermian aplasia the clinical symptoms are static.

Recurrent episodes of ataxia are seen in certain inborn errors of metabolism viz. maple syrup urine disease, hartnup disease and pyruvate dehydrogenase deficiency. Also seen in children with basilar migraine and certain autosomal dominant ataxias. In case of intermittent ataxia enquire if it is precipitated by infection, stress or high carbohydrate diet.This is observed in case of pyruvate dehydrogenase deficiency.

Accompanying symptoms:

Ask for any recent viral infection or cough. Varicella is the most common acute infectious cause of ataxia.

Ask for symptoms such as fever, nausea, vomiting, lethargy, headache and head tilting. Early morning headache with vomiting and change in mental status are symptoms of raised intracranial tension. Does the child develop any skin rash after exposure to sunlight? This phenomenon is seen in cases of Hartnup disease.

Visual loss, vertigo, tinnitus, paresthesias of fingers and toes with severe throbbing occipital headache would suggest basilar migraine.

Recurrent loose fatty stools with vomiting isseen in abetalipoproteinemia.

Ingestion of drugs and toxins:

Toddlers are very susceptible to accidental ingestion of drugs.

One must enquire whether child is receiving an antiepileptic drug for convulsions or antihistaminics for cold. An overdose of these drugs can give rise to ataxia. At times some member in the family may be receiving drugs which little children may consume accidentally during play.

History of recent immunizations:

Has the child received any vaccines in the recent past?

The only vaccine which could be the preceding cause of acute cerebellar ataxia is varicella vaccine. No other vaccine has been linked to cerebellar ataxia.

Head trauma:

Do ask the parents whether the child sustained any head injury.

Mild head injuries are sustained by toddlers on a daily basis, but most of the times there are no after effects. However, at times ataxia may follow even mild head injuries, mostly as part of post-concussion syndrome. Ataxia may also follow cervical injuries.

Family history:

Does anybody in the family have a similar illness?

Progressive ataxias can be hereditary. They are either autosomal dominant or recessive. Certain in-born errors of metabolism viz. Maple syrup urine disease and Hartnup disease are also inherited and can present as intermittent episodes of ataxia.

Illness in the neonatal period:

How was the neonatal period? Did the child suffer from any illness in the newborn period? Certain inborn errors of metabolism such as maple syrup urine disease present with seizures in the neonatal period. Pyruvate dehydrogenase deficiency can present with severe lactic acidosis.

Psychomotor development:

How is the development of the child?

Is it normal for his age? Has the child developed any mental changes?

Children with in-born errors of metabolism do show mild to moderate developmental delay. Mental changes ranging from emotional instability to altered sensorium does occur in some of them.

Patients with congenital malformations such as hypoplasia of the cerebellum and vermal aplasia often present with developmental delay and hypotonia. Delayed development can also be a feature of hereditary ataxias.

B. Examination

After taking the relevant history, it is essential to do a thorough examination to arrive at a working diagnosis. True ataxia is a sign of cerebellar dysfunction, however, loss of balance or abnormal gait can occur for several reasons such as vestibular dysfunction, musculoskeletal or psychiatric abnormalities. Physical examination can help to differentiate true ataxia from other causes of abnormal gait. After having confirmed that the child does have ataxia, the next step is to determine whether it is a cerebellar or sensory ataxia. In case of cerebellar ataxia one must assess whether the pathology is in the vermis or cerebellar hemisphere.

Physical findings

- General examination
- Mental status
- Gait
- Ophthalmic examination
- Cranial nerve dysfunction
- Tone, power and reflexes
- Cerebellar signs
- Sensations
- Abdomen

General examination:

One must observe whether the child is awake, alert or in acute distress. Does he have dysmorphicfeatures ? Joubert syndrome has a characteristic facies. The skin must be examined for presence of scars or crusted lesions which would indicate varicella infection.

Look for telengiectasia in the eyes and other parts of the body which would indicate ataxia telengiectasia.

The ears must be examined for the presence of fluid in the middle ear as acute labyrinthitis can give rise to an unsteady gait.

Growth should be assessed, failure to thrive is seen in ataxia due to abetalipoproteinemia.

Look for kyphoscoliosis seen in case of Freidrich's ataxia.

Mental status:

A child brought with acute cerebellar ataxia should be assessed for his mental status. Is he fully conscious or is his consciousness altered ? Children with acute cerebellar ataxia are always conscious, even if ataxia is severe and this helps in differentiating causes due

---

to drug ingestion, hemorrhage in a brain tumor and encephalitis which are characterized by declining consciousness. Seizures may also appear in encephalitis.

In a child brought with chronic or progressive ataxia in which the cause is congenital abnormalities there is some degree of mental deficiency.

Gait:

In a fully conscious child one must observe his gait. In cerebellar lesions gait is wide based lurching and staggering. While in case of disease of the peripheral nerves or posterior column gait is wide based but is not so much lurching as careful. The foot raises high with each step and slaps down heavily on the ground (high stepping gait).

Hysterical gait disturbances are often extreme. Child appears to sit without difficulty but when brought to standing immediately begins to sway from the waist. Ataxia varies from mild unsteadiness while walking to complete inability to stand or walk. Ataxia is maximal at onset in acute cerebellar ataxia. It is marked in children who have ingested toxic dose of anticonvulsants such as phenytoin.

Speech:

Listen carefully to the speech of the child. In case of cerebellar ataxia there is dysarthria which means there is fluctuation in rhythm, tone, volume and clarity. It is also known as scanning speech.

The speech is normal in children with sensory ataxia.

Ophthalmic examination:

Look for nystagmus. Note the position of the eye when nystagmus appears, its character and direction of fast component. Horizontal nystagmus indicates cerebellar lesions. It is marked in cases who have ingested toxic doses of anticonvulsants. Also look for paralysis of the sixth cranial nerve which would result in internal squint. Paralysis of this nerve indicates increased incracranial tension and is a false localizing sign.

The fundus must be examined for papilloedema. Increased intracranial tension in a child with ataxia would indicate an intracranial space occupying lesion or hydrocephalus.

Examine the pupils. Pupillary abnormalities would indicate mass lesions and intoxication.

Examination of cranial nerves:

Cranial nerves dysfunction associated with ataxia is seen in brainstem encephalitis.

Examination of motor system:

Examine the power, tone and reflexes.

One must differentiate poor coordination from weakness.

Cerebellar involvement leads to hypotonia of muscles. The deep tendon reflexes are usually present. Typically the knee jerk is pendular.

In case of peripheral neuropathy there is hypotonia of muscles, areflexia and also loss of vibration sense below the level of the lesion on the same side.

Asymmetry is uncommon in acute cerebellar ataxia.

Hyperreflexia / areflexiasuggests causes other than cerebellar ataxia.

Cerebellar signs:

Carefully examine for cerebellar signs which include the following:

- Observe the gait. It is wide based and lurching in cerebellar lesions. In severe ataxia child may not be able to sit.

In lesions affecting the vermis child cannot sit still and moves the body constantly to and fro and bobs the head (titubation). Disturbances of cerebellar hemisphere results in swaying in the direction of the affected hemisphere. Gait can be observed by asking the child to move around a chair.

- Dysarthria. Scanning or slurring speech.
- Dysmetria. Look for poor coordination of voluntary movements.

  Finger to nose test – for upper extremity.

  Heel to shin test – for lower extremity.
- Dysdiadochokinesia – inability to perform alternating movements with speed and precision viz. supination and pronation.
- Rebound phenomenon. This is done by extending the patient's elbow and then releasing the wrist suddenly, the hand may jerk back and hit the face.
- Romberg's sign. A positive Romberg indicates sensory ataxia. This test assesses the loss of position sense in the legs. The child is asked to stand with feet together and arms outstretched. He is then asked to close his eyes. If he becomes unsteady the test is positive. In case of cerebellar ataxia the child will be unsteady with both eyes open and closed.

Examination of sensations:

Examination of the sensory system should be done. Test for stereognosis. Information for sense of position, weight, shape, size and vibration are carried in the posterior column of the same side. Involvement of these fibers would lead to sensory ataxia. Also test for touch, pain and temperature.

Examination of abdomen:

Palpate the abdomen for presence of organomegaly and any masses. If a mass is felt or there is a hepatomegaly think of neuroblastoma.

Table: **Differences between sensory and cerebellar ataxia**

Characteristics	Sensory ataxia	Cerebellar ataxia
• Location and lesion	Peripheral nerves or posterior column disease	Cerebellar disease
• Gait	Wide based, high stepping	Lurching, staggering
• On examination	Can look normal on sitting, loss of peripheral position and vibration sense, positive Romberg	Unable to stay balanced sitting Worse if legs are crossed Worse with running and standing
• Associated findings	Loss of position and vibration sense in lower extremities	Intention tremors Ocular and limb dysmetria
• Speech	Normal	Slurred

Clues from general examination

Clinical clue	Diagnosis
Short stature & Telangiectasia	Ataxia telangiectasia
Cataract	Sjogren syndrome
Deafness	Friedrich's, refsum disease, mitochondrium
Icthyosis	Refsum disease
Spine / foot deformity	Friedrich's ataxia, ataxia with Vitamin E deficiency

Which investigations to be done?

All of the investigations are not indicated in every child with ataxia. They would depend upon the most probable cause after a thorough clinical examination. Acute cerebellar ataxia post infectious is the commonest cause of ataxia in children. Diagnosis is always by excluding other conditions mimicking post viral ataxia. Metabolic screen is indicated in children suspected to be suffering from in-born errors of metabolism. Neuroimaging is diagnostic in cases with raised intracranial tension.

Investigations

- Blood – complete blood count
- Cerebrospinal fluid examination
- Neuroimaging
- Toxicology screen
- Electrolytes and blood gases
- Metabolic screen
- Immunoglobulins
- Fibroblast culture
- Electroencephalogram
- Molecular diagnosis

Complete blood count:

Complete blood count indicated where the cause is infection.

Cerebrospinal fluid examination:

CSF examination is indicated in cases of viral encephalitis. CSF reveals mononuclear leucocytes with or without protein elevation.

Neuroimaging of the brain:

MRI of the brain is indicated in all intracranial space occupying lesions. Also in children with hydrocephalous and brain trauma. It is also very useful in congenital malformations. It is the best method to visualize the cervicomedullary junction and associated Arnold's Chiari malformation. MRI is the study of choice in congenital cerebellar hypoplasia and also in aplasia of the vermis.

Toxicology screen:

In children suspected to have consumed anticonvulsants their level in serum and urine must be estimated.

Electrolytes and blood gases:

In pyruvate dehydrogenase deficiency, there is acidosis and levels of lactate & pyruvate concentration are always elevated during attacks. Blood concentration of lactate may be elevated between attacks.

Metabolic screen:

Indicated in suspected in-born errors of metabolism. In Hartnup disease constant feature is aminoaciduria involving neutral monoamino carboxylic amino acids. In Maple Syrup urine disease, the odor of urine is like that of maple syrup. During attack blood and urine have elevated concentration of branch chain amino acids and ketoacids. Between attacks the concentration is normal.

Immunoglobulins:

In ataxia telangiectasia there is increased level of alfa-fetoprotein and decreased IgA, IgG2 and CD4 counts.

Fibroblast culture:

In order to confirm the diagnosis in cases of in-born errors of metabolism the enzyme activity is estimated in cultured fibroblast.

Electroencephalogram:

It should be done in suspected basilar migraine. The EEG shows occipital intermittent delta activity during and just after an attack in basilar migraine.

Molecular diagnosis

Can be considered in cases of hereditary ataxias.

Clues from investigations

Investigations	Conditions and findings
1. Urine and/or serum toxic screening	All cases acute or intermittent ataxia
2. Neuroimaging CT / MRI brain	Acute cerebellar ataxia - Normal
	Congenital ataxias - Hypoplasia of vermis or cerebellar hemispheres
	Arnold Chiari malformations - Herniation of cerebellar tonsils and medulla
	Dandy Walker malformations - Posterior fossa cyst communicating with IV ventricle
	ADEM – Multiple asymmetrical foci of demyelination in cerebellum, basal ganglia and cerebrum
	Vascular causes - Infarcts, hemorrhage
	Ataxia telangiectasia - Cerebellar atrophy Friedrich's, abetalipoproteinemia, Refsum's disease - Normal cerebellum
CT / MRI abdomen chest	Opsoclonus myoclonus syndrome - to rule out neuroblastoma
3. Nerve conduction studies	Peripheral neuropathies in hereditary ataxia
4. Visual evoked potentials	Demyelinating disorders (ADEM)
5. ECG, ECHO	Friedrich's ataxia, mitrochondrial disorders
6. Genetic testing	Ataxia telangiectasia - mutation in ATM gene Friedrich's ataxia - GAA repeats
7. Metabolic workup	In-born errors of metabolism
8. Biomarkers	Associated with autosomal recessive ataxia

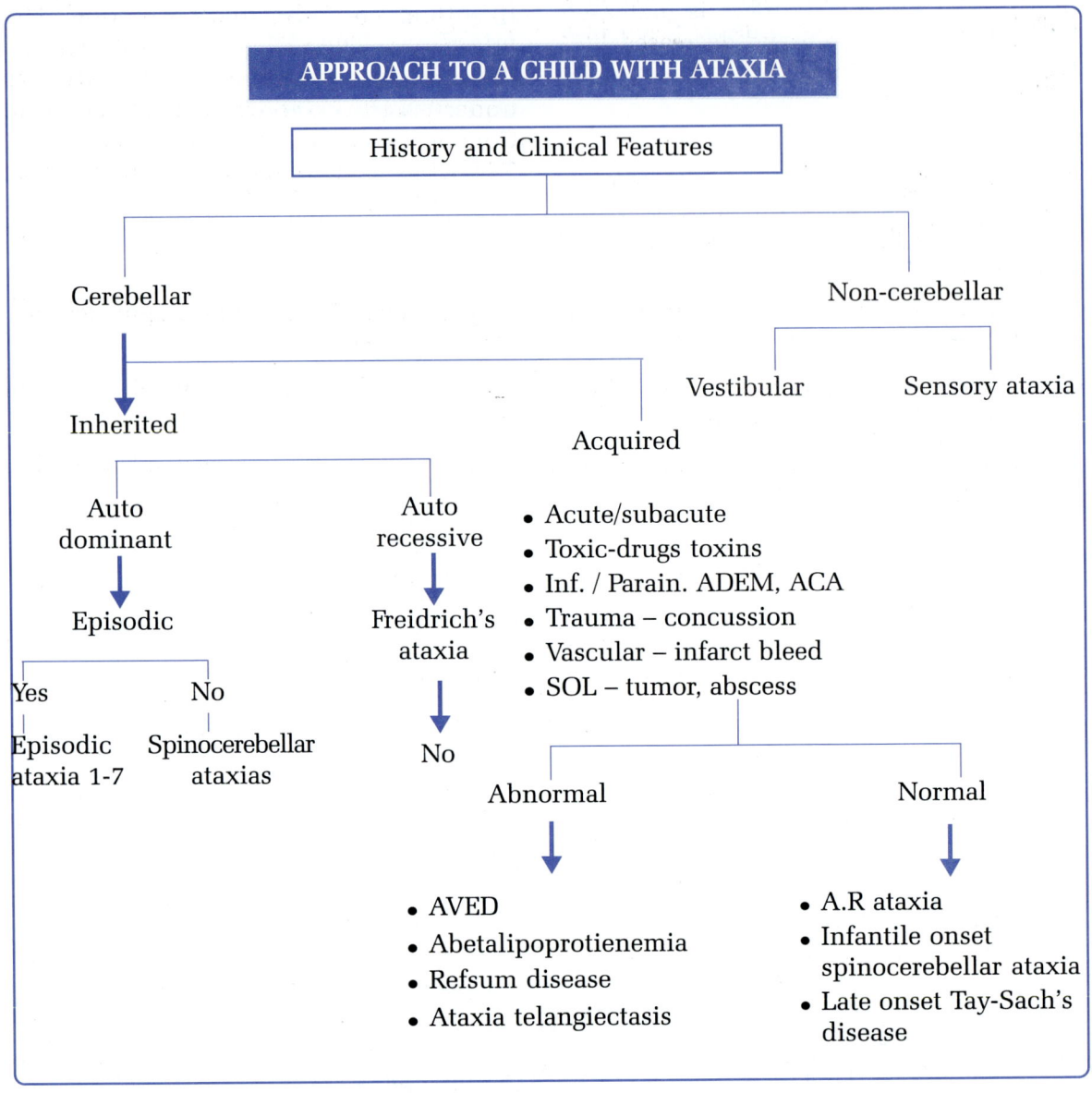

APPROACH TO A CHILD WITH ATAXIA

History and Clinical Features

Cerebellar

Non-cerebellar

Vestibular   Sensory ataxia

Inherited

Acquired

Auto dominant

Auto recessive

- Acute/subacute
- Toxic-drugs toxins
- Inf. / Parain. ADEM, ACA
- Trauma – concussion
- Vascular – infarct bleed
- SOL – tumor, abscess

Episodic

Freidrich's ataxia

Yes   No

No

Episodic ataxia 1-7   Spinocerebellar ataxias

Abnormal   Normal

- AVED
- Abetalipoprotienemia
- Refsum disease
- Ataxia telangiectasis

- A.R ataxia
- Infantile onset spinocerebellar ataxia
- Late onset Tay-Sach's disease

SUMMARY

Ataxia in children is a manifestation of a range of disorders. One must proceed in a systematic manner based on mode of onset, whether it is of an acute onset, recurrent or chronic.

In childhood acute ataxia is the most common cause either due to drug ingestion or post-infectious cerebellar demyelination. The infection usually responsible is chicken pox. Intermittent ataxia is usually due to underlying in-born errors of metabolism. Common causes of inherited ataxias are Friedrich's ataxia and ataxia telangiectasia.

SUGGESTED READING

1. Fenichal Gerald M. Clinical Pediatric Neurolog. A signs and symptoms approach. 5th Edition. Ataxia: 219-237.

2. Leema Pauline C, Saravanan R, Ravi LA. Approach to a child with ataxia: Indian Jour. of Pract. Pediatr. 2016;18(2):109-121.

3. Sivasamy L. Approach to acute ataxia in childhood. Diagnosis and evaluation. Pediatr Ann 2014;45:153-159.

DELAYED PUBERTY

INTRODUCTION

Delayed onset of puberty in a child female or male is a cause of concern for parents. In a normal population of girls and boys 2.5 percent of individuals will mature at a time beyond 2 standard deviation (SD) from the mean most of them having a physiological or constitutional delay in growth and adolescence. Majority of the children have no endocrine abnormality.

DEFINITION

Puberty is said to be delayed if pubertal changes do not start by the age of 14 years in boys and 13 years in girls or if more than 5 years have elapsed between the first signs of puberty and completion of genital growth/menarche.

ETIOLOGY OF DELAYED PUBERTY (Girls and Boys)

Table: Causes of delayed puberty (Girls and Boys)

1. Constitutional delay in puberty.

2. Hypogonadotropic hypogonadism:

   Functional: Chronic infection, systemic diseases, protein energy malnutrition, psychosocial deprivation, excess energy expenditure as in athletes, exogenous obesity.

   Developmental or acquiredlesions: Idiopathichypogonadotrophichypogonadism, intrasellar and suprasellar tumors. Prader-Willi syndrome, Lawrence-Moon-Biedl syndrome, cranial surgery, irradiation, trauma.

   Endocrinopathies: Hypothyroidism, glucocorticoid excess, poorly controlled diabetes mellitus, panhypopituitarism isolated growth hormone deficiency, hyperprolactinemia.

3. Hypergonadotrophic hypogonadism:
   Congenital:

   - Ovarian and testicular dysgenesis-Klinefelter and Noonan syndrome, Turner syndrome
   - Disorders of steroid biosynthesis
   - Androgen insensitivity. Acquired:
   - Irradiation or chemotherapy, trauma or torsion of gonads, surgical resection, orchitis, oophoritis, premature ovarian failure.

4. Miscellaneous: Mullerian duct failure.

Before proceeding to the evaluation of a child with delayed puberty, it is important to know the normal physical changes taking place during puberty.

NORMAL PUBERTAL DEVELOPMENT

Pubertal development and progress are best ascertained by Tanner's staging.

Boys: The first sign of puberty in boys is an increase in the size of the testis. This is followed by penile and scrotal changes. Testicular size is documented as a measurement of the longest axis or by testicular volume using the Prader's orchidometer. Volume of 4 ml or length of 2.5 cm (1 inch) defines the onset of puberty. Presence of axillary hair and other changes such as that of the voice and an increase in growth velocity only occur in mid to late puberty. Facial hair does not appear until late puberty.

Girls: The first demonstrable sign of puberty in females is breast development. Caution must be exercised in examination of breast tissue in obese girls as simple fat may be mistaken for breast tissue. Pubic and axillary hair, acne and body odour develop as a result of androgens secreted from the adrenal gland. Peak growth spurt occurs in Tanner's stage 3 and menarche occurs in Tanner's stage 4 breast development.

Changes in body size: Height velocity increases during puberty with resultant epiphyseal cartilage fusion leading to achievement of adult height. A boy gains in height by 7 to 12 cms in a year, while a girl gains 6 to 11 cms at the time of peak height velocity.

EVALUATION

While evaluating a child with delayed puberty one must first exclude constitutional delay, which is a physiological state and is the commonest cause of delayed puberty in office practice. The next step would be to decide whether the cause is central, i.e. in the hypothalamic pituitary axis or in the gonads.

A. History

Points in History

- Family history of delayed puberty
- What was the birth weight?
- Developmental milestones

- Record of growth velocity
- History of chronic illness
- Nutritional history
- Past history of viral infections, especially mumps
- Symptoms of raised intracranial tension
- History of central nervous system (CNS) infections/trauma/ radiation
- History of anosmia

Family history

Enquire whether puberty was delayed in other family members. In constitutional delay, there can be a history of delayed pubertal growth spurt in either a parent or sibling. The spurt is less pronounced and more delayed. History of hypogonadism or infertility in the family is also important for hereditary form of disorder.

Birth weight

In case of constitutional delay the birth weight is normal, but subsequently growth falters.

In chromosomal aberrations and other syndromes the child usually has a low birth weight. Children with Turner syndrome have a low birth weight, but children with Noonan syndrome are usually large at birth.

Developmental milestones

In case of constitutional delay the milestones are normal.

Record of growth

If growth records are available one must analyze the growth velocity. Again in case of constitutional delay although the birth weight is normal, growth slows down from early childhood and onset of puberty is also delayed.

History of chronic illness

Any history of malabsorption, chronic infections such as tuberculosis, chronic anemia, metabolic illness especially renal failure, congenital or rheumatic heart disease. Any psychological illness must also be enquired.

CNS illness

Enquire about meningitis, encephalitis, intracranial tumors (intrasellar&suprasellar), head trauma, cranial irradiation, neuro surgery which could affect the hypothalamic pituitary axis leading to delayed puberty.

Exposure of gonads to irradiation and drugs can also lead to delayed puberty.

History of anosmia

History of anosmia in a male child would suggest Kallmann syndrome.

History of infection

Mumps in prepubertal boys can lead to orchitis in turn, which can lead to pubertal delay.

B.   Examination

Points on examination
• Anthropometric measurements
• Signs of pubertal development
• Stigmata of various syndromes
• Midline defects
• Central nervous system check-up including fundus examination and visual fields

Anthropometric measurements

The first thing that should be done in a child presenting with delayed puberty is to record anthropometric measurements including body proportions and fat distribution.

Growth assessment often helps in distinguishing the cause of delayed puberty and is an important part of the evaluation. The height of those with primary gonadal failure is usually normal unless associated with syndromes. In isolated gonadotropin deficiency childhood growth is normal but pubertal growth spurt does not occur.

Short stature would be present in constitutional delay, hypothyroidism, panhypopituitarism, Turner syndrome. Boys with Klinefelter syndrome usually have a tall stature with eunuchoid proportions, i.e. upper segment to lower segment ratio less than 0.09 and arm span more than height. Weight related to height is decreased in malnutrition and chronic disease and increased in most hormonal disorders. Obesity is a feature of many syndromes associated with hypogonadism, viz. Prader-Willi syndrome, Angelman syndrome and Lawrence- Moon-Biedl syndrome.

Pubertal developments

After recording the anthropometric measurements, one should look for signs of pubertal development. Penile, scrotal and testicular development should be assessed in boys. Stretched phallic length is measured in cm from the mons to the tip of the glans. Scrotal rugosities are one of the initial manifestations of puberty and should be looked for. Testicular volume can be measured by calipers or with the Praderorchidometer. A volume of more than 4 mL indicates gonadotropin stimulation.

In case of Klinefelter syndrome there is microphallus, cryptorchidism and gynecomastia. If orchitis occurs in prepubertal boys they present with underdeveloped external genitalia and lack of virilising signs.

Male babies born with congenital gonadotropin deficiency have normal sexual differentiation but micropenis.

In girls any evidence of pubertal development should be looked for. In case of constitutional delay, all stages of sexual maturity are delayed, but ultimately attained.

Stigmata of various syndromes

In children presenting with delayed pubertal development, stigmata of various syndromes must be looked for. In Noonan syndrome apart from short stature they have a webbed neck, downslanting palpebral fissures and low set ears. In Prader-Willi syndrome apart from obesity the child has small hands and feet, mental retardation and hypogonadism. Kallmann syndrome has microphallus, undescended testis and hyposmia or anosmia. A typical patient with Turner syndrome has distinct facies with micrognathia, epicanthal folds, low set and rotated or deformed ears, fish like mouth and narrow, high-arched palate. Other features are webbing of the neck, shield shaped chest and widely spaced nipples.

Central nervous system examination

Examination of the nervous system is important. Whenever there are symptoms and signs of raised intracranial tension the fundus should be examined for papilledema and visual fields recorded to rule out lesions in hypothalamic pituitary region. Anosmia or hyposmia should be checked as it is a feature of Kallmann syndrome.

C. Investigations

After a proper history and clinical examination one tentatively thinks that the cause is either a constitutional delay, which is very common or the cause is due to lesion in the hypothalamic pituitary region or lastly due to direct affection of the gonads.

Depending upon the provisional cause investigations should be planned.

Table: Showing investigations and probable diagnosis

Sr. No.	Investigations	Probable Diagnosis
1.	Bone age (x-ray of wrist with tips of finger included) Less than chronological age	Constitutional delay Hypothyroidism Hypopituitarism
2.	Complete blood count Leucocytosis anemia	Chronic anemia
3.	Liver function testsDeranged	Liver dysfunction
4.	Renal function testsDeranged	Renal failure
5.	Plasma testosterone / oestradiolLow levels	Primary gonadal dysfunction
6.	Gonadotropins (FSH / LH) High levels Low levels or normal	Hypergonadotropichypogonadism Hypogonadotropichypogonadism
7.	Karyotyping indicated in	Chromosomal disorders
8.	MRI / CT brain indicated in suspected	Intracranial lesion especially hypothalamic pituitary region
9.	Pelvic ultrasonography in girls, to assess	Uterus, endometrial thickness, ovaries, etc.

Assessment of skeletal age

In all cases of delayed puberty skeletal age must be assessed. If skeletal age is less than chronological age one has to consider various endocrinopathies viz. hypopituitarism and hypothyroidism. In constitutional delay also bone age is less than chronological, but is equal to the height age.

Complete blood count

Complete blood count is indicated in cases, where delayed puberty appears to be due to systemic illness, chronic infections, long standing anemia or malnutrition.

Liver function and renal function test

Girls above 13 years and boys above 14 years, who have no evidence of systemic illness or dysmorphic features should undergo routine liver and renal function tests in addition to complete blood count.

Screening for chronic infections

Since chronic infections such as tuberculosis and acquired immunodeficiency syndrome (AIDS) are common in this country necessary test should be done if there is clinical evidence of infection.

Hormonal assays

Following are the indications for hormonal assay:

- Girls and boys with a bone age less than 13 or 14 years
- With dysmorphic features
- Evidence of maldevelopment
- Associated short stature.

Basal and GnRH stimulated gonadotropin status

These will be of great help when biologic age reaches the adolescent age range and bone age has reached the pubertal age of close to 11 years in girls and 12 to 13 years in boys. High gonadotropin levels or excessive response to LH, FSH to GnRH stimulation at this point, are indicative of primary gonadal failure. If LH and FSH are low or normal, it may be difficult to differentiate between constitutional delay in puberty and hypogonadotropic hypogonadism.

Other hormones estimation

Testosterones, estradiol and prolactin levels are also estimated. Low levels of these hormones also indicate primary gonadal dysfunction. In Klinefelter syndrome testosterone levels are low, but oestrogen secretion from testis is increased. FSH and LH are elevated.

In idiopathic hypogonadotropichypo-gonadism plasma, LH, FSH and gonadal steroids are below the normal range.

Assessment of growth hormone or thyroid function is indicated if previous growth rate is subnormal. The human chorionic gonadotropic (HCG) test is also used in boys if the testis are not palpable or testicular defect is suspected and gonadotropin levels are not elevated.

Karyotyping

Karyotyping is indicated if there is stigmata of chromosomal disorder or FSH and LH are high.

Neuroimaging

Magnetic resonance imaging of the brain is indicated, whenever there is suspicion of an intrasellar or extrasellar tumor or any intracranial lesion especially in the hypothalamic pituitary region.

An ultrasound scan of the abdomen is very helpful in girls to study the uterus, cervix, endometrial thickening and the ovaries.

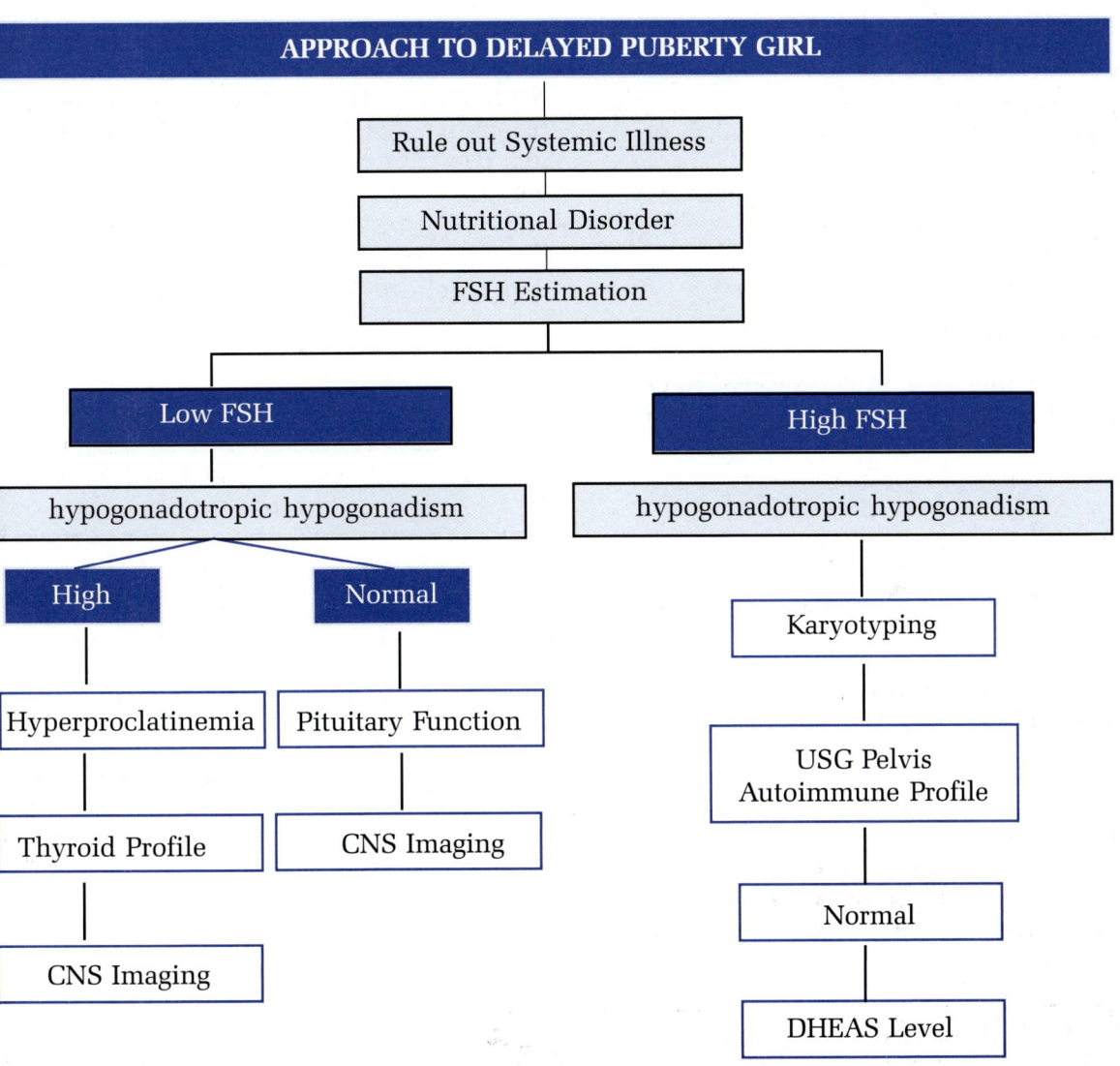

APPROACH TO DELAYED PUBERTY GIRL

Rule out Systemic Illness

Nutritional Disorder

FSH Estimation

Low FSH → hypogonadotropic hypogonadism

High FSH → hypogonadotropic hypogonadism

Low FSH branch:
- High → Hyperproclatinemia → Thyroid Profile → CNS Imaging
- Normal → Pituitary Function → CNS Imaging

High FSH branch:
- Karyotyping → USG Pelvis Autoimmune Profile → Normal → DHEAS Level

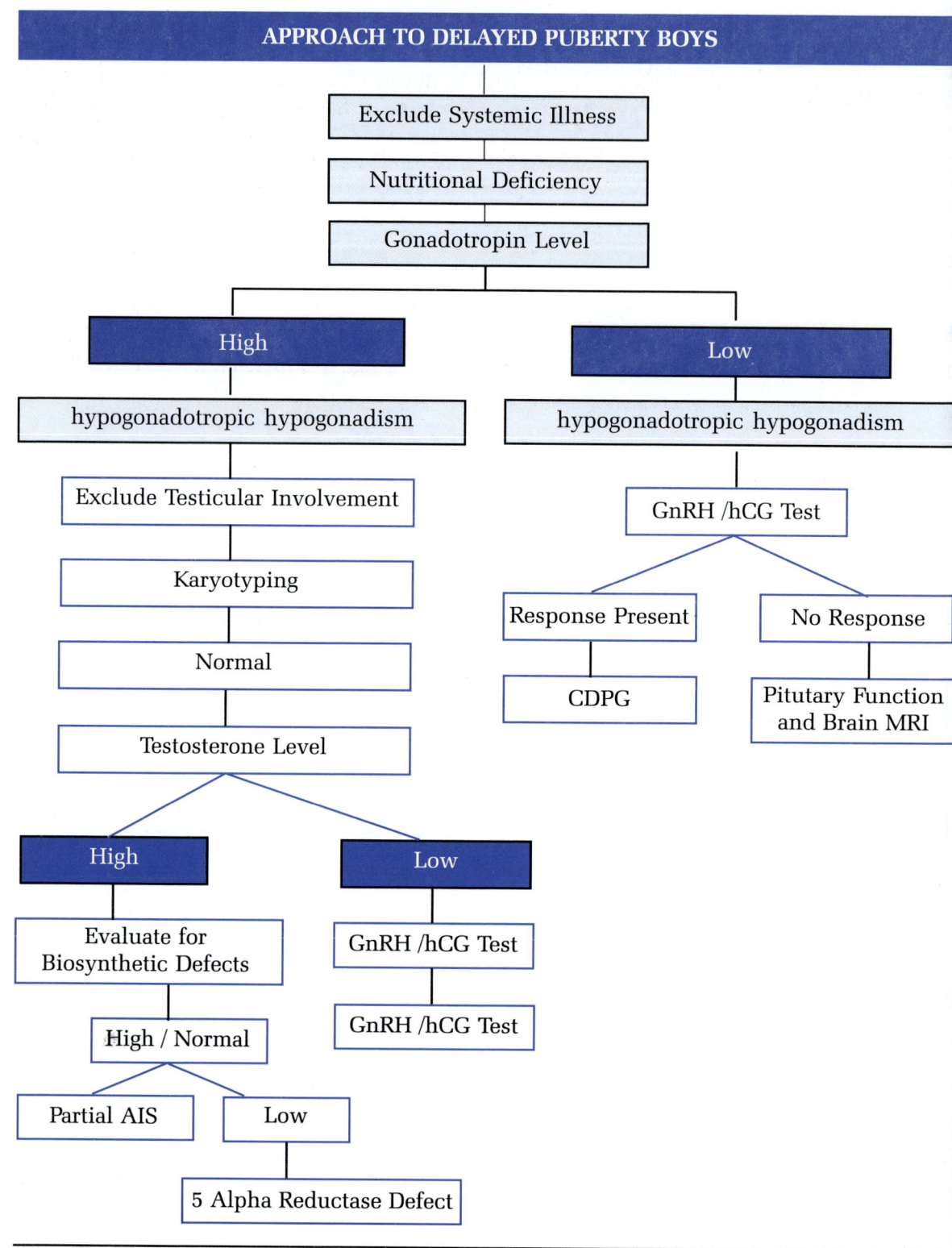

APPROACH TO DELAYED PUBERTY BOYS

Exclude Systemic Illness

Nutritional Deficiency

Gonadotropin Level

High — hypogonadotropic hypogonadism

Exclude Testicular Involvement

Karyotyping

Normal

Testosterone Level

High — Evaluate for Biosynthetic Defects — High / Normal — Partial AIS, Low — 5 Alpha Reductase Defect

Low — GnRH /hCG Test — GnRH /hCG Test

Low — hypogonadotropic hypogonadism

GnRH /hCG Test

Response Present — CDPG

No Response — Pitutary Function and Brain MRI

SUMMARY

The commonest cause of delayed puberty is 'constitutional delay' where children mature late. They are otherwise normal and do not have any systemic or endocrine pathology. In such children history of delayed puberty is often present in parents or sibs. Only after excluding a physiological cause one must consider pathological causes.

Lack of appearance of secondary sex characters by 13 years in girls and 14 years in boys indicates delayed puberty. In a girl, absence of menarche by the age of 16 years or 5 years after puberty onset also indicates pubertal delay.

SUGGESTED READING

1. Delayed puberty. Textbook of Pediatrics, 2013 Ed. Piyush Gupta. 1st Edition 525-526.

2. Colaco Prisca: Disorders of Puberty. IAP. Textbook of Pediatrics (2013) 5th Ed. 768-769.

32

PRECOCIOUS PUBERTY

INTRODUCTION

Puberty is a phase of growth through which a physically and sexually immature child transforms into a physically and sexually mature adult capable of independent existence and procreation. The process should start at an appropriate age and should proceed at normal rate so as to result in normal physique and function at an appropriate age. The average age of onset of puberty is 11 years in girls though it can start as early as 8.5 years and as late as 13 years. In boys average age of onset of puberty is 12 years with normal range extending from 9 to 14 years.

Precocious puberty denotes early pubertal development. It is generally defined as appearance of clinical features of onset of puberty (i.e. appearance of breast bud in girls and testicular enlargement to > 3 ml in boys) earlier than 8 years in girls and 9 years in boys.

ETIOLOGY

Early onset of puberty is common in girls and may represent normal variation in the age at onset of puberty. In most cases puberty is slowly progressive and there is no pathological cause. A detail workup is indicated in those girls with progressive forms of precocious puberty.

Causes of precocious puberty can be classified as central (gonadotrophin dependent GDPP) or peripheral (gonadotrophin-independent precocious puberty (GIPP)).

Central precocious puberty (CPP) is due to activation of the hypothalamic-pituitary-gonadal axis and is therefore gonadotropin dependent. It is also called as true precocious puberty. Peripheral or gonadotrophin releasing hormone (GnRH) independent precocious puberty results from the production of sex steroids. The sources of sex steroids may be gonadal or extragonadal. It is also called pseudoprecocious puberty. Central precocious puberty is more common than peripheral. GDPP is idiopathic in more than 90% of cases.

Table: Causes of precocious puberty

A. **Central precocious puberty** (GDPP)

- Idiopathic
- Tumors:hamartoma, glioma, craniopharyngioma
- Infections:neurotuberculosis, meningitis
- Malformations:hydrocephalus, arachnoid cyst
- Head trauma, neurosurgery, perinatal insult
- Cranial irradiation

B. **Peripheral precocious puberty** (GIPP):

- Autonomous gonadal activation - Ovarian cyst - McCune-Albright syndrome - Testotoxicosis
- Tumors of ovary or testis- Granulosa cell tumor, androgen producing ovarian tumor, hCG producing tumors

- Adrenal disorders: Congenital adrenal hyperplasia, adrenal tumor
- Exposure to exogenous sex steroids
- Severe untreated primary hypothyroidism

C. **Pubertal variants:**
- Premature thelarche
- Premature pubarche
- Premature menarche

PRECOCIOUS PUBERTY

Central cause or	Peripheral cause or
Gonadotropin dependent GDPP	Gonadotropin independent GIPP
↓	↓
Female : Almost always idiopathic	Female: McCune Albright
Male: Look for central cause	USG Pelvis
CT / MRI	Male: Testotoxicosis or androgens
	17 OHP Genetic Testing

Central or GDPP is due to premature activation of the hypothalamic-pituitary-gonadal (HPG) axis and therefore is isosexual. Peripheral or GIPP results from the production of sex steroids independent of the HPG axis. May be isosexual or heterosexual.

Before proceeding to the evaluation of a child with precocious puberty, it is important to know the normal physical changes taking place during puberty (ref.chap.31)

extensive investigations, although an underlying cause such as a tumor should always be considered and excluded.

Central precocious puberty (CPP) is the most common form of precocious puberty and is five times more common in girls and is most often idiopathic. In $2/3^{rd}$ of boys CPP is secondary to CNS pathology. Younger the child greater are the chances of a pathological cause.

EVALUATION

A careful history and clinical examination should be performed. An accurate height, pubertal staging and bone age should be recorded. Follow-up of height velocity and pubertal progress is most important for differentiating various aetiologies and deciding the need for therapeutic intervention. Many patients do not require

A. History

Points in history
- Age of onset of puberty
- History of vaginal bleeding
- Rate of progression
- Family history of precocious puberty
- History of birth asphyxia or any injury in the neonatal and postneonatal period

- History of neurotuberculosis or meningitis
- Symptoms of raised intracranial pressure
- History of neurosurgery head trauma radiotherapy
- History of administration of drugs or hormones
- Symptoms of hypothyroidism
- History of seizures

Age of onset:

Assessment should initially include a detailed history for the onset of secondary sexual characteristics, the pattern of development and onset of menarche in girls.

When was the first sign of puberty noticed? Premature thelarche is commonly noted at 2 age periods. Significant breast enlargement can occur in the first 2 to 4 years of life. Occasionally, persistence or progression of breast tissue may be noted from birth.

Second peak usually occurs around 6 years. It may be asymmetric to begin with and often unilateral.

Both the situations are benign, but need close follow-up.

Idiopathic gonadotropin-dependent precocious puberty has an onset between 6 and 7 years of age and has slow progression. Hypothalamic hamartoma on the other hand has an early onset in the first 3 to 4 years and rapid progression. Earlier the onset greater the chances of an underlying organic cause.

Progression of puberty:

Enquire about the progress of puberty from the time of onset. On an average completion of puberty from onset takes about 5 years. A slowly progressive puberty with an early onset usually represents a normal variation. Puberty that progresses rapidly needs to be investigated. In idiopathic CPP the rate of progression may sometimes be very slow with menarche occurring upto 5 years after breast development. Very rapid progression of puberty is seen in androgen producing tumors, ovarian cysts and some CNS tumors such as hypothalamic hamaratomas. Accelerated growth is a feature of both central and peripheral precocious puberty, but is not seen in pubertal variants.

Family history:

History of precocious puberty in other family members must be enquired. Early onset of menarche in the mother indicates idiopathic central precocious puberty in girls or familial testotoxicosis in boys. A history of precocious puberty in boys and genital ambiguity in girls of the same family would suggest CAH.

Neurologic disorders:

Neurotuberculosis and meningitis are quite common in our country. They can lead to damage in the hypothalamic pituitary region. Similarly, one must enquire for any history of birth asphyxia, head trauma, neurosurgery or cranial irradiation. Symptoms of raised intracranial tension, such as headache, vomiting, blurring of vision, seizures which would suggest raised intracranial tension due to space occupying lesions. History of episodes of uncontrolled laughter (gelastic epilepsy) is a feature of CPP commonly due to hypothalamic hamaratoma.

History of drug administration:

Is the child receiving any drugs such as steroids, estrogens and androgens?

B. Clinical Examination

Assessment of puberty is the cornerstone for approaching a child with precocious puberty. Pubertal development is usually assessed by Tanner's stages also known as sexual maturity rating, SMR. Tanner Stage 1 is prepubertal, while Tanner Stage 5 is adult maturity. In boys, penis and testis development, as well as pubic hair growth are assessed. In girls, breast development and pubic hair growth are assessed. In girls, puberty usually begins with breast development but occasionally with the appearance of pubic hair. Menarche usually occurs 2 years after breast development begins. In boys testicular enlargement > 3 ml marks the onset of puberty and is followed by appearance of pubic hair and development of external genitalia. The pubertal growth spurt is an early event in girls usually at Tanner Stage B2, while in boys the growth appears late, usually at the time when testicular volume of 10 ml is attained.

Points on examination

- Evaluate growth
- Androgen effects
- Oestrogen effects
- Pubertal staging
- Abdominal and rectal examination
- Testicular palpation
- Signs of McCune-Albright syndrome
- Signs of hypothyroidism
- Neurologic examination

Assessment of growth:

Growth of the child should be assessed by various anthropometric measurements, viz height, weight, arm span and body proportions.

Advanced growth is characteristic of precocious puberty, growth retardation is indicative of hypothyroidism or concomitant growth hormone deficiency. Features of hypothyroidism should also be assessed.

Extent of precocious development:

Pubertal staging should be done according to Tanner's criteria.

The vaginal mucosa should be inspected. Glistening red appearance is consistent with non-estrogenized mucosa while a pink, dull mucosa with secretions is indicative of estrogenization.

Clitoral size should be assessed. Breasts should be carefully palpated for galactorrhea.

Androgenic effects:

Look for androgen effects such as acne, hirsutism, increased muscle mass and clitoromegaly.

Oestrogen effects:

Breast development and changes in vaginal mucosa.

Abdominal and rectal examination for uterine size, ovarian masses and adrenal tumors.

Testicular palpation in boys:

Testicular volume (using an orchidometer) greater than 3 ml indicates the onset of CPP. Prepubertal testicular volume (less than 4 ml) is characteristic of CAH and adrenal tumor. Scrotal masses usually unilateral suggest testicular tumors. Pointers to CAH are hypertension and hyperpigmentation.

Signs of McCune Albright syndrome:

Presence of Café-au-lait spots, fibrous dysplasia.

Neurologic examination:

It should include fundus examination and perimetry.

C. Investigations

All boys with precocious pubertal development and all girls with following features should be evaluated.

- Precocious puberty stage 3 or higher
- Stage 2 with additional criteria such as increased growth velocity
- Evidence of CNS dysfunction

There are 2 sets of investigations done in any child presenting with precocious puberty viz. radiological investigations and hormonal evaluation.

Girls: In girls initial investigations should include bone age and basal gonadotropin levels.

1. Advanced bone age (more than 2 years ahead of chronological age) is suggestive of progressive precocious puberty while normal bone age indicates slowly

progressive puberty – retarded bone age is diagnostic of hypothyroidism.

2. Gonadotropins: Pooled gonadotropin levels are preferred due to their pulsatile secretion. LH is a better indicator of pubertal status than FSH. LH levels in the pubertal range and LH and FSH ratio more than 1 are suggestive of onset of puberty. In equivocal cases, LH levels should be measured after GnRH stimulation test.

Pubertal LH levels are suggestive of central precocious puberty. In these girls MRI brain should be done for evidence of an organic lesion.

Prepubertal levels of LH following GnRH stimulation test suggest peripheral precocious puberty. These girls should be subjected to USG of ovaries and adrenals (for ovarian cyst and adrenal tumor). Also a skeletal survey done for fibrosis dysplasia.

APPROACH TO PRECOCIOUS PUBERTY IN GIRLS

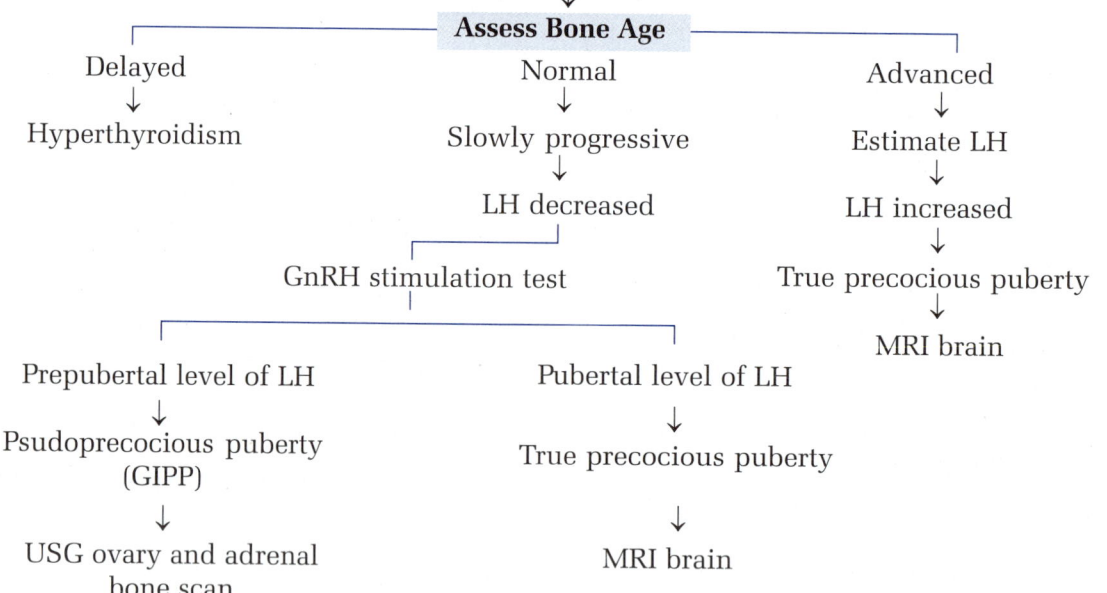

Boys: In boys initial investigations should include bone age, LH, FSH and testosterone levels. All boys with pubertal LH levels should undergo visual field examination and MRI of brain. Prepubertal LH levels suggests GIPP. In these cases adrenal imaging and estimation of serum 17OHP levels should be done. Levels of hCG should be done if these investigations are non-contributory.

Precocious Puberty   234

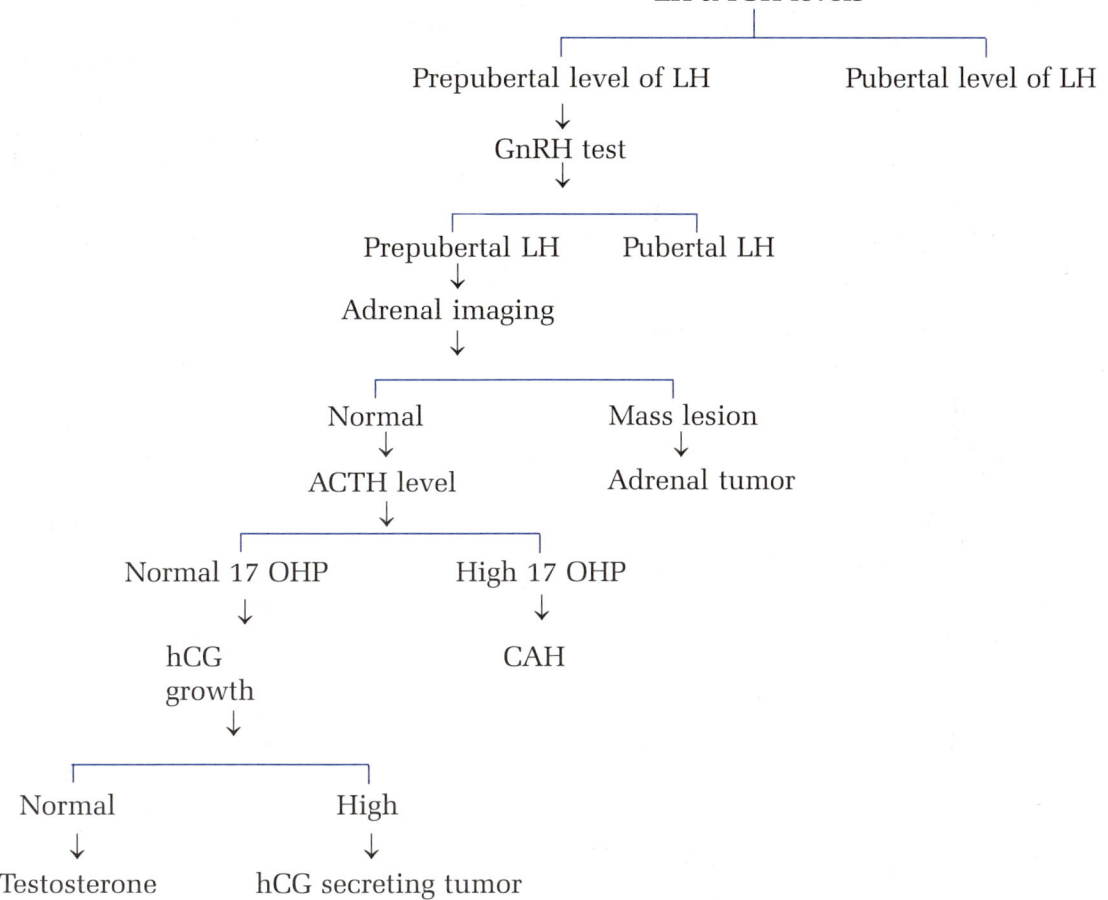

SUMMARY

Appearance of secondary sexual characters before the age of 8 years in girls and 9 years in boys is considered precocious. It is commoner in girls.

Clinical features in girls are: Rapid gain in height and of development of breasts, axillary and pubic hair and early appearance of menarche.In boys: Acne, voice change, rapid enlargement of penis, scrotum and testis and erections with ejaculation.

Causes of precocious puberty can be central due to affection of hypothalamic pituitary gonadal axis or peripheral due to involvement of gonads.

Extensive investigations are indicated if growth is accelerated, skeletal age is advanced, more than one sign of puberty is present and levels of sex hormones are high

SUGGESTED READING

1. Precocious puberty. Diagnostic approach 2016, BMJ. Best Practice.
2. Colaco Prisca Disorders of Puberty. IAP Textbook of Pediatrics, 5th Edition 2013 p. 764-768.

Chapter

33

CHEST PAIN

INTRODUCTION

Whenever a child complains of chest pain the parents are extremely worried and rush to the physician for advise and management. Fortunately, in majority of cases, the etiology is benign. However, in 25% of the cases the cause can be pathological. Therefore, the clinician's aim would be to identify if the cause of chest pain is organic.

ETIOLOGY

There are numerous causes for pediatric chest pain which are listed in table.

The most frequently reported cause is musculoskeletal pain, followed by respiratory causes.

Table: **Causes of chest pain**

A. **Non-cardiac**

1. Musculoskeletal and chest wall
   - Trauma (contusion / rib fracture)
   - Costochondritis/ Tietze syndrome
   - Chest wall strain (exercise, forceful coughing, over use injury)
   - Cutaneous (e.g. Herpes zoster)
   - Breast tenderness
   - Skeletal anomaly
2. Respiratory:
   - Pneumonia
   - Pleuritis
   - Pleurodynia
   - Severe cough

   - Asthma
   - Pneumothorax
   - Pulmonary embolism
3. Gastrointestinal
   - Oesophageal foreign body
   - Gastroesophageal reflux disease
4. Hematologic and oncologic
   - Sickle cell disease
   - Tumor (chest wall, thoracic or mediastinal)
5. Neurologic
   - Spinal nerve root compression
6. Psychiatric
   - Stress-related pain

B. **Cardiac**
   - Pericarditis
   - Myocarditis
   - Endocarditis
   - Structural viz
   - Hypertrophic cardiomyopathy, valvular stenosis, mitral valve prolapse
   - Coronary artery disease
     - Kawasaki disease
     - Anomalous coronary arteries
     - Premature atherosclerosis
   - Arrhythmias
   - Aortic aneurysm
     - Marfan's syndrome
     - Turner
     - Noonan's syndrome

C. **Idiopathic**

EVALUATION

Evaluation of pediatric patients presenting with chest pain includes a thorough history and physical examination.

A. History

While eliciting history it is essential to focus on the points given in the box.

Points in history
• Age
• Onset of pain
• Nature of pain
• Fever
• Associated symptoms
• History of trauma
• Associated conditions

Age:

Younger children are more likely to have a cardiorespiratory source for their chest pain whereas an adolescent is more likely to have a psychogenic cause.

Onset of pain:

Children having an organic cause of pain are more likely to have acute pain. On the other hand children with non-organic chest pain are more likely to have pain for a longer duration.

Nature of pain:

Children often have difficulty in localising and qualifying their pain. In instances where the child is able to localize chest pain (e.g. right sided, left sided and sternal), no specific relationship to a particular diagnosis has been found. Pericarditis usually presents with sharp substernal pain which is alleviated by leaning forward.

Fever:

Presence of fever with chest pain points towards an infectious aetiology such as pneumonia, pleuritis, myocarditis pericarditis.

Associated symptoms:

When pain wakes up a child from sleep the cause of pain is organic. Pain associated with exertion, syncope is more likely to be cardiac in nature, or exercise-induced asthma.

Midsternal burning pain which worsens on lying down indicates gastrooesophageal reflux.

Trauma:

Trauma can lead to chest wall injury. Severe trauma can cause pneumothorax or pneumomediastinum.

History of heart disease:

Pain can be due to an underlying cardiac disease. At times although there is no fresh pathology in the underlying disease the child complains of chest pain due to anxiety of the underlying condition.

Associated conditions:

Children suffering from certain serious conditions such as Kawasaki disease, asthma, Marfan's syndrome and Lupus are at risk of complications such as ischemia, pneumothorax, pleural effusion.

Stressful events:

One should enquire whether the child is under stress.

B. Physical examination

Points on examination

- Vital signs
- Respiratory system
- Cardiovascular system
- Evidence of trauma
- Drooling in a young child

Vital signs:

As soon as a child with chest pain is brought one must assess whether the child looks sick or does he appear normal. Vital signs should be checked to assess whether the child is febrile, has tachycardia, tachypnea, respiratory distress. Is the blood pressure normal.

Any signs of shock.

If a young child has drooling then one must suspect foreign body aspiration usually a coin.

Respiratory system:

Respiratory system should be examined in detail. Look for respiratory distress. If there is crepitus i.e. palpable subcutaneous air also called subcutaneous emphysema, auscultate for decreased breath sounds. One must consider pneumonia and pneumothorax.

Presence of bilateral wheeze suggests asthma and chest pain could be due to complications like pneumomediastinum and pneumothorax.

Cardiovascular system:

Presence of pathological murmur, pericardial rub, arrhythmia, one must consider pericarditis, myocarditis, supraventricular tachycardia or structural heart diseases.

Red flag signs in a child with chest pain

- Young age
- Acute onset
- Associated with trauma
- Syncope
- Respiratory distress
- Palpitation
- Abnormal cardiorespiratory findings
- Trauma
- Precipitated by exercise

If a child with pain has any of the associated signs and symptoms enumerated in the box, the child is likely to have an organic cause for the chest pain. Such children need investigations, close monitoring and if need be, hospitalization.

C. Investigations

Table: Indications for investigations

Investigation	Symptoms	Signs
Chest x-ray	• Fever	• Tachypnoea, rales and distress
	• Cough	• Ill appearance
	• Breathlessness	• Tachycardia
	• Acute onset of pain	• Abnormal cardiac findings
	• Pain affecting sleep	• Decreased breath sounds
	• Pain associated with exercise	• Subcutaneous emphysema
	• H/O foreign body ingestion	• Drooling
	• Associated medical conditions	

Electrocardiogram	• Pain precipitated by exercise	• Tachycardia
	• Syncope, palpitation	• Abnormal cardiac findings
	• Fever	• Ill look
	• Underlying serious medical problems	• Fever

X-ray chest:

Hypertrophic cardiomyopathy patients usually give a history of increased chest pain with exertion. Arrhythmias can cause chest pain in the pediatric patient. Premature ventricular tachycardia can present as a fleeting sharp pain. Myocardial infarction is rare in children. But when they get an attack they present with severe substernal chest pain with radiation to the left arm or jaw.

It is indicated in all children with history of trauma. Also in cases with respiratory symptomatology viz. pneumonia, pneumothorax, pneumomediastinum and subcutaneous emphysema, X-ray chest is also done in children with myocarditis, pericarditis and structural heart disease.

Electrocardiogram and echocardiography:

In abnormal cardiac examination, ECG and ECHO must be done.

CT Scan of chest:

In suspected pulmonary embolism scan of the chest should be done.

Holter monitor if arrhythmia is suspected.

SUMMARY

Chest pain is a worrisome symptom that often causes parents to bring their children to the emergency department for evaluation. In majority of cases, the etiology of chest pain is benign. Children having an organic cause of chest pain are more likely to have acute pain, sleep disturbance due to pain, and associated fever or abnormal examination findings. Chest radiograph is required in some, especially in patients with history of trauma. In children, myocardial ischemia is rare, thus routine ECG is not required on every patient.

SUGGESTED READING

1. Massin MM, Bourguinont A, Coremans C, et al. Chest pain pediatric patients presenting to an emergency department. Clin Pediatr 2004.

2. Evangelista JA, Parsons M, Renneburg AK. Chest pain in children: diagnosis through history and physical examination. J Pediatr Health Care. 2000;14:3-8.

CLINICAL PHOTOGRAPHS

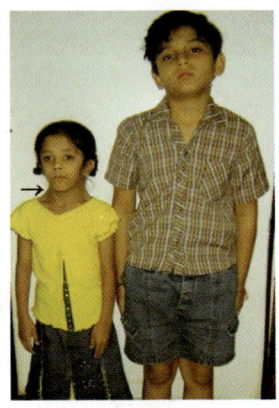

Two eight year old children. The girl on left has short stature & webbing of neck - Turner's syndrome

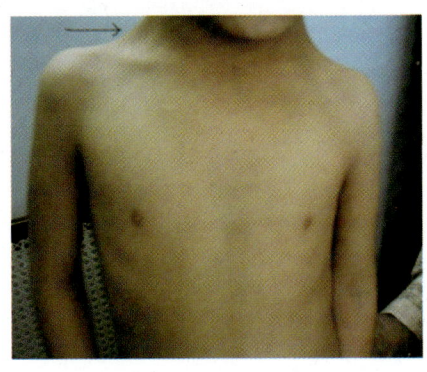

Turner's syndrome - Note the webbed neck & shield shaped chest with widely spaced nipples

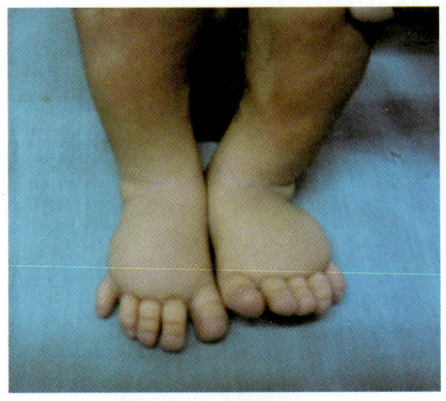

Turner's syndrome - oedema over dorsum of feet

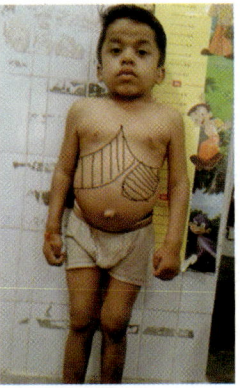

Storage disorder - short stature with massive hepatosplenomegaly

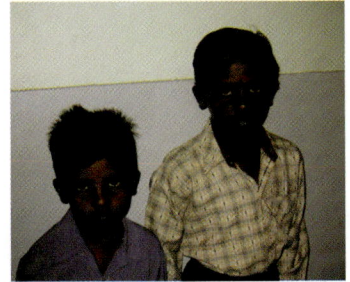

Siblings with Addison's disease

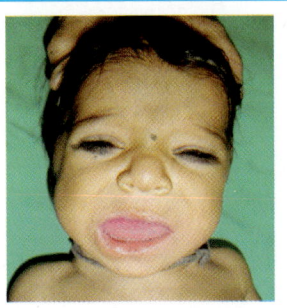

Cretinism

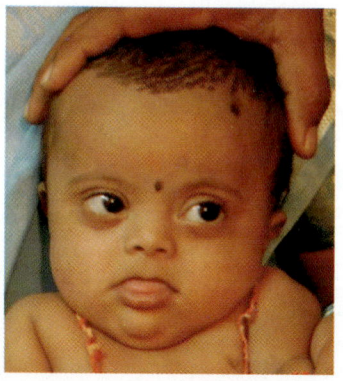

Down's syndrome

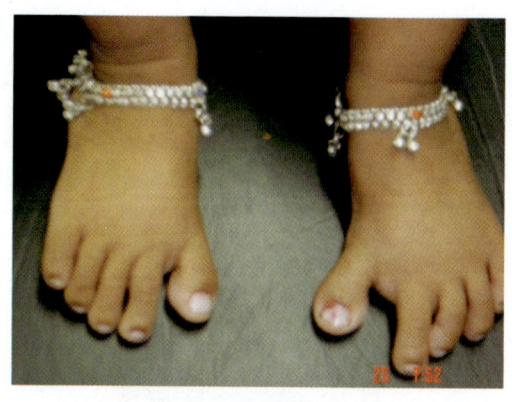

Down's syndrome - increased distance between great toe and first toe

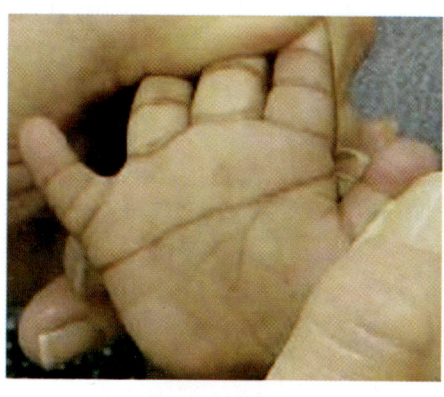

Down's syndrome - Transverse palmar crease (Simian crease)

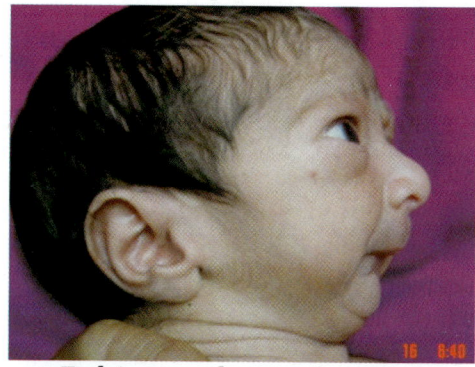

Pierre Robin syndrome (sequence) - a condition in which the infant has an unusual small lower jaw and a tongue that falls back in the throat causing difficulty in breathing

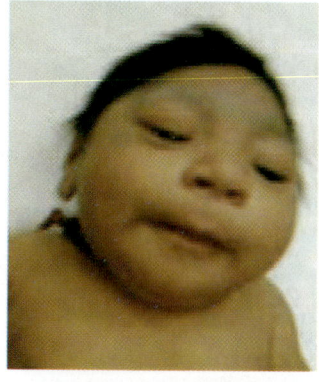

Primary Microcephaly

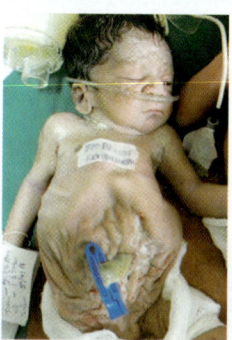

Prune Belly syndrome (Eagle Barret syndrome) - Triad of lax, redundant & wrinkled abdominal wall, undescended testes, and urological abnormalities

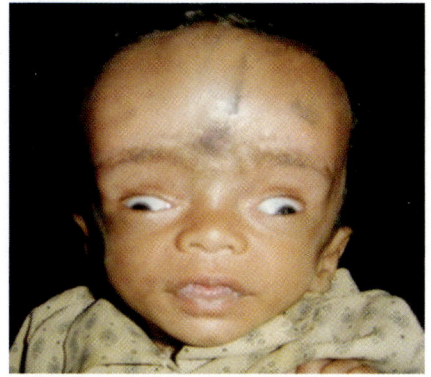

Hydrocephalus - note the sun-set appearance of the eyes

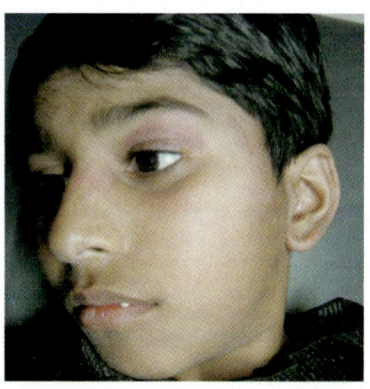

Dermatomyositis - note the heliotrope discoloration over upper eyelid

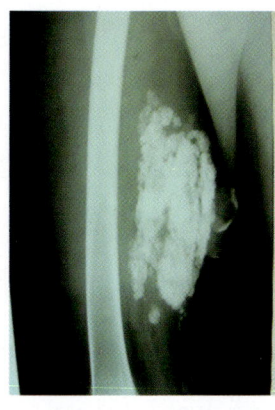

Dermatomyositis - skiagram showing calcification within the muscle

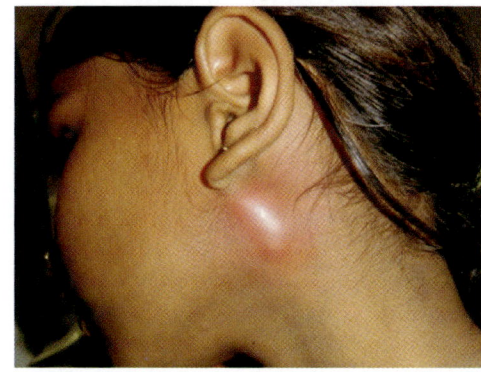

Acute pyogenic cervical lymphadenitis

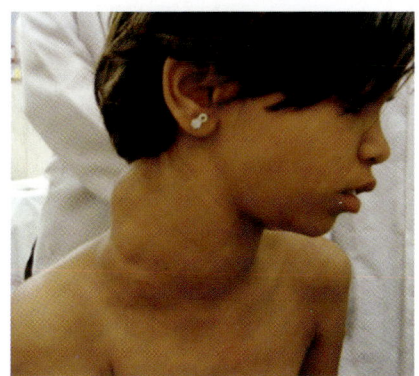

Hodgkin's Lymphoma

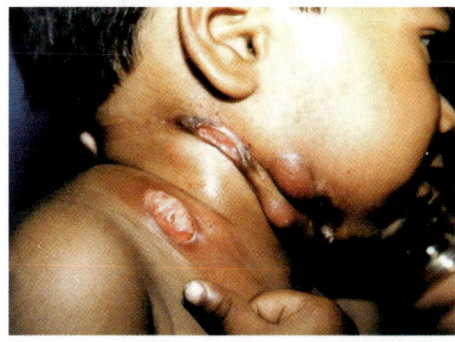

Tubercular lymphadenitis with multiple discharging sinuses in neck

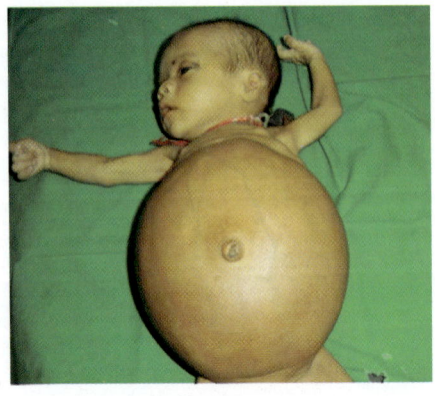

Gross Biliary ascitis in a case of Cirrhosis
of liver in late stage of Biliary Atresia

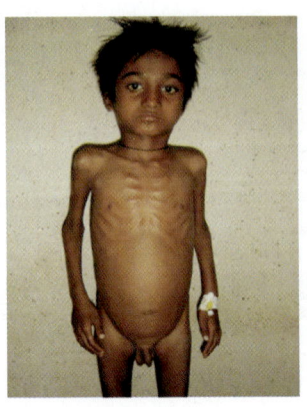

Tubercular ascitis

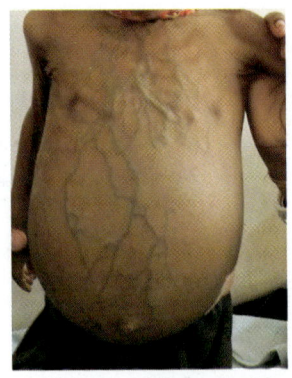

Cirrhosis of liver with portal hypertension

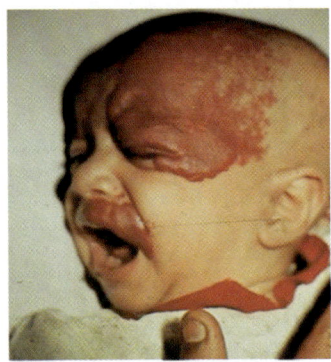

Sturge-Weber syndrome. Note the
haemangioma over forehead, scalp, upper
eyelid & upper lip. The child presented
with seizures

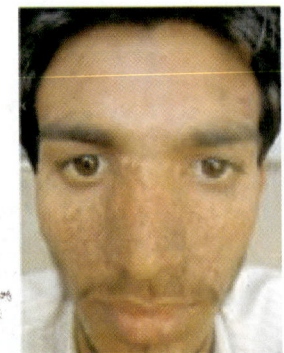

Neurofibromatosis. Apart from the freckles,
the child also had multiple café-au-lait spots
over body

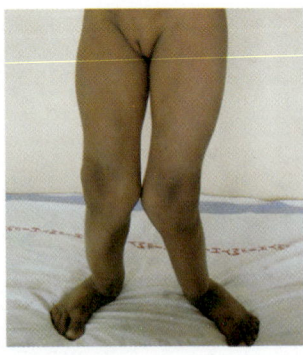

Skeletal Fluorosis leading to knock-knees

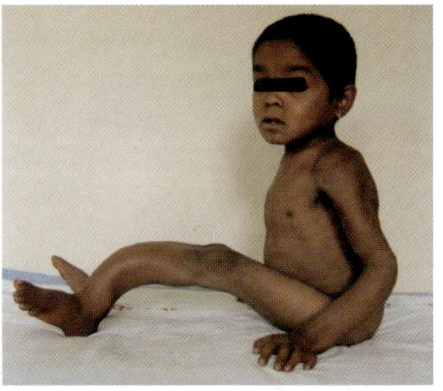

Skeletal Fluorosis leading to bending of tibia and fibula

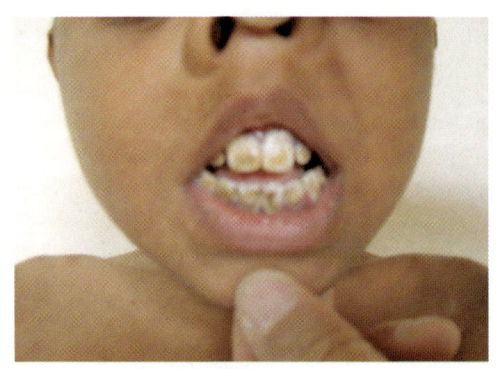

Dental fluorosis. Note yellowish brown discolouration over the tooth surface

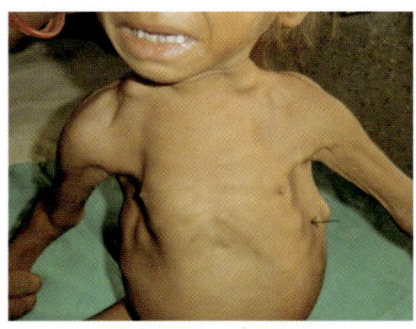

Scurvy. Note the scorbutic beading

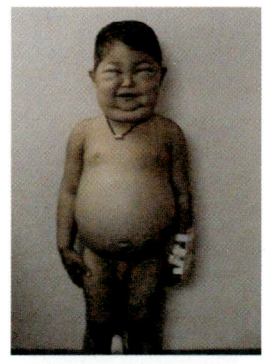

Nephrotic syndrome with massive generalised oedema

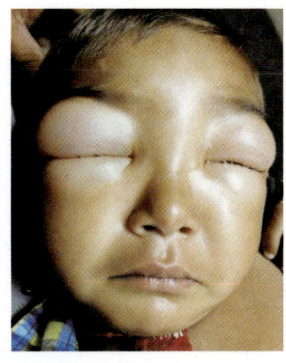

Nephrotic syndrome with massive facial oedema leading to moon facies

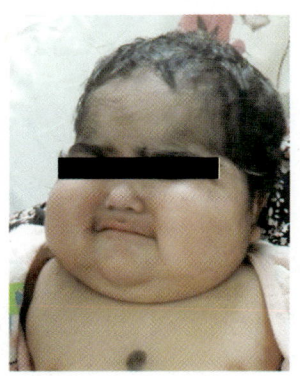

Steroid toxicity. Moon facies due to prolonged administration of steroids. Also note hirsutism over the forehead

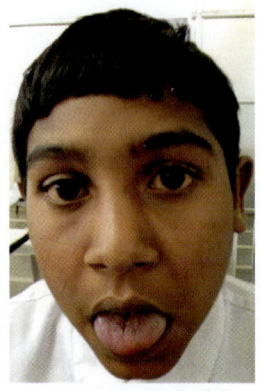

Central cyanosis in a child with Cyanotic Heart Disease. Note the suffused conjunctiva and blue tongue

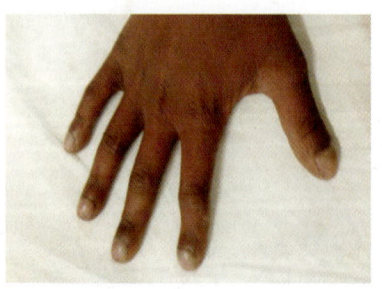

Clubbing of nails

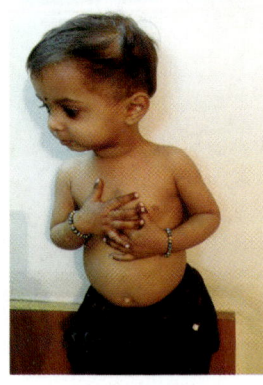

Sibling (1) with congenital Megaloblastic anaenia. Note pigmentation of knuckles

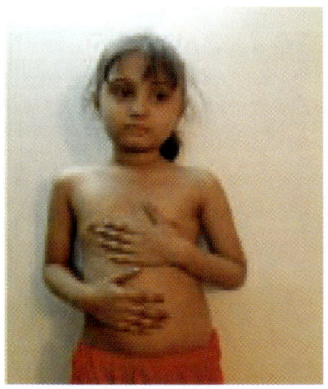

Sibling (2) with congenital Megaloblastic anaenia. Note pigmentation of knuckles

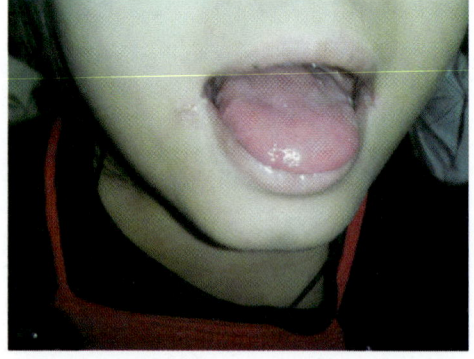

Bald tongue with angular stomatitis

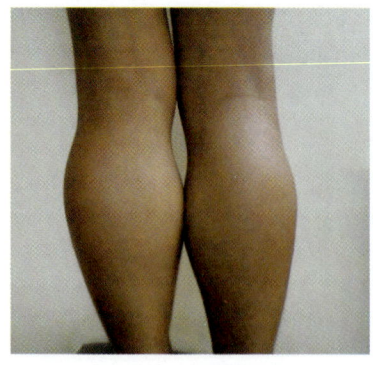

Duchenne Muscular Dystrophy. Note the hypertrophied calf muscles

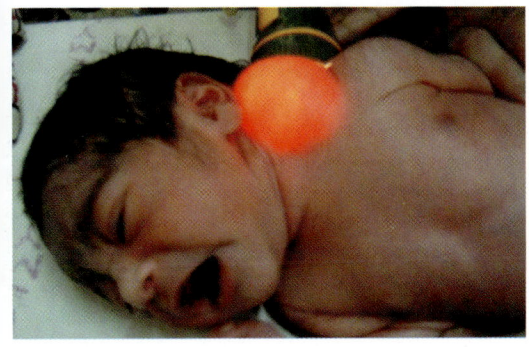

Cystic Hygroma, a cystic lesion that is brilliantly translucent

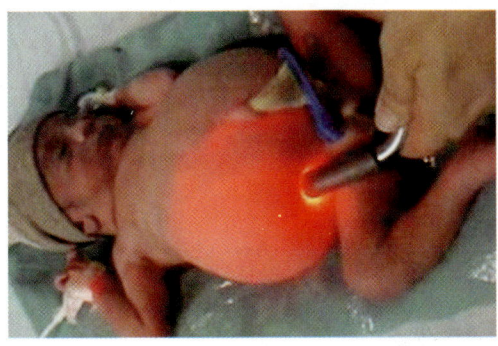

G. I. perforation in a newborn baby

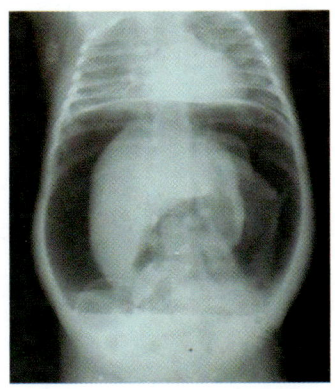

Skiagram of G. I. perforation in a newborn baby with characteristic Football-sign

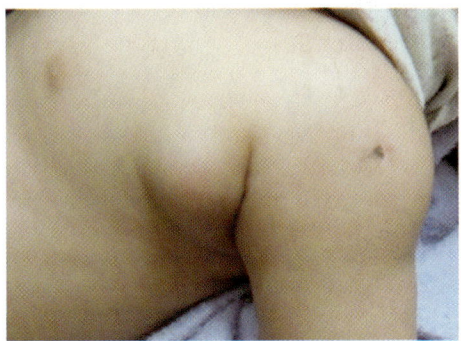

Post-BCG adenitis in left axilla

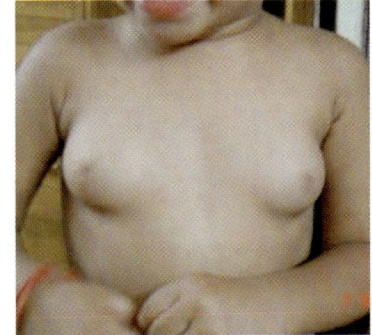

Premature Thelarche (bilateral) in a 2 year old girl

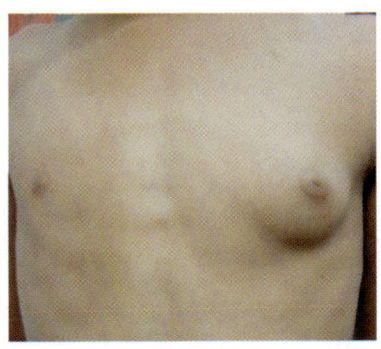

Premature Thelarche (unilateral)

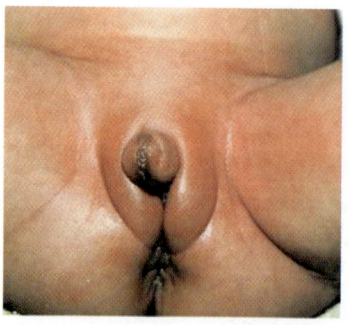

Ambiguous external genitalia in a case of Female Pseudohermaphroditism

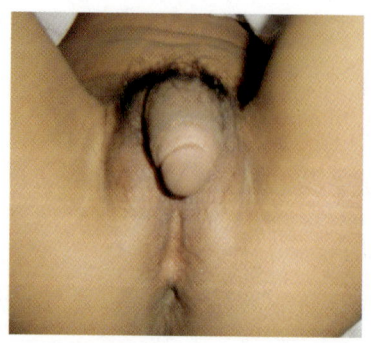

Ambiguous external genitalia in a case of Female Pseudohermaphroditism. Note marked clitoral hypertrophy and empty labio scrotal folds

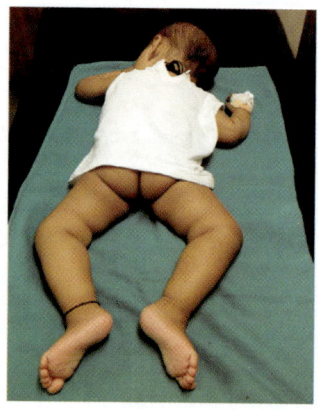

Floppy infant - note the frog-like posture

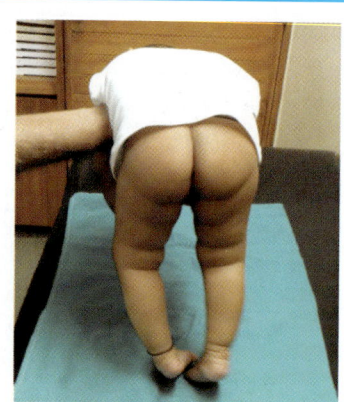

Floppy infant

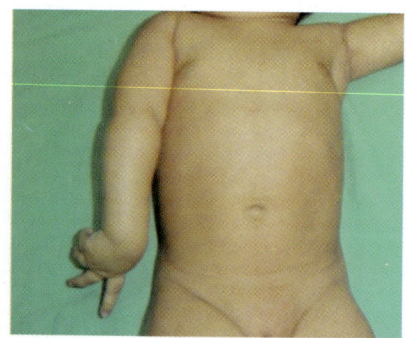

Erb's Palsy

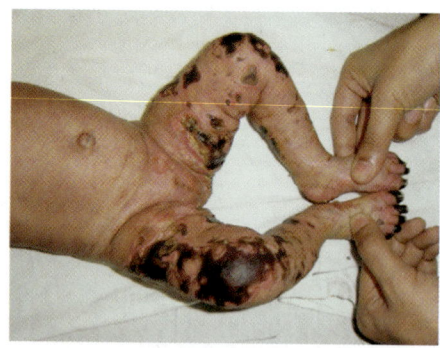

Purpura Fulminans

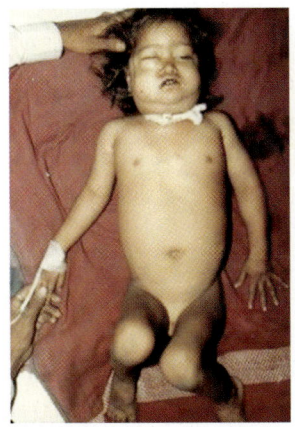

Massive Surgical Emphysema

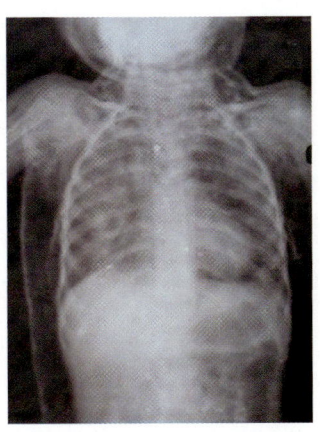

Skiagram showing air in subcutaneous tissues in a surgical emphysema

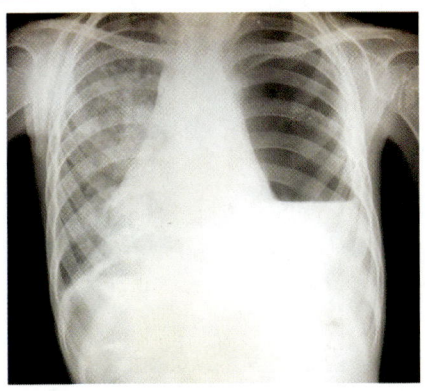

Skiagram of Hydropneumothorax

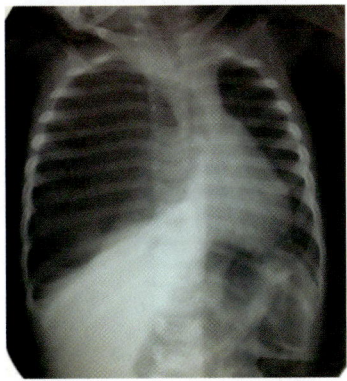

Skiagram of Tension Pneumothorax showing herniation of pleura onto the opposite side

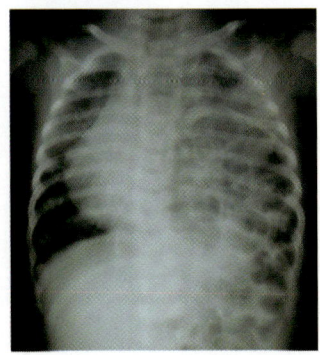

Skiagram of Diaphragmatic hernia

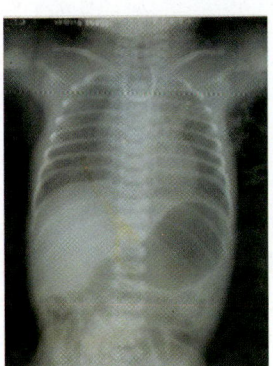

Skiagram of Oesophageal atresia with distal tracheo-oesophageal fistula. Note the curled up catheter in the upper pouch

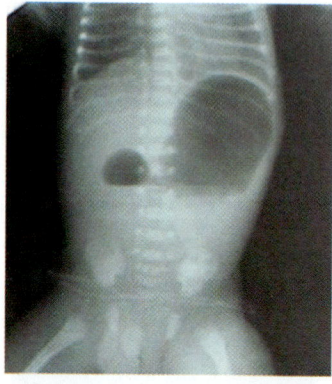

Duodenal atresia with characteristic Double-bubble sign in abdominal skiagram

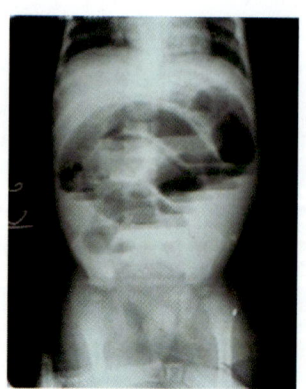

Jejuno-ileal atresia showing multiple air-flui levels in skiagram

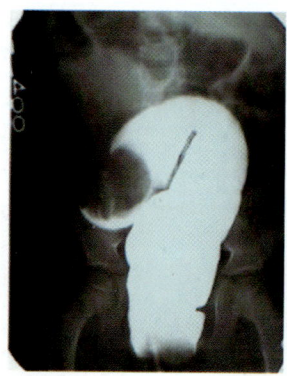

Intussusception showing 'coiled spring' appearance in contrast Barium enema

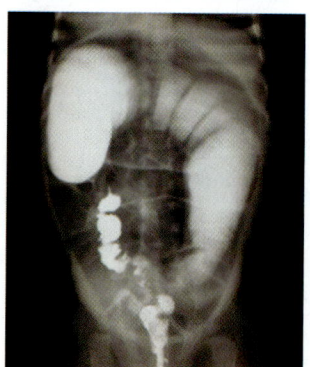

Hirschprung's disease

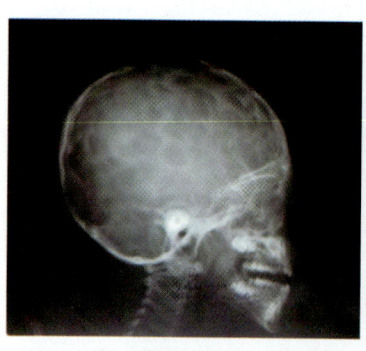

Silver-beaten appearance of skull

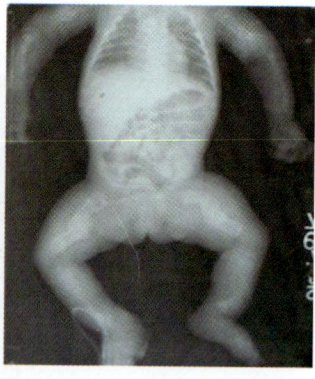

Osteogenesis Imperfecta - note multiple fractures of long bones

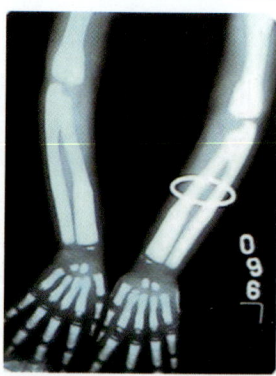

Osteopetrosis (Albers - Schonberg disease) also known as Marble Bone disease. Note increased bone density No distinction between cortical and medullary bone